# ASTHMA AND RESPIRATORY INFECTIONS

# LUNG BIOLOGY IN HEALTH AND DISEASE

*Executive Editor*

**Claude Lenfant**
*Director, National Heart, Lung and Blood Institute*
*National Institutes of Health*
*Bethesda, Maryland*

## ADDITIONAL VOLUMES IN PREPARATION

Airway Remodeling, *edited by P. H. Howarth, J. W. Wilson, J. Bousquet, S. Rak, and R. Pauwels*

Respiratory-Circulatory Interactions in Health and Disease, *edited by S. M. Scharf, M. R. Pinsky, and S. Magder*

The Lung at High Altitudes, *edited by T. F. Hornbein and R. B. Schoene*

Genetic Models in Cardiorespiratory Biology, *edited by G. G. Haddad and T. Xu*

*The opinions expressed in these volumes do not necessarily represent the views of the National Institutes of Health.*

# ASTHMA AND RESPIRATORY INFECTIONS

*Edited by*

## David P. Skoner

*Children's Hospital of Pittsburgh
University of Pittsburgh School of Medicine
Pittsburgh, Pennsylvania*

MARCEL DEKKER, INC.

NEW YORK · BASEL

**ISBN: 0-8247-7710-7**

This book is printed on acid-free paper.

**Headquarters**
Marcel Dekker, Inc.
270 Madison Avenue, New York, NY 10016
tel: 212-696-9000; fax: 212-685-4540

**Eastern Hemisphere Distribution**
Marcel Dekker AG
Hutgasse 4, Postfach 812, CH-4001 Basel, Switzerland
tel: 41-61-261-8482; fax: 41-61-261-8896

**World Wide Web**
http://www.dekker.com

The publisher offers discounts on this book when ordered in bulk quantities. For
more information, write to Special Sales/Professional Marketing at the headquarters address above.

Current printing (last digit):
10 9 8 7 6 5 4 3 2 1

**PRINTED IN THE UNITED STATES OF AMERICA**

# INTRODUCTION

*Asthma and Respiratory Infection* is much more than the title of this volume; it is an issue of major importance to the understanding of asthma, its pathogenesis, as well as the reasons for its development. Indeed, rhinoviral infections, lower respiratory tract infections, allergic rhinitis, and asthma are all pathologies that are sometimes interconnected and sometimes unrelated.

Today, a large body of evidence links these pathologies in one way or another, but seemingly contradictory questions persist. For example, do viral respiratory infections actually trigger the development of asthma, or do they merely exacerbate it? Conversely, are individuals with a history of asthma more likely to become infected, especially with rhinovirus? Regardless of the sequence of events that relate respiratory infection and asthma, much is to be learned about the cellular, subcellular, and molecular mechanisms that may bind these pathologies.

The complexity of this relationship is heightened by the observation that exposure to respiratory viral infections in very early life may protect a child from developing asthma. This notion provokes a bit of knee-jerk skepticism . . . but not so fast! The so-called "hygiene hypothesis" suggests that a reduction of respiratory infectious disease, or increased use of antibiotics in early life, has led to increased prevalence of allergic disease, including asthma. Although the biological mechanisms of this hypothesis are not yet fully understood, its epidemiological basis is hard to challenge.

This volume, edited by David P. Skoner, does not address the possibility of asthma prevention by early respiratory infection, but it does open the window on the interplay between asthma and respiratory infection in childhood and adult life. The Lung Biology in Health and Disease series of monographs has introduced a large number of volumes about asthma, each focusing on a specific aspect of this disease. And here and there, the role of respiratory infection has been touched upon; however, this volume is the first to present a comprehensive discussion of how asthma and respiratory infections relate to each other. Thus, it is an important addition to the series.

Dr. Skoner and the expert contributors he has assembled present to the readership—basic researcher and clinician as well—what we know today and what we do not know. It is clear that much additional work needs to be done to illuminate further this very important area of lung disease. In Dr. Skoner's words in his Preface, "ultimately the patients will be the beneficiaries."

As the Executive Editor of this series of monographs, I thank the editor and the authors for this major contribution to our understanding of a complex and elusive topic.

**Claude Lenfant, M.D.**
**Bethesda, Maryland**

# PREFACE

Healthy individuals experience many upper respiratory tract infections per year, commonly referred to as "colds." Asthma has also become an increasingly prevalent and costly disorder in our society. A link between these two disorders has been postulated for the last few decades, but has now been solidified based on recent information.

Patients who experience acute asthma attacks often report the presence of a cold in the days preceding the attack. Since approximately 1957, respiratory viruses have been implicated as the cause of such colds in asthmatic patients. However, the magnitude of the virus–asthma link and the cellular and biochemical mechanisms by which viruses could trigger asthma have only recently become the subject of intense investigation in a number of laboratories across the world. This accumulating base of evidence collected through modern technology prompted the publication of this volume in the prestigious Lung Biology in Health and Disease series.

The discovery and isolation of viruses were pivotal to investigating the virus–asthma relationship. Influenza viruses were first isolated in 1933 and the discovery of other respiratory viruses, such as parainfluenza virus and respiratory syncytial virus, followed in the 1940s and 1950s. It was not until 1960 that David Tyrrell and colleagues at the Common Cold Research Unit of Salisbury, England, discovered rhinoviruses, which are now recognized as the most common precipitants of acute asthma attacks. Rhinoviruses have also been associated with exacerbations of chronic bronchitis and acute otitis media; however, this book focuses exclusively upon their role in asthma.

The list of contributors to this volume is impressive. It includes both clinical and basic scientists, which fosters a bench-to-bedside approach, an approach that is warranted more than ever due to the rapid and unprecedented development of new vaccines and antiviral agents with the potential to modify the development and/or expression of asthma, and the publication of national and international guidelines on the diagnosis and management of adult and pediatric asthma.

This comprehensive and timely review of the relationship between respiratory viruses and asthma is unique and should be of great interest to basic scientists, virologists, clinicians and clinical investigators with an interest in asthma (e.g., allergists/immunologists, pulmonologists, pediatricians, internists, and general practitioners), as well as individuals in the pharmaceutical industry. In addition to incorporating a wide body of recent research, this state-of-the-art volume should illuminate future pathways of research in this important field, with the goal of ultimately benefiting affected patients.

I would like to acknowledge the assistance and support of a number of individuals, including Mary Beth Wesesky; Betty Angelini, R.N., B.S.N.; William J. Doyle, Ph.D.; and Mark Sperling, M.D. To my parents, Peter and Helen, my wife, Janet, my children, Jessica, Alison, Jonathan, Amanda, and Julianne, siblings Barbara, Peter, and John, and special friends Joseph Kenneth Skoner and Rev. John T. Boyle, I express my sincere gratitude. Finally, I acknowledge the contribution of the eminent editor of this series, Dr. Claude Lenfant, whose enthusiasm, support, and gentle, but firm, direction made the completion of this volume possible.

*David P. Skoner*

# CONTRIBUTORS

**Robert L. Atmar, M.D.**  Associate Professor of Medicine, Microbiology and Immunology, and Molecular Virology, Department of Medicine, Baylor College of Medicine, Houston, Texas

**Richard Beasley, M.B.Ch.B., D.M., F.R.A.C.P.**  Professor of Medicine, Department of Medicine, Wellington School of Medicine, Wellington, New Zealand

**William W. Busse, M.D.**  Professor, Department of Medicine, University of Wisconsin Medical School, Madison, Wisconsin

**A. J. Chauhan**  University of Southampton, Southampton, England

**Sheldon Cohen, Ph.D.**  Professor, Department of Psychology, Carnegie Mellon University, Pittsburgh, Pennsylvania

**Jonathan M. Corne, M.A., M.R.C.P.**  University Medicine, University of Southampton, Southampton, England

**Floyd W. Denny, Jr., M.D.**   Emeritus Professor of Pediatrics, University of North Carolina School of Medicine, Chapel Hill, North Carolina

**Elliott F. Ellis, M.D.**   Former Medical Director, MURO Pharmaceutical, Tewksbury, Massachusetts

**Gert Folkerts, Ph.D.**   Associate Professor, Department of Pharmacology and Pathophysiology, Faculty of Pharmacy, Utrecht University, Utrecht, The Netherlands

**Deborah A. Gentile, M.D.**   Assistant Professor, Department of Pediatrics, Children's Hospital of Pittsburgh, Pittsburgh, Pennsylvania

**James E. Gern, M.D.**   Associate Professor, Department of Pediatrics, University of Wisconsin Medical School, Madison, Wisconsin

**Jack M. Gwaltney, Jr., M.D.**   Head, Division of Epidemiology and Virology, and Professor, Department of Internal Medicine, University of Virginia Health Sciences Center, Charlottesville, Virginia

**Richard G. Hegele, M.D., F.R.C.P.(C), Ph.D.**   Associate Professor, Department of Pathology and Laboratory Medicine, University of British Columbia, Vancouver, British Columbia, Canada

**James C. Hogg, M.D., Ph.D., F.R.C.P.(C)**   Professor of Pathology, Pulmonary Research Laboratory, University of British Columbia, Vancouver, British Columbia, Canada

**Sebastian L. Johnston, M.B., B.S., M.R.C.P., Ph.D.**   Senior Lecturer, University Medicine, University of Southampton, Southampton, England

**Michael Kabesch, M.D.**   University Children's Hospital, Munich, Germany

**Robert F. Lemanske, Jr., M.D.**   Professor, Departments of Pediatrics and Medicine, University of Wisconsin Medical School, Madison, Wisconsin

**Frans P. Nijkamp, Ph.D.**   Professor of Pharmacology and Pathophysiology, Utrecht University, Utrecht, The Netherlands

**Mario Rodriguez**   Assistant Professor, Department of Medicine, Medical College of Pennsylvania, Hahnemann University, Philadelphia, Pennsylvania

**David P. Skoner, M.D.**   Chief, Allergy and Immunology Section, Children's Hospital of Pittsburgh, and Associate Professor of Pediatrics and Otolaryngology, University of Pittsburgh School of Medicine, Pittsburgh, Pennsylvania

**Ronald B. Turner, M.D.**   Professor of Pediatrics, Department of Pediatrics, Medical University of South Carolina, Charleston, South Carolina

**David Tyrrell, M.D., F.R.C.P., F.R.C.Path, F.R.S.**   Former Director, Common Cold Unit, Salisbury, Wiltshire, England

**Henk J. Van der Linde**   Utrecht University, Utrecht, The Netherlands

**Erika von Mutius, M.D.**   Head, Allergy and Outpatient Clinic, University Children's Hospital, Munich, Germany

**Theodore J. Witek, Jr.**   Boehringer Ingelheim Pharmaceuticals, Ridgefield, Connecticut

# CONTENTS

# 1

# The Impact of Respiratory Virus Infections on the World's Children

**FLOYD W. DENNY, Jr.**

University of North Carolina
School of Medicine
Chapel Hill, North Carolina

## I. Introduction

Acute infections of the respiratory tract are the most common affliction of the human host. In developed or industrialized countries infections of the upper and lower respiratory tract are important causes of disability and days lost from work or school, but the case fatality rate is small, except in certain patients at high risk. In developing countries respiratory infections are also a leading cause of disability; in children under 5 years of age they are the leading cause of death. In keeping with the topic of this book, it is the purpose of this chapter to paint a picture of the clinical impact of the respiratory viruses of humans. All classes of microorganisms are capable of infecting the respiratory tract, but only viruses and bacteria are common causes; since both of these microorganisms are inextricably involved in some respiratory infections, both will be addressed when appropriate. No effort will be made to make this a review of more unusual causes of respiratory infections.

---

This chapter is adapted in large part with permission from Denny FW, Jr. The clinical impact of human respiratory virus infections. Am J Respir Crit Care Med 1995; 152:S4–S12.

*1*

Because of the complexity of acute respiratory infections (ARIs), an effort will be made to simplify the presentation by presenting first a classification of ARIs. This will be followed by a review of the common infectious agents and the clinical diseases they cause, including the interaction of viruses and bacteria in causing infections and the risk factors associated with severe and fatal ARIs. The first part of this chapter will highlight studies from developed countries, where numerous reports have elucidated many aspects of the etiology, epidemiology, clinical features, and management of childhood respiratory infections.

ARIs present very different problems in developed and developing countries. The second part of the paper will highlight studies reported from developing countries and compare these studies with those from developed nations.

## II.  Classification of Acute Respiratory Infections

Acute respiratory infections can be classified conveniently by separating the upper from the lower tracts at the epiglottis, although it is recognized that infection involves both areas in some patients (Fig. 1).

### A.  Upper Respiratory Tract Infections

The majority of acute upper respiratory tract infections (AURIs) are not complicated by any of the listed entities. The most common complication is otitis media. The proportion of patients with upper respiratory tract infections (URIs) in whom otitis media develops depends on several factors, including the age of the child and the agent causing the upper respiratory tract infection, and varies from 15 to 25% in children younger than 1 year of age, and 2 to 5% in those of early school age (1). The other complications are less frequent. Our present knowledge of the etiology of upper respiratory tract infections suggests that among uncomplicated cases it is usually important only to identify those patients infected with the group A streptococcus, with the assumption that most of those remaining are caused by respiratory viruses or rarely to other bacteria. Although the upper respiratory clinical syndromes of herpetic gingivostomatitis, pharyngoconjunctival fever, herpangina, lymphonodular pharyngitis, and hand, foot, and mouth disease may suggest a viral etiology, the specific, infecting virus is usually not apparent. Many terms have been used to classify acute upper respiratory tract infections: URI, either afebrile or febrile; pharyngitis; tonsillitis; and pharyngotonsillitis. Because of the vagueness of most of these terms, it is probably best to concentrate primarily on differentiating group A streptococcal upper respiratory tract infections from all others, presumably due mostly to viruses.

### B.  Lower Respiratory Tract Infections

The majority of acute lower respiratory tract infections (ALRIs) are not complicated and can be classified by the anatomical area of the respiratory tract primarily

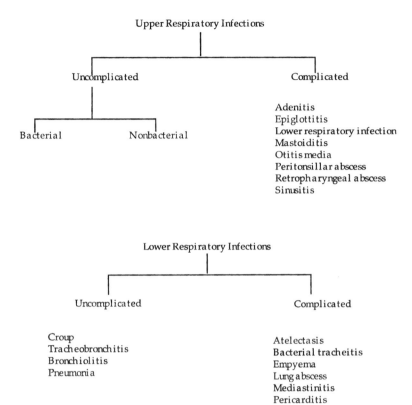

**Figure 1** Classification of acute upper and lower respiratory infections.

affected (Fig. 1). Infection may involve more than one site of the lower tract, but most infected children have a single site of major involvement. This classification of lower respiratory tract infection syndromes has been especially useful because there is close association between the syndrome and other associated factors, including causative agents.

## III.  Etiology of Acute Respiratory Tract Infections

The causative agents associated with acute respiratory infections are relatively well understood and are similar everywhere in the world where studies have been done. All classes of microorganisms, including viruses, bacteria, fungi, parasites, and protozoa, are capable of infecting the respiratory tract. Only certain viruses

**Table 1**  Viruses and Bacteria as Causes of Acute Upper Respiratory Infections

| Viruses | Bacteria |
| --- | --- |
| Adenoviruses | Group A streptococci |
| Coronaviruses | Groups C and G streptococci |
| Enteroviruses | *Arcanobacterium hemolyticum* |
| Herpes simplex virus | *Chlamydia pneumoniae* |
| Influenza viruses | *Mycoplasma pneumoniae* |
| Parainfluenza viruses | |
| Respiratory syncytial virus | |
| Rhinoviruses | |

and bacteria are common causes—these are listed in Tables 1 and 2 and are representative of several reported studies (2–7). A comparison of the tables shows that the same agents are involved generally in infections in both sites but vary in their relative roles. The group A streptococcus is the prime bacterial cause of upper respiratory infections. The other bacteria listed are either infrequent causes of AURIs or, in the case of *Arcanobacterium hemolyticum*, a controversial cause (8). The listed viruses are far more common causes of AURIs. All of these viruses can infect all parts of the respiratory tract, but the coronaviruses, the enteroviruses, the herpes simplex virus, and the rhinoviruses are found primarily in upper respiratory infections. The viruses that are usually involved in ALRIs are the adenoviruses, the influenza viruses, the parainfluenza viruses, and the respiratory syncytial viruses. All of the listed bacteria are widely accepted as causative agents of ALRIs. *Mycoplasma pneumoniae* is an important cause of tracheobronchitis and pneumonia in older children and young adults but an infrequent cause of illness in young children, when viruses are much more common (9). *Chlamydia pneumoniae* has been recognized as a cause of similar illnesses but much less frequently than *M. pneumoniae* (10).

**Table 2**  Viruses and Bacteria as Causes of Acute Lower Respiratory Infections

| Viruses | Bacteria |
| --- | --- |
| Adenoviruses | *Chlamydia pneumoniae* |
| Enteroviruses | *Haemophilus influenzae* |
| Influenza viruses | *Mycoplasma pneumoniae* |
| Parainfluenza viruses | *Streptococcus pneumoniae* |
| Respiratory syncytial virus | |

The roles of *Streptococcus pneumoniae* and *Haemophilus influenzae* cannot be dispatched so easily. Both are recognized causes of lower respiratory tract infections but pose special problems in diagnosis. Although type b *H. influenzae* is associated commonly with acute epiglottitis and *S. pneumoniae* with lobar pneumonia in the older child, these two bacteria have not been associated closely with any of the syndromes listed in Figure 1, and they are not recognized causes of uncomplicated upper respiratory tract infections. This makes the clinical diagnosis of lower respiratory tract infections caused by these agents difficult. This problem is compounded by the carriage of *H. influenzae* and *S. pneumoniae* in the upper respiratory tract in a high percentage (up to 20% and 50%, respectively) of normal children at certain ages and during certain seasons (11,12). The failure of anticapsular polysaccharide antibodies to develop in young children has also hampered etiological studies. At the present time, in the absence of epiglottitis or lobar pneumonia in the older child, the only way to associate *H. influenzae* or *S. pneumoniae* with lower respiratory tract infection is to isolate the bacterium from the blood or pleural space or directly from the lung by percutaneous aspiration. Because of these problems, the roles of these two bacteria as causes of lower respiratory tract infections in patients are largely unknown. Although studies suggest that the organisms are infrequent causes in the United States, especially when compared with viruses and *M. pneumoniae*, there is widespread belief, and some evidence, that they play a major role in the increased morbidity and mortality associated with lower respiratory tract infections in developing countries (13,14).

Although it is clear that viruses are far more frequent causes of ARIs than are bacteria, precise data regarding their relative roles are not available. It is a common assumption by nonmedical and medical personnel alike that patients with viral infections of the respiratory tract have frequent superimposed bacterial infections. While this is correct in some complications of ARIs, the data are far from clear in most situations. Several scenarios of the interrelations of viruses and bacteria can be proposed:

> Scenario 1: Simultaneous infections of the respiratory tract by viruses and bacteria are not related except by temporal circumstance.
> Scenario 2: Viral infections alter the host in a manner that promotes superinfection with a bacterium.
> Scenario 3: Bacteria alter the virus in a manner that promotes increased severity of the virus infection.

Scenario 3 has been proposed, but its clinical significance is not clear; it will not be discussed further (15). In upper respiratory infections both scenarios 1 and 2 are reasonable possibilities. Bacterial and viral AURIs are so frequent that simultaneous or closely related occurrence certainly occurs. Scenario 2 is probably applicable to otitis media and sinusitis, but it is not clear if this is due

**Table 3**  Isolation of Bacteria from Lung Aspirates
of Children with Untreated Pneumonia

|  | Age (yr) | Positive culture (%) |
|---|---|---|
| Recife, Brazil | 0–4 | 60.0 |
| Sao Paulo, Brazil | 0–7 | 54.1 |
| Zaria, Nigeria | 0–8 | 61.3 |
| Goroka, PNG | 0–5 | 57.8 |
| Newark, NJ | 0–15 | 11.1 |

*Source*: Adapted from Ref. 13.

to obstruction to the drainage systems of these cavities or to virus changes in the respiratory epithelium.

In the lower respiratory tract the situation is far more complex. With only a few exceptions, bacteria do not appear to cause infections of the larynx, trachea, bronchi, or bronchiole. At the level of the alveolus information is not available that allows clarification of this matter. It has been documented that bacterial superinfections occur in patients with influenza virus infections but data are lacking to support scenario 2 with the other respiratory viruses (16). Indeed, Hall has reported on the infrequency of bacterial infections in small children with respiratory syncytial virus (RSV) infections (17). Representative studies from developed and developing countries (Table 3) suggest that bacterial infections of the lung are far less common in advantaged populations (13). In studies of lung aspirates bacteria were isolated in 54.1–61.3% in children from Brazil, Nigeria, and Papua, New Guinea, as compared to 11.1% in New Jersey. Over 80% of these isolates were *S. pneumoniae* or *H. influenzae* (Table 4). The role of preceding virus infec-

**Table 4**  Bacteria Isolated from Lung Aspirates
of Untreated Children[a]

|  | Percent of total positive cultures |
|---|---|
| *Streptococcus pneumoniae* | 45.0 |
| *Haemophilus influenzae* | 22.8 |
| *S. pneumoniae* plus *H. influenzae* | 12.9 |
| *Staphylococcus aureus* | 8.7 |
| Other | 10.6 |

[a] 171 of 339 (50.5%) positive.
*Source*: Adapted from Ref. 13.

tions in those children with increased occurrence of bacterial pneumonia is unknown.

## IV. Role of Respiratory Viruses and Bacteria as Causes of Acute Respiratory Infections

Much is known of the roles of group A streptococci, *M. pneumoniae*, and viruses
as causes of childhood acute respiratory infections. In most instances, the isolation of these agents from the upper respiratory tract can be correlated with active
infections; with few exceptions, the most notable being the group A streptococcus, they are not isolated from the throats of well children. Furthermore, specific
clinical syndromes are associated frequently with specific agents. These associations have been confirmed by accurate serological tests that demonstrate specific
antibody responses. The occurrence of acute respiratory infections is associated
with several important factors: the age of the patient, season of the year, clinical
syndrome, infecting agent, and the extent of contact (crowding).

### A. Upper Respiratory Tract

One of the most comprehensive studies on the incidence of respiratory infections
was reported from Cleveland, Ohio (Fig. 2) (18). Results of these studies show

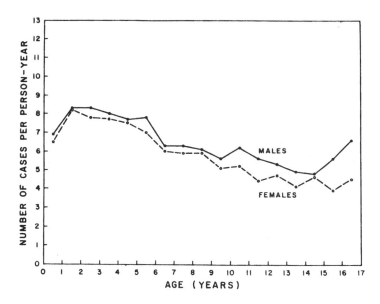

**Figure 2** Incidence of the common respiratory diseases by age and gender, Cleveland,
OH. (From Ref. 18.)

that acute respiratory infections, mostly AURIs, are common in children, occurring at a rate of four to more than eight per year, depending on age and contact. Close contacts increased the incidence. Adults usually have four to five respiratory infections per year.

Bacteria are unusual causes of uncomplicated AURIs in children less than 2–3 years of age. Group A streptococcal infections are more frequent in school-age children, but even at this age most AURIs are not caused by bacteria.

### B. Lower Respiratory Tract

Only a small proportion of acute respiratory infections involve the lower respiratory tract in developed countries. Results from the Chapel Hill day-care studies (Fig. 3) show that less than 10% of infections involved the lower tract; the proportion was higher in young children (11). These data can be compared with those obtained from a study in a private pediatric practice in Chapel Hill where various factors have been associated with the occurrence of ALRIs. The data and illustrations are considered representative of similar studies reported by others (4,19,20).

#### Age and Gender Incidence

The age- and gender-specific attack rates for total lower respiratory tract infections and four respiratory syndromes are shown in Figure 4; several important aspects of ALRIs are demonstrated. Lower respiratory tract infections are com-

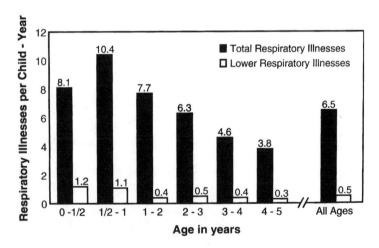

**Figure 3** Frequency of respiratory illnesses by age. (Courtesy of Frank Porter Graham Child Development Center, Chapel Hill, NC.)

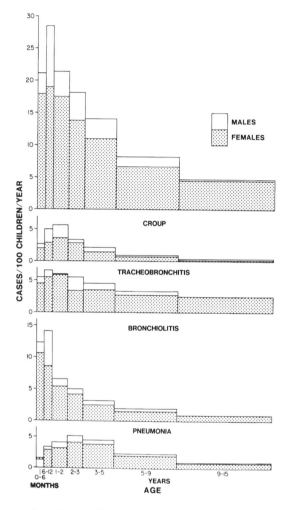

**Figure 4** Age- and gender-specific attack rates for total lower respiratory illnesses and four respiratory syndromes, 1964–1975. Rate for boys is represented by entire column, that for girls by stippled portion. Overall rate not shown. (From Ref. 41.)

mon; in this study one of every four or five children younger than 1 year of age was taken to the pediatrician each year because of a lower respiratory tract infection (4,20). This rate declined until the late elementary school ages. Lower respiratory tract infections occurred more frequently in young boys than girls, and this persisted through the lower elementary school ages, both for total lower respiratory tract infections and the specific syndromes. Of the syndromes, croup is the most likely to occur in boys, with a male-to-female ratio of 1.73 in 6- to 12-month-old infants. As shown in the four lower frames of Figure 4, with the exception of bronchiolitis, the age-specific attack rates for the clinical syndromes were different from those of total lower respiratory tract infections and also different from each other. All syndromes occurred less frequently during the first 6 months of life. The incidence of bronchiolitis most nearly resembled the overall incidence of lower respiratory tract infections, peaking in 6- to 12-month-old infants and declining sharply thereafter. Croup peaked in the second year and pneumonia in the third year. Of all the syndromes, tracheobronchitis was most likely to be found in children after the first few years of life.

### Association of Respiratory Agents and Syndromes

The association between respiratory syndromes and infecting agents is well established and is demonstrated in Figure 5 (4,20). These data show associations across all age groups; with corrections for age, these associations become more dramatic. Croup was caused most frequently by the parainfluenza viruses, especially type 1. Tracheobronchitis was associated with respiratory syncytial virus, *M. pneumoniae*, and the influenza viruses. The cause of bronchiolitis was most frequently respiratory syncytial virus. Respiratory syncytial virus and *M. pneumon-*

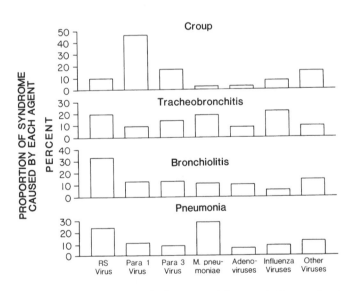

**Figure 5** Association between principal agents and four respiratory syndromes. RS virus, respiratory syncytial virus; para 1 virus, parainfluenza virus type 1; para 3 virus, parainfluenza virus type 3. (From Ref. 4.)

*iae* were common causes of pneumonia. In our studies, the influenza viruses were not prominent causes of pneumonia, as reported by Glezen (21,22). Influenza A virus was not isolated as frequently by us, probably because of the relatively insensitive isolation system used.

### Age Distribution of Lower Respiratory Tract Infections Caused by Specific Infecting Agents

As has been shown, the respiratory infecting agents are associated to some degree with all respiratory syndromes. The age-specific incidence of lower respiratory

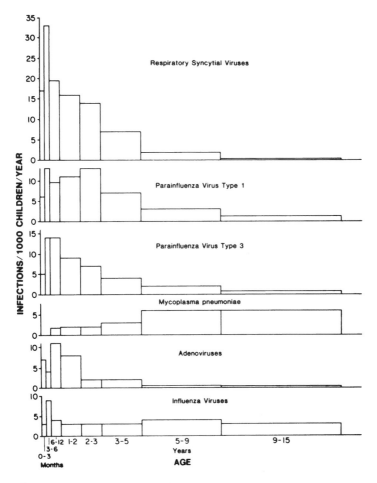

**Figure 6** Age-specific attack rates of lower respiratory infections caused by certain agents. (From Ref. 41.)

tract infections caused by specific agents differs, at times to a marked degree, and is shown in Figure 6 (4,20). In all instances, with the exception of the adenoviruses, rates during the first 3 months of life were lower than in later months. The patterns of the curves for respiratory syncytial virus and parainfluenza type 3 are similar except that respiratory syncytial virus rates were higher in the first few years. By comparison, parainfluenza virus type 1 occurred in slightly older children, and adenovirus infections occurred almost exclusively in the first 5 years of life. The influenza viruses occurred commonly in all age groups. The rates for *M. pneumoniae* infections show an entirely different age distribution; no isolates were made in children younger than 3 months of age, and the peak rates occurred in school-aged children.

### Seasonal Occurrence of Syndromes and Agents

The respiratory agents, and consequently the associated syndromes, frequently have characteristic seasonal patterns (4,20). An example of this (Fig. 7) shows the monthly occurrence of various agents in relationship to occurrence of total lower respiratory tract infections in Chapel Hill (1963–1971). Respiratory syncytial virus infections occurred in yearly outbreaks in the winter and early spring. Parainfluenza type 1 viruses occurred in the fall. Not shown here is that small outbreaks of type 2 parainfluenza viruses occurred in the years when type 1 was absent. Parainfluenza type 3 viruses occurred in a very different pattern. They were the most ubiquitous of the isolates and could be isolated in all seasons.

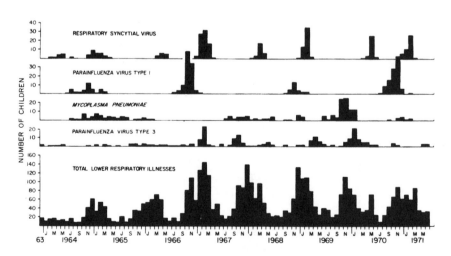

**Figure 7** Number of isolations according to month of four major respiratory pathogens from children with lower respiratory illnesses, Chapel Hill, NC. (From Ref. 23.)

*Mycoplasma pneumoniae* also had a very different pattern of occurrence. Outbreaks were unpredictable, usually starting in late summer or fall, and were long-lasting. The general aspects of seasonal occurrence are as follows. There is a close association between the seasonal incidence of bronchiolitis and the isolation of respiratory syncytial virus, both occurring in the winter to early spring. The occurrence of croup, which is closely associated with the isolation of the parainfluenza viruses, especially type 1, is predominantly in the fall and early winter. As observed earlier, the most common causes of pneumonia are respiratory syncytial virus and *M. pneumoniae*, but because these agents occur usually in different seasons and in different age groups, the seasonal occurrence of pneumonia can differ markedly. Tracheobronchitis also occurs in seasonal patterns according to the causative agent but is most closely associated with the influenzae viruses, which occur in winter and spring.

## V. Role of Various Risk Factors in the Occurrence of Acute Respiratory Infections

Several risk factors that cause increased incidences and/or severity of respiratory infections have been identified and are discussed below (20,24).

### A. Age of the Host

ARIs are a greater problem for the very young and the elderly. As already discussed, all respiratory infections are more frequent in small children and are generally more severe, as indicated by more frequent involvement of the lower respiratory tract. The severity of ARIs is also a problem in the elderly, in whom they are a major cause of morbidity and death.

### B. Crowding

Respiratory infections are, for the most part, spread by direct contact or large droplets from the respiratory tract and are thus more likely to occur during conditions that foster close contact. This has been demonstrated for all forms of crowding—number of siblings, room occupancy, population density, and probably day-care attendance. The role of day care has not been defined as clearly as is desirable, but presently available data suggest higher incidence figures for day-care attendees (11,19). Most crowding would be expected to increase incidence primarily but might play a role in increasing severity as well as in situations in which crowding is so intense that the infecting dose of microorganisms is large. It is speculated that this might play a role in the increase in severity of acute respiratory infections in developing countries.

### C. Gender

The role of gender as a risk factor has received little attention. Data suggest only slight and probably insignificant differences in incidences between boys and girls for upper respiratory tract infections. There are clear-cut gender differences for acute lower respiratory tract infections, with a preponderance of disease occurring in boys, suggesting that the risk is to increased severity. These differences may have pathogenic significance but are of little help to the physician in managing children with acute respiratory infections.

### D. Inhaled Pollutants

Inhaled pollutants have received much attention in the past few years (25,26). Although studies vary somewhat in the degree of risk caused by passive tobacco smoking, both for increased incidence and for increased severity, there is increasingly strong evidence that passive smoking is an important risk factor. The impact of passive smoking appears to be greatest in the child younger than 1 year of age and is related most closely with maternal smoking. There is also evidence that wood-burning stoves and possibly the use of gas for cooking are responsible for increasing the risk of acute respiratory infections (27,28).

### E. Anatomical Abnormalities, Metabolic and Genetic Disease, and Immunological Deficiencies

It is clear that abnormalities such as tracheoesophageal fistulas, cystic fibrosis, congenital heart disease, and immunodeficiency syndromes are associated to varying degrees with increased risk for respiratory infections, both in incidence and severity. It is beyond the scope of this chapter to consider these further. The role of atopy and/or reactive airways in increasing the risk for respiratory infection is controversial (29). There seems to be a relationship between respiratory infections and asthma, but the "chicken-and-egg" relationship is unclear. The same is true for the relationship between atopy and bronchiolitis. It is commonly believed that the atopic child has more frequent bouts of otitis media and sinusitis, but prospective studies to prove this point have not been reported.

### F. Nutrition, Including Breast Feeding

It seems probable that malnutrition is important in increasing the risk for acute respiratory infections, especially in developing countries. Because malnutrition is often associated with other risk factors such as crowding and inhaled pollutants, it has not been possible to define clearly its role. The recent report of the role of vitamin A deficiency in increasing risk for acute respiratory infections is of interest but needs further study to assess its importance (30). Breast feeding appears to be important in developing countries in reducing the risk for acute respiratory infections, but the data relating to a protective effect of breast-feeding in developed countries are contradictory (31). Results of studies show only small or no reductions in the incidence of all respiratory infections, but do suggest that the severity of infections might be decreased in young breast-fed infants. It is clear that the effect of nutrition on the risk for acute respiratory infections, including breast and other forms of feeding, needs increased attention.

### G. Social and Economic Factors

It is difficult, if not impossible, to separate the various social and economic factors that may have an impact on the occurrence of acute respiratory infections, but low social class is linked clearly with increased risk (32). Crowding, malnutrition, and inhaled pollutants, all found in low socioeconomic class, especially in developing countries, are contributing factors. The role of stress could be a contributing factor, particularly the stress that is associated with being poor (33).

## VI. Role of Acute Respiratory Infections in Developing Countries

The impact of ARIs in developing countries is much greater than that described above for developed nations (34–38). Several aspects of nonindustrialized populations contribute to the magnitude of this problem. One of these is the increased numbers of small children in whom ARIs are a larger problem. For example, in 1991, 89.4% of the 164 million of the world's births were in the developing world, but 98.2% of deaths occurred there (39). The annual causes of the deaths of children under 5 are shown in Table 5 (40). Respiratory infections and diarrhea

**Table 5**  Annual Deaths of Children Under 5 Years of Age

| | Deaths (millions) | |
|---|---|---|
| Cause of death | No | Percent |
| Respiratory infections | | |
| Pertussis | 0.51 | 4 |
| Measles | 1.52 | 11 |
| Other acute respiratory infections | 2.2 | 15 |
| Neonatal tetanus | 0.79 | 6 |
| Diarrhea | 4.0 | 28 |
| Malaria | 1.0 | 7 |
| Other | 4.2 | 29 |
| Total | 14.22 | 100 |

*Source*: Adapted from Ref. 39.

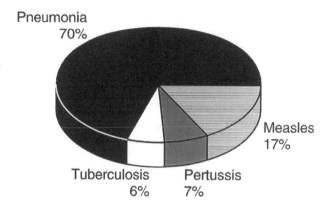

**Figure 8**  Percentage distribution of ARI-related deaths of children under 5. (Adapted from Ref. 38.)

accounted for over one-half of all deaths. The percentage distribution of the ARI-related deaths of children under 5 is shown in Figure 8 (39). Pneumonia, responsible for 70% of the ALRI-related deaths, is clearly the big problem in children in the developing world. Further examples of the problems presented by ARIs in these children are shown in the next three tables (13). The proportion of children presenting with ARIs in outpatient services varied from 30 to 60% (Table 6). The proportion of admissions into hospital due to ARIs varied from 31.5 to 35.8% (Table 7), and the case fatality rate of children admitted to the hospital because of ARIs was as high as 12.3% (Table 8).

The agents causing ARIs are the same all over the world, wherever studies have been done. Thus, RSV, the parainfluenza viruses, the adenoviruses, and the influenza viruses are the principal respiratory viruses found in children with se-

**Table 6**  Proportion of Children in Outpatient Services with Acute Respiratory Infections

| Country | Percent |
|---------|---------|
| Brazil | 41.8 |
| Nigeria | 30.1 |
| Thailand | 60.7 |
| Iraq | 39.3 |

*Source*: Adapted from Ref. 13.

**Table 7** Proportion of
Admissions to Hospital Due
to Acute Respiratory Infections
of Children Under 15 Years
of Age

| Country | Percent |
| --- | --- |
| Bangladesh | 35.8 |
| Burma | 31.5 |
| Pakistan | 33.6 |
| Zambia | 34.0 |

*Source*: Adapted from Ref. 13.

vere ARIs; of these RSV appears to be the most important. The rhinoviruses, doubtless a huge problem as a cause of AURIs, do not appear to be a major cause of ALRIs. As mentioned above, available data from developing and developed countries (Table 3) suggest that bacteria infections of the lung are far more common in disadvantaged populations (13). In studies of lung aspirates, bacteria were isolated in 54.1–61.3% in children from developing countries as compared to 11.1% in New Jersey. Over 80% of these isolates were *S. pneumoniae* or *H. influenzae* (Table 4).

One of the most startling aspects of ARIs in developing nations is that the incidence of total ARIs is very similar all over the world where studies have been done (13). Examples of this are shown in Table 9; the incidence rates for India, Costa Rica, Michigan, and Washington are remarkably similar. In sharp contrast are the marked differences in the incidence of severe and fatal ARIs in developing and developed countries (13). Table 10 compares the incidence for

**Table 8** Case Fatality of
Children Admitted to Hospitals
Because of Acute Respiratory
Infections

| Country | Percent |
| --- | --- |
| Bangladesh | 12.3 |
| Brazil | 10.2 |
| Burma | 8.1 |
| Malaysia | 2.7 |
| Pakistan | 7.3 |

*Source*: Adapted from Ref. 13.

**Table 9**  Incidence of Acute Respiratory Illnesses

|  | Episodes per year | | |
|---|---|---|---|
|  | Infants | 1–2 years | 3–5 years |
| Costa Rica | 5.9 | 7.2 | 4.2 |
| India | 5.6 | 5.3 | 4.8 |
| Michigan | 6.1 | 6.1 | 4.7 |
| Washington | 4.5 | 4.5 | 4.8 |

*Source*: Adapted from Ref. 13.

pneumonia in several advantaged and disadvantaged populations. The rates for pneumonia in Native American children in the Southwest and in children in the Peoples Republic of China and Papua, New Guinea, were up to eightfold greater than in children in North Carolina and Washington. The rates for deaths due to pneumonia in developing world children are even more remarkable, being up to several hundred times greater in Egypt and Guatemala than in France and the Netherlands (Table 11) (13).

The epidemiology of ARIs in children in developing countries is similar in most ways to that in children in developed countries. As mentioned above, the incidence of total ARIs is very similar in both locations but the severity is far greater in developing nations. The greatest impact is on small children all over the world, and in general boys are affected slightly more frequently than girls. The occurrence of the various clinical syndromes—croup, tracheobronchitis, bronchiolitis, and pneumonia—has not been studied extensively in developing countries. It is clear, however, that pneumonia is the syndrome of greatest importance, and it would appear that croup is relatively unusual. The seasonal occurrence of agents and their associated clinical syndromes in developing coun-

**Table 10**  Annual Incidence of Pneumonia in Children

|  | Cases per 1000 children | | |
|---|---|---|---|
|  | Total | Infants | 1–4 Years |
| North Carolina | 36 | — | 40 |
| Washington | 30 | — | 36 |
| Navajos, New Mexico, and Arizona | 91.2 | 291.4 | 49.9 |
| China | 74.6 | 95.2 | 53.5 |
| Tari Basin, PNG | — | 256 | 62 |

*Source*: Adapted from Ref. 13.

**Table 11**   Deaths from Pneumonia and
Influenza in Children 1–4 Years of Age

| Country | Year | No. per 100,000 |
|---|---|---|
| France | 1980 | 0.7 |
| Netherlands | 1981 | 1.1 |
| Egypt | 1979 | 173.6 |
| Guatemala | 1979 | 251.0 |

*Source*: Adapted from Ref. 13.

tries in temperate climates is similar to that described above in the United States. The seasonal occurrence of outbreaks of ARIs in tropical climates, however, is frequently variable, but outbreaks tend to occur during rainy seasons.

Risk factors, as with epidemiology, have many similarities in all countries but are more important in developing nations. Young age is a risk factor everywhere. Crowding, inhaled pollutants, low birthweight, and malnutrition (including breast-feeding and vitamin A and micronutrient deficiency) are probably important, but their precise roles in increased severity have not been well documented. Since all are associated with low social and economical conditions, it has been difficult to pinpoint the risk factor or factors that are most important.

## VII.   Summary and Conclusions

Acute respiratory infections are the most frequent illnesses of the human host. Most infections are caused by viruses and bacteria; the proportion caused by viruses is much greater. The viruses most frequently involved are adenoviruses, influenza viruses, parainfluenza viruses, respiratory syncytial viruses, and rhinoviruses. Acute respiratory infections are more common in young children and have rather specific seasonal occurrences, and some agents are associated with specific respiratory syndromes. Risk factors associated with increased incidence or severity of respiratory infections are occurrence in the very young or the elderly; crowding; being male; inhaled pollutants; anatomical, metabolic, genetic, or immunological disorders; and malnutrition, including vitamin or micronutrient deficiency. Respiratory infections are a much greater problem in developing countries than in developed countries; they are the leading causes of death in children under 5. The same agents cause infections, and the incidence of total respiratory infections is the same as in the developed countries. The precise causes of increased morbidity and mortality in the developing world are unclear, but crowding, inhaled pollutants, and malnutrition are likely candidates. The interactive role of viruses and bacteria is not clear but may play a role in increased severity of respiratory infections.

### References

1. Henderson FW, Collier AM, Sanyal MA, Watkins JM, Fairclough DL, Clyde WA Jr., Denny FW. A longitudinal study of respiratory viruses and bacteria in the etiology of acute otitis media with effusion. N Engl J Med 1983; 306:1377–1383.
2. Glezen WP, Clyde WA, Jr., Senior RJ, Sheaffer CI, Denny FW. Group A streptococci, mycoplasms and viruses associated with pharyngitis. JAMA 1967; 202:119–124.
3. Loda FA, Clyde WA Jr., Glezen WP, Senior RJ, Sheaffer CI, Denny FW Jr. Studies on the role of viruses, bacteria and *M. pneumoniae* as causes of lower respiratory tract infections in children. J Pediatr 1968; 72:161–176.
4. Denny, FW, Clyde WA Jr. Acute lower respiratory tract infections in non-hospitalized children. J Pediatr 1986; 108:635–646.
5. Foy, HM, Cooney MK, Maletzky AJ, Grayston JT. Incidence and etiology of pneumonia, croup and bronchiolitis in preschool children belonging to a prepaid medical care group over a four-year period. Am J Epidemiol 1973; 97:80–92.
6. Monto AS, Cavallaro JJ. The Tecumseh study of respiratory illness. II. Patterns of occurrence of infection with respiratory pathogens, 1965–1969. Am J Epidemiol 1971; 94:280–289.
7. Monto AS, Ultman BM. Acute respiratory illness in an American community. JAMA 1974; 227:164–169.
8. Karpathios T, Drakonaki S, Zervoudaki A, Caupari G, Fretzayas A, Kremastinos J, Thomaidis T. *Arcanobacterium hemolyticum* in children with presumed streptococcal pharyngotonsillitis or scarlet fever. J Pediatr 1992; 121:735–737.
9. Denny, FW, Clyde WA Jr., Glezen WP. *Mycoplasma pneumoniae* disease: clinical spectrum, pathophysiology, epidemiology and control. J Infect Dis 1971; 123:74–92.
10. Grayston JT. *Chlamydia pneumoniae* (TWAR) infections in children. Pediatr Infect Dis J 1994; 13:675–685.
11. Loda FA, Glezen WP, Clyde WA Jr. Respiratory disease in group day care. Pediatrics 1972; 49:428–437.
12. Loda FA, Collins AM, Glezen WP, Strangert K, Clyde WA Jr, Denny FW. Occurrence of *Diplococcus pneumoniae* in the upper respiratory tract of children. J Pediatr 1975; 87:1087–1093.
13. Pio A, Leowski J, ten Dam HG. The magnitude of the problem of acute respiratory infections. In: Douglas RM, Kerby-Eaton E, eds. *Acute Respiratory Infections in Childhood*, Proceedings of an International Workshop, Syndey, August 1984, University of Adelaide, pp. 3–17.
14. Graham NMH. The epidemiology of acute respiratory infections in children and adults.: A global perspective (review). Epidemiol Rev 1990; 12:149–178.
15. Scheiblauer H, Reinacher M, Tashiro M, Rott R. Interactions between bacteria and

influenza A virus in the development of influenza pneumonia. J Infect Dis 1992; 166:783–791.

16. Leigh MW, Carson JL, Denny FW Jr. Pathogenesis of respiratory infections due to influenza virus: Implications for developing countries (review). Rev Infect Dis 1991; 13(suppl 6):S501–S508.

17. Hall CB, Powell KR, Schnabel KC, Gala CL, Pincus PH. Risk of secondary bacterial infection in infants hospitalized with respiratory syncytial viral infection. J Pediatr 1988; 13:266–271.

18. Dingle JH, Badger GF, Jordon WS Jr. *Illness in the Home. A Study of 25,000 Illnesses in a Group of Cleveland Families*. Cleveland: The Press of Western Reserve University, 1964.

19. Denny FW, Collier AM, Henderson FW. Acute respiratory infections in day care. Rev Infect Dis 1986; 8:527–532.

20. Denny FW. Acute respiratory infections in children: etiology and epidemiology (review). Pediatr Rev 1987; 9:135–146.

21. Glezen WP. Viral pneumonia as a cause and result of hospitalization. J Infect Dis 1983; 147:765–770.

22. Glezen WP. Serious morbidity and mortality associated with influenza epidemics. Epidemiol Res 1982; 4:25–44.

23. Glezen WP, Denny FW. Epidemiology of acute lower respiratory disease in children. N Engl J Med 1973; 288:498–505.

24. Strope GL, Stempel DA. Risk factors associated with the development of chronic lung disease in children. Pediatr Clin North Am 1984; 31:757–771.

25. Health effects of environmental tobacco smoke exposure. In: The Health Consequences of Involuntary Smoking: A Report of the Surgeon General. Rockville, MD: U.S. Department of Health and Human Services, 1986:17–118.

26. Committee on Passive Smoking, Board of Environmental Studies and Toxicology, National Research Council. Effects of Exposure to Environmental Tobacco Smoke on Lung Function and Respiratory Symptoms in Environmental Tobacco Smoke: Measuring Exposures and Assessing Health Effects. Washington, DC: National Academy Press, 1986:202–209.

27. Honicky RE, Osborne JS III, Akpom CA. Symptoms of respiratory illness in young children and the use of wood-burning stoves for indoor heating. Pediatrics 1985; 75:587–593.

28. Melia RJW, Florey CV, Altman DG, Swan AV. Association between gas cooking and respiratory disease in children. Br Med J 1977; 2:149–152.

29. McIntosh K. Bronchiolitis and asthma: possible common pathogenetic pathways. J Allergy Clin Immunol 1976; 57:595–604.

30. Sommer A, Katz J, Tarwatjo I. Increased risk of respiratory disease and diarrhea in children with preexisting mild vitamin A deficiency. Am J Clin Nutr 1984; 40:1090–1095.

31. Frank AL, Taber LH, Glezen WP, Kasel GL, Wells CR, Paredes A. Breastfeeding and respiratory virus infection. Pediatrics 1982; 70:239–245.

32. Gardner G, Frank AL, Tabor LH. Effects of social and family factors on viral respiratory infection and illness in the first year of life. J Epidemiol Commun Health 1984; 38:42–48.

33. Graham NMH, Douglas RM, Ryan P. Stress and acute respiratory infection. Am J Epidemiol 1986; 124:389–401.
34. McIntosh K, Halonen P, Ruuskanen O. Report of a workshop on respiratory viral infection; epidemiology, diagnosis, treatment, and prevention. Clin Infect Dis 1993; 16:151–164.
35. Denny, FW, Loda FA. Acute respiratory infections are the leading cause of death in children in developing countries. Am J Trop Med Hyg 1986; 35:1–2.
36. Berman S. Epidemiology of acute respiratory infections in children in developing countries (review). Rev Infect Dis 1991; 3(suppl 6):S454–S462.
37. Selwyn BJ, on behalf of the Coordinated Data Group of BOSTID Researchers. The epidemiology of acute respiratory tract infections in young children: comparison of findings from several developing countries. Rev Infect Dis 1990; 12(suppl 8):S870–S888.
38. McIntosh K. Etiology and epidemiology of acute respiratory tract infections in children in developing countries. Overview of the symposium. J Infect Dis 1990; 12(suppl 8):867–S869.
39. Grant JP. *The State of the World's Children, 1993*. New York: Oxford University Press, 1993.
40. Grant JP. *The State of the World's Children, 1990*. New York: Oxford University Press, 1990.
41. Denny FW, Clyde WA Jr. Acute respiratory tract infections: an overview. Pediatr Res 1983; 17:1026–1029.

# 2

## Respiratory Viruses and Asthma
Epidemiological Considerations in Evaluating
Their Association

**THEODORE J. WITEK, Jr.**

Boehringer Ingelheim Pharmaceuticals
Ridgefield, Connecticut

## I. Introduction

Epidemiology can be defined as the differential distribution of disease and the factors that affect this distribution. Asthma can be defined as a chronic inflammatory disorder of the airway whose inflammation causes an associated increase in airway responsiveness to a variety of stimuli (1).

Among the factors associated with precipitation of asthmatic symptoms is upper respiratory infection (URI). The association of URIs with asthma is based on clinical observation (e.g., a mother presents her child to the clinic with worsening asthma symptoms "that really got worse when the child's cold started"), extensive epidemiological studies (e.g., clinical and virological work-ups prompted by increased symptoms and decreased lung function in a community-based setting), and unique retrospective accounts in a variety of clinical settings (e.g., over 75% of children in an emergency room trial of bronchodilators note upper respiratory infection as a precipitating cause). While such observations do not establish causality, they do provide a working hypothesis for understanding one aspect of the complexities of asthma, and they help suggest opportunities and focus strategies to address a significant public health problem.

This chapter will begin with a brief review of the viruses that have been associated with asthma exacerbation, focusing on methods of detection, incubation period, and clinical manifestations. The value and limitations of epidemiology will be reviewed through a discussion of basic principles, including sources of data, establishing exposure, defining effect, and assessing temporal relationships. Finally, some of the host and environmental factors that may influence our observed associations of infection and asthma will be discussed.

## II. Respiratory Viruses Associated with Asthma

Numerous types of viral infections have been reported to be associated with asthmatic symptoms. In an extensive review by Pattemore and colleagues (2), viruses associated with asthmatic symptoms (wheezy episodes) were tabulated by "cross-sectional" and prospective studies. These viruses include rhinovirus (RV), coronavirus, respiratory syncytial virus (RSV), parainfluenza virus, influenza virus, adenovirus, and enterovirus (and mycoplasma). Overall viral identification rates were calculated to be 24% in the "cross-sectional" studies and 32% in the prospective studies. As will be discussed in greater detail later in this chapter, there are numerous clinical and laboratory factors that affect the identification of virus (as well as the documentation of "asthma").

Among the most studied viruses in the context of asthma are rhinovirus and RSV and, to a lesser degree, influenza, parainfluenza, and adenovirus. The methods of detection, incubation period, and clinical manifestations of these viruses will be summarized (see Table 1).

### A. Rhinovirus

Rhinovirus was first discovered in 1956 (3) and is one of the best characterized human viruses. It has many antigenic types and is responsible for the majority of common cold illness. In 1989, intracellular adhesion molecule-1 (ICAM-1) was identified as the cellular receptor for the majority of RV types (4,5). Rhinoviruses grow well in human embryonic lung fibroblasts (MRC-5 strain, WI-38 strain) and certain strains of HeLa cells. This process can take from 48 hours up to one week (6). Therefore, the development of the polymerase chain reaction (PCR) for RV detection (7,8) has been a welcomed tool for clinical epidemiology.

The clinical course of RV illness has been well characterized (9–11), with symptoms emerging approximately 2 days after infection and lasting about a week. Viral shedding peaks around the second day after infection. Upper respiratory symptoms of sore throat, rhinorrhea, and nasal congestion predominate (11). The frequency of RV infection is greater in children than adults, and adults with children get more colds than adults without children.

**Table 1** Key Features of Common Respiratory Viruses

| Virus | Incubation period | Seasonality | Common clinical manifestations | Cell culture isolation period (days) | Detection methods | | | | | | |
|---|---|---|---|---|---|---|---|---|---|---|---|
| | | | | | EIA | IF | PCR | CF | HAI | ELISA | NT |
| Rhinovirus | ~2 days | Year-round with late spring and early fall | Common cold syndrome | 2–7 | | | √ (RT) | | | | √ |
| Respiratory syncytial virus | 2–8 days | Winter | Bronchiolitis and viral pneumonia are the most serious manifestations in young children Older children and adults Common cold syndrome, bronchitis | 3–14 | √ | √ | √ (RT) | √ | | √ | √ |
| Influenza | ~2 days | Winter | Flu syndrome: chills, fever, aches, and respiratory symptoms | 3–5 | √ | √ | √ (RT) | √ | √ | √ | √ |
| Parainfluenza | 2–8 days | Late fall | Croup syndrome and bronchiolitis | 3–8 | | √ | √ (RT) | √ | √ | √ | √ |
| Adenovirus | 5–7 days | | Febrile pharyngitis and bronchitis | 2–10 | √ | √ | √ | √ | √ | √ | √ |

EIA = Enzyme immune assay; IF = immunofluorescence; PCR = polymerase chain reaction; CF = complement fixation; HAI = hemoglutination-inhibition; ELISA = enzyme-linked immunosorbent assay; NT = neutralization; RT = reverse transcriptase.

## B. Respiratory Syncytial Virus

RSV was isolated in 1956 (12) and was soon recognized as a major respiratory pathogen in infants and younger children. Virus isolation is accomplished by its growth in several human heteroploid cell lines (HEp-2, HeLa), where it results in the syncytial cytopathic effect (reflected in its name).

Virus can be grown within a week from clinical specimens. Good collection technique, rapid transport to the lab, and diligent control of cell culture (to maintain subconfluent monolayer) is required. Nasal wash or pharyngeal aspirates provide the best specimens. Rapid enzyme immunoassay kits for viral antigen detection (13) have been utilized in clinical surveys. Immunofluorescence and enzyme immunoassays are very sensitive and specific—more so with adult specimens than with pediatric specimens. A variety of tests can be utilized for serum antibody measurement.

Surveillance data indicate widespread RSV activity beginning each fall, peaking in the winter months, and returning to baseline in the spring. RSV can remain infective on inanimate objects for hours, and outbreaks can result in very high attack rates (14). Viral incubation is usually within 1 week and can involve the entire respiratory tract.

Bronchiolitis and viral pneumonia are among the most serious manifestations of RSV infection. Hospitalization can result, particularly in younger children. The risk for severe infection and mortality is increased in those with congenital heart disease, prematurity, bronchopulmonary dysplasia, or cystic fibrosis (15).

## C. Influenza

Influenza is a primary culprit in overall respiratory morbidity. The respiratory mucosa is the principal site of infection. Illness severity ranges from a common cold-like illness to the typical flu syndrome to severe viral or secondary bacterial pneumonia. With an incubation period of about 2 days and a respiratory mode of transmission, rapid spread and explosive outbreaks can be observed (16). Respiratory specimens (nasal, throat, lower respiratory) are useful for viral isolation, and several mammalian cell lines afford detection in 3–5 days. Shell vial centrifugation culture techniques can afford a more rapid diagnosis (17). Immunofluorescence assays and ELISA are also available and have been used in large epidemiological surveys (18).

## D. Parainfluenza

Parainfluenza, isolated in the mid-1950s, is associated with symptomatic respiratory illness ranging from common cold symptoms to lower respiratory illnesses in children. The croup syndrome (laryngeo-tracheal bronchitis) is often precipitated by parainfluenza. Parainfluenza 3 is the second most prevalent cause of bronchiolitis or pneumonia in infants after RSV. Incubation ranges from 2 to 8 days (16).

Viral isolation is possible between 3 and 8 days after cell culture inoculation with respiratory specimens. Again, shell vial techniques can be used (17). Rapid diagnosis can also be afforded by documentation of parainfluenza antigen.

### E. Adenovirus

Adenoviruses were recognized in 1953 (20) and have been associated with respiratory illness in both children and adults. It is regarded as a minor contributor to total common cold illness but is associated frequently with febrile pharyngitis and bronchitis. Additionally there is some evidence that persistent or latent adenoviral infection may contribute to the pathogenesis of childhood asthma (21). Respiratory tract infection has an incubation period of 5–7 days. A variety of respiratory specimens are useful for viral isolation.

### III. Basic Observations

Important basic observations in the association between viral illness and asthma include (1) the higher viral identification rates during symptomatic (i.e., wheezy) versus asymptomatic periods, and (2) the temporal association of asthma following URI onset. Additionally, age-specific susceptibilities to certain viruses are important to consider in studying the association.

There are typically higher rates of viral isolation during periods of wheezing than during asymptomatic periods. Although across-study direct comparisons are difficult due to variations in the techniques of virus isolation and definitions of asthma (discussed later), general trends remain evident (22–36) (Fig. 1). Bacteria, on the other hand, can be identified equally as often with and without symptoms. The most extensive evidence for this comes from a hospitalized cohort of asthmatic children where no differences were detected in isolation of five bacterial pathogens among cultures from those wheezing ($n = 65$) and not wheezing ($n = 178$) (27).

The frequent occurrence of a clinic presentation of asthma exacerbation with a history of recent URI is also demonstrated in prospective studies. This temporal relationship has been nicely demonstrated in the extensive observations by Johnston et al. (22), where virus isolation coincided with objective dips in peak expiratory flow. Similar trends between virus isolation and asthma symptom scores (28) and daily medication score (27) have been reported. The specific interval between URI onset and asthma "events" has not been extensively described. In one group of children, wheezing began within 2 days of URI symptoms (mean 43 hours) and lasted 4 days (29).

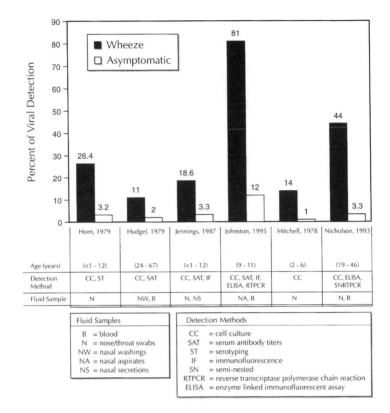

**Figure 1**  Rates of viral identification in periods of wheezy illness and in periods free of symptoms. Despite across-study variations in virus isolation technique and illness/symptom definitions, the trend remains consistent. (Illustrations prepared by Leigh Rondano, copyright © Boehringer Ingelheim Pharmaceuticals, Inc., 1996. All rights reserved. Used with permission.)

As alluded to in the overview of specific respiratory viruses, there are age-specific manifestations among the numerous viruses, and these also need to be considered when attempting to study the association of asthma and URI. For example, RSV can result in severe bronchiolitis during first infection in infancy with milder illnesses later in life. Rhinovirus, on the other hand, produces a more "uniform" milder illness throughout life. This, coupled with the fact that rhinovirus, is the most common cause of URI, makes rhinovirus a useful model in evaluating the association of URIs and asthma. Most of the examples used in this chapter focus on human rhinovirus infection.

## A.  Sources of Data

Optimal characterization of "exposure" and "effect" (or outcome) will strengthen the study of the association of URIs and asthma. In this case, exposure can be regarded as the URI and effect can be viewed as the manifestation of asthma.

There are numerous sources of data to explore the association of URI and asthma. They range in complexity, and each has obvious advantages and disadvantages. These sources include (1) the individual patient; (2) a cohort involved in an outbreak of infection or, on the other hand, an exacerbation of asthma; and (3) surveys that prospectively characterize infectious illness and pattern of asthma symptoms and lung function. Table 2 lists some examples (with varying degrees of robustness) of the methods associated with different data sources.

The association of URI and asthmatic symptoms is commonly described by individual patients among the case load of the general practitioner. Patients who present with asthma often note a history of a cold illness or upper respiratory symptoms some days prior to the onset of wheezing. While this patient history, at present, does not have a direct impact on subsequent therapy, it can suggest to the practitioner and public health specialist that typical periods of URI outbreaks can be expected to relate to an increase in asthma symptoms. Consequently, appropriate outpatient care may be stepped up.

**Table 2**  The Spectrum of Methods Utilized to Assess "Exposure" and "Effect" in the Association of Respiratory Viral Illness and Asthma

| Type of observation | Exposure assessment | Outcome assessment | Comment |
|---|---|---|---|
| Community-based survey of children | Mother's assessment of child's "wheeze with cold"[+] | Mother's assessment of child's wheeze with and without cold[+] | Increase risk of "wheeze with cold" with increasing ETS exposure observed |
| Community-based study of children | Viral infections by PCR or conventional cell culture[+++] | Reported exacerbations of respiratory symptoms PEFR[+++] | URI associated with 80–85% of asthma exacerbations in children |
| Controlled clinical trial of broncho-dilators in ER asthma | List precipitators of asthma attack[+] | Presentation to emergency department for acute asthma treatment[+++] | 3/4 of exacerbations associated with URI |

ETS = Environmental tobacco smoke; PEFR = peak expiratory flow rate; URI = upper respiratory infection.
Value of method for assessing factors is rated from low (+) to high (+++).

Beyond the individual patient history, the association of respiratory infection with asthma can be supported by examination of particular outbreaks. This has been highlighted in a series of camp outbreaks such as the Boy Scout Jamboree in 1957, where about 4% of influenza cases had associated asthma (30), and a similar rate was noted in a Canadian girl's camp that same year (31). Another approach is to utilize a cohort of known active asthmatics, such as those presenting to the emergency ward. For example, in a clinical trial of emergency room (ER) bronchodilator therapy in children, more than three-quarters of the children were noted to have had an URI within the previous 7 days (32). In a survey of adults presenting for asthma, about 56% noted a history consistent with viral syndrome (33).

The previously mentioned data sources establish either the infectious outbreak (e.g., flu outbreak) or clinical asthma (e.g., presentation to ER in need of therapy), but it is difficult to provide a source of data that does both. This is, in fact, one of the limitations of epidemiology in that such characterization is optimally done in a prospective fashion that is time and resource draining. Nevertheless, such studies have been performed, among the most extensive being that of Johnston and coworkers (22). In their 13-month prospective trial, diary cards and peak expiratory flow rates were monitored to allow for early viral sampling by both PCR and conventional methods. Figure 2 provides a time-course scenario from this study and illustrates the association of well-documented infection with well-documented asthma monitoring.

## B.  Exposure and Effect

Assessments of exposure and effect can utilize objective and subjective measures. For example, URI can be characterized by symptom diaries, some of which have been standardized (34), as well as documentation of the infection through a variety of clinical virological techniques. Objective measures of physiological function such as rhinomamometry to measure airflow (9,11,35), laser Doppler velocimetry to measure nasal blood flow (36,37), and tympanometry to measure ear pressures (35) have limited value in defining illness. Nasal lavage, however, is an extremely useful tool to evaluate virology (38) as well as mediators of inflammation. Obviously, multiple interventions are limited in large field trials. Likewise, asthma can be surveyed through symptom diaries or questionnaires, (some of which have been computerized for larger field trials), as well as objectively surveyed with portable peak flow meters or computerized spirometers.

The degree of rigor in these measures can impact the quality and interpretation of the observed association. Some of the methodological factors associated with these measurements are illustrated in Figure 3 and will be briefly reviewed here.

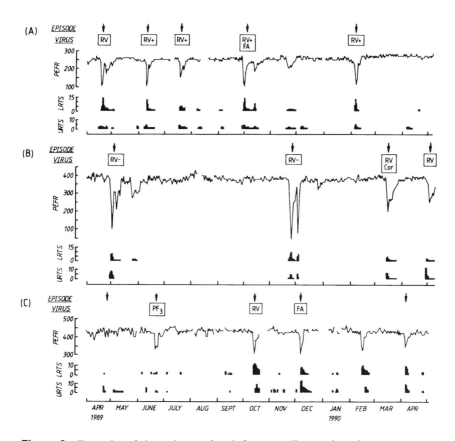

**Figure 2** Examples of charts drawn of peak flow recordings and respiratory symptoms for three 9- to 11-year-old children with virus-induced asthma exacerbation. The horizontal axis represents time. On the vertical axis, URTs and LRTS = upper and lower respiratory symptom scores, respectively: PEFR = morning peak expiratory flow rate. Reported episodes are indicated by vertical arrows, and viruses detected by the following symbols: RV = rhinovirus (+ = major group, − = minor group; others are ungrouped); FA = influenza virus type A; Cor = coronavirus; PF = parainfluenza virus; the absence of a symbol below an arrow indicates that no virus was detected for that reported episode. For each child there is one episode of a fall in peak flow accompanied by respiratory symptoms, which was not reported to the investigators (no arrow present). (From Ref. 22.)

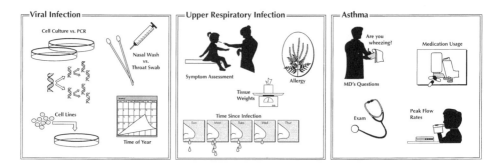

**Figure 3**  Factors associated with the evaluation of upper respiratory illness, virus isolation, and asthma. (Illustrations prepared by Leigh Rondano, copyright © Boehringer Ingelheim Pharmaceuticals, Inc., 1996. All rights reserved. Used with permission.)

### URI Symptoms

Documentation of upper respiratory infection is primarily through assessment of symptoms. With common cold illness, the symptom profile can change over the course of the active acute illness; however, the spectrum of nasopharyngeal symptoms is usually present over a period of a week or so. The type and severity of symptoms will also be affected if one prospectively evaluates a cohort for the development of symptoms or attempts to recruit patients with recent onset (e.g., 48 hours). In the latter group, early symptoms such as sore throat can be missed, but the overall severity at presentation will be greater as patients are now at the peak of their symptoms. This has been illustrated when symptoms were profiled in a group of subjects presenting with a natural cold of recent onset and compared to a group who were similarly surveyed following a controlled challenge with rhinovirus (Fig. 4).

One limitation of prospective evaluation of cohorts is the difficulty ensuring a true episode of URI against background symptoms such as a dry throat, sneeze, cough, or headache. There are no formal symptomatic criteria that clearly establish infection early on; however, the presence and relative persistence of upper airway symptoms such as sore throat and rhinorrhea can be useful. Here, rapid methods of viral detection become particularly valuable to corroborate symptoms and help rule out irritation from environmental pollutants and allergic symptomology. Establishing infection in field trials used to evaluate antiviral therapy becomes particularly important, as limiting the number of true nonillnesses will strengthen the trial's ability to demonstrate efficacy.

Retrospective recall of URI symptoms is commonly utilized in cohorts of asthmatics or bronchitic who present with acute symptoms. Here the potential problems are twofold. First, patients with a chronic illness may be less likely to

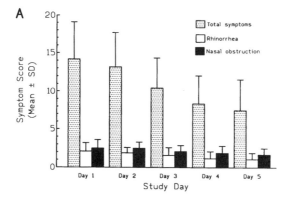

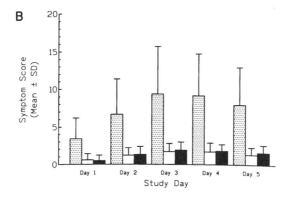

**Figure 4** Mean total, rhinorrhea, and nasal obstruction symptom scores reported by study day in the natural (A) and induced (B) colds. (From Ref. 9).

be affected by symptoms that may be more bothersome (e.g., rhinorrhea) than limiting (e.g., dyspnea); therefore, recall of the symptoms such as rhinorrhea can be compromised. Second, recall, in general, may be less, particularly as the time from onset of URI symptoms to presentation with lower airway symptoms is prolonged. In one survey of adult asthmatics presenting to the emergency ward (33), over half of the patients noted symptoms of viral illness, with an average duration of symptoms upon presentation to the hospital of 4 days. In this cohort, however, there was limited documentation of the presence of virus.

Whether this is more reflective of vigor of recall, the sensitivity and resolution of the questions, or the issues surrounding viral culture is difficult to determine; however, rhinovirus detection is more successful when specimens are collected during peak viral shedding early in the illness. Specimens collected late in the illness are less likely to yield the true occurrence of virus and therefore are less useful in determining the association between URI and asthma. These issues will be discussed in greater detail in the following section.

### Documenting Viral Illness

Documentation of respiratory viruses clearly strengthens the association between the URI illness and asthma. For example, viral identification allows for stronger partitioning of viral versus allergic symptoms. However, there are many technical points that limit study to study comparisons and thus, the overall interpretation of the association. These include (1) timing of specimen collection relative to illness onset; (2) spectrum of viruses one can evaluate; and (3) techniques for both collection and analysis of virus.

Technical details associated with viral identification are beyond the scope of this chapter; nevertheless, some basic issues are identified to alert the reader to their potential impact on epidemiological observations. First, timing of specimen sampling relative to common cold illness is extremely important because viral shedding decreases after acute illness. As noted above, one cannot expect high viral identification rates much after acute URI illness subsides. This point is illustrated in a large emergency ward study of asthma and URI (39), where rhinovirus was detected by PCR in 25 out of 131 specimens; 23 of the 25 were from those presenting within 4 days of URI symptom onset. In those subjects who presented after 5 days of symptom onset, only 2 of 31 specimens had virus detected.

Another methodological consideration is the comparative susceptibilities of cell lines for virus isolation. Rhinovirus isolation, for example, is not uniform among commonly used cell types (40). Additionally, rhinovirus was detected in a single cell type in only 20–35% of positive samples tested in multiple cell types, suggesting that utilization of a combination of susceptible cell lines is necessary for optimal recovery. The practical impact of these observations relates to the availability of the sophisticated laboratories involved in viral isolation in large field trials and the resources associated with more extensive methods. This is also the case when attempting to isolate numerous viruses, where a variety of techniques can be employed.

Finally, evolving methods such as PCR have improved isolation rates. For example, rhinovirus detection by PCR has resulted in isolation rates in the range of 80% during rhinovirus season (41) and during exacerbations of asthma in children (22) and adults (42). In employing these methods, however, it is important to evaluate viral detection rates during symptom-free periods in order to establish baseline rates of detection in symptom-free asthmatics. Careful evaluation of the sensitivity of the entire assay system should be made in order to assess and compare results. For instance, using nasal aspirates as their source of RNA,

Johnston et al. (22) reported picornavirus detection in 12% of pediatric patients evaluated while symptom-free, at a timepoint 2 weeks after onset of cold and asthma symptoms. However, no virus was detected in samples prepared from nose and throat swabs taken from symptom-free adult asthmatics by Nicholson et al. (42). As mentioned previously, differences in detection have been shown between adults and children, possibly due to quantity of viral shedding. Differences between sample sources may result in varying detection rates, although PCR may be less affected by this process than conventional methods, since amplification of very small amounts of RNA by the PCR process is possible. This extreme sensitivity necessitates that care be taken to avoid cross-contamination of samples. Also, vehicles such as transport medium can be routinely tested for false-positive results with each PCR procedure. These methods are described elsewhere and are beyond the scope of this chapter.

### Defining Asthma

There are a number of well-established measures of asthma symptoms (43) and physiological function (44) that can be applied to epidemiological studies. Both spirometry, which provides a useful "snapshot" of degree and severity of airway obstruction, and peak flow or portable spirometry, which are useful for serial testing, have a role in disease characterization (43). Other tests that examine airway responsiveness provide more information, but at the expense of time. Bronchial challenge test procedures can be modified for large-scale application (45).

While such objective tests can be used in epidemiological surveys to identify asthma, their application requires refinement when studying the association of asthma with viral illness. Typically, one must define a change in objective function that is reflective of true decompensation against the normal variability of the measure.

For example, the approach utilized by Johnston et al. (22) involved symptom variations around the median for a given child and considered PEF drops indicative of an "episode" when they fell to or below the 10th percentile. Similar criteria were also considered in the duration of an episode. As illustrated in Figure 2, PEFs were stable with sudden drops associated with viral infection. The median maximal fall in PEFR was 80 L/m for the reported episodes and 50 L/m for unreported episodes.

In the prospective study of adults by Nicholson and coworkers (42), subjects were given categorical clinical classifications based on upper and lower symptoms (Table 3). To characterize the episode with objective measures, they compared PEFs for 2 weeks after symptom onset with the corresponding period during the previous month. Asthma was classified as present if there was a significant difference between these periods (days 1–7) and the mean decrease relative to control period was ≥50 L/m.

**Table 3**  Classification of Symptomatic Episodes in a Prospective Trial of Adults

| | | |
|---|---|---|
| Symptom rating: | 0—Absent | |
| | 1—Mild | |
| | 2—Moderately severe | |
| | 3—Severe | |
| Categories: | Runny nose | Muscle aches |
| | Stuffy nose | Chills |
| | Sneezing | Cough |
| | Sore throat | Painful swollen neck glands |
| | Hoarseness | Increase use of tissues |
| | Red or water eyes | Chest tightness |
| | Face ache or earache | Wheeze |
| | Feeling unwell | Breathless |
| Classification: | Doubtful cold | Symptoms scoring no more than 1 (mild) or in only one of categories nose, throat, and cough |
| | Cold | Symptoms of two or more of the categories nose, throat, cough, and systemic features, with at least one symptom scoring 2 (moderately severe) or more |
| | Subjective exacerbation of asthma | Increase in one or more symptoms of wheeze, chest tightness, and breathlessness in association with an increase in bronchodilator use; or subject was noted to be wheezing on clinical examination; or subject was admitted to hospital for asthma |
| | Cold with asthma | Symptoms of cold and subjective exacerbation combined |
| | Doubtful cold plus asthma | Symptoms of doubtful cold and subjective exacerbation of asthma together |

*Source*: Ref. 42.

Symptoms can be assessed through a variety of instruments, many of which are designed to detect the presence of asthma. In evaluating the relationship between one event such as viral infection and asthma, it is useful to be able to assess variations in established disease as they relate to intensity and frequency of symptoms. In evaluating asthma symptomology over time, short symptom-reporting intervals are necessary. For URI symptoms, daily recordings are optimal. Thus, the extent of questioning needs to be balanced with the requirement for frequent assessments.

## IV. Host and Environmental Factors

### A. Age

Extensive surveys conducted several decades ago, such as those in the small rural American town of Tecumseh, Michigan (46–48), provide a backdrop of the occurrence of URI in a general population. As seen in Figure 5, more than five episodes per year can be expected in the first years of life, with an average of about two to three per year throughout a lifetime. The slight increase in frequency noted in the third decade is commonly associated with increased transmission to parents from preschool- and school-aged children. This pattern has been observed in other adult (49) and pediatric (50) cohorts.

The decreasing frequency of upper respiratory infection with age is paralleled by the decreasing frequency of lower respiratory tract infection with age. In a 1979 report (50) of a cohort of North Carolina children presenting with symptoms and signs of respiratory illness, there was a steady decline over the

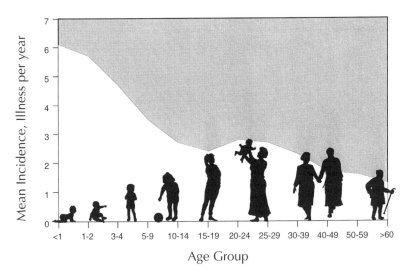

**Figure 5** Mean annual illness frequency for total respiratory illness as observed in the studies by Monto and colleagues in Tecumseh, Michigan. (Illustrations prepared by Leigh Rondano, copyright © Boehringer Ingelheim Pharmaceuticals, Inc., 1996. All rights reserved. Used with permission.)

first 6 years of life. The wheezing associated respiratory illness among these infections was highest during the first year (11.4 cases per 100 children per year), fell to about half of this (6.0 per 100) in the second year, and gradually declined thereafter.

Numerous viruses are responsible across all age groups with some obvious age-specific viral illnesses evident. Most notable is the higher prevalence of RSV infection in younger children. In the North Carolina cohort (50), RSV was the most important cause of wheezing in infants and preschool children. Here, RSV accounted for 44% of the isolates among the cases with wheezing infections from age 0–2 and 31% of the isolates among wheezing infections in those 2–5 years old. In each of the 11 years of this investigation, the incidence of wheezing illness peaked simultaneously with RSV-documented infections.

### B. Gender

Overall, females have been observed to have higher acute upper respiratory tract illness rates than males. The incidence of respiratory infections has been observed to be greater in males than in females during the first 3 years of life, with a reverse pattern noted after age 3 (46). The largest differences between males and females in the 1976–1981 Tecumseh survey occurred in the period of ages 20–34 (47).

There are limited data to examine the potential pattern shifts based on current family and work practices. Data from 20 years ago, however, pointed to a higher incidence rate in nonemployed women (47).

Family composition can also impact infection rates in the mother and father. For example, the presence of one child sharply increases rates in both parents; thereafter, rates gradually decline in both parents as the age of the oldest child increases. The return to those illness rates associated with having no children occurs slightly sooner for the father (oldest child 10–14 years) than for the mother (oldest child 15–19 years) (48).

Gender differences impacting the association of respiratory infection and asthma are not clear. In one of the largest pediatric surveys, "wheezing-associated respiratory illness" (WARI) occurred more frequently in boys, with a relative risk of 1.35. Attack rates were higher throughout preschool and elementary school years, after which time risks for WARI were equal for both sexes (50). In older patients with respiratory disease, it has been observed that both males and females with chronic bronchitis had more rhinovirus infections than do control subjects, with the difference between the male groups being statistically significant (51).

### C. Environmental Tobacco Smoke

Observation studies have associated environmental tobacco smoke (ETS) exposure with "wheeze with colds," which serves to highlight environment as a potentially important variable in the association of URI and asthma. For example, in a cohort of over 11,000 school-aged children, Cunningham and colleagues (52) reported that approximately 8% had wheezing without a cold. These data were provided in an interview with the child's biological mother, and there were no differences in wheezing without a cold between those currently exposed to ETS and those not. The prevalence of wheezing with colds was higher, affecting 16.5% of the cohort. When evaluated with respect to ETS exposure, significantly more children were reported to wheeze with colds (19.7%) if exposed to ETS than if not (13.4%). The relative odds for wheezing with colds (1.65) demonstrated significant upward trends for the number of smokers at home as well as the number of cigarettes smoked per day in the home.

### D. Exercise

Beyond the well-described bronchoprovocation of exercise, there may be an interaction among asthma, URI, and exercise. The working hypothesis to describe this potential interaction can be derived from the immune alterations observed with acute and chronic exercise (53).

The risk of URI appears to be lessened in those engaged in moderate types of exercise and increased with heavy exertion (54). Several components of immune function can be suppressed for several hours following prolonged heavy exercise. These include increased neutrophil/lymphocyte ratio, decreased T-cell function, and decreased natural killer cell activity. While this does not offer succinct reasons for increased risk of infection, it may be related to these observations.

While the increased risk of infection associated with exercise observed in athletes has not concentrated on a relationship of exercise-related URI to asthma risk, one cannot rule out the possibility that certain immune modulations associated with exercise could influence the association of URI and asthma.

### V. Summary

Asthma exacerbations are associated with upper respiratory viral infections. Viral identification is higher during symptomatic periods of asthma than during asymptomatic periods, and a close temporal relationship between colds and increased asthma symptoms can be observed.

In studying the association of URI with asthma in population studies, symptoms, virology, and physiological alterations can all be utilized to characterize both the URI and asthma. Studies that prospectively monitor symptoms and lung function are best but are resource draining. Furthermore, it is necessary to consider several methodological aspects to optimize interpretation of results. For example, time of study must be sufficiently long (to capture seasonal trends in viral illness), a true illness episode must be considered against background symptoms (to ensure a true illness has emerged), and timing and methods of specimen collection for viral documentation must be optimized (to capture viral shedding when it is likely to occur and to ensure results are not influenced by variations in specimen collection). In addition to optimizing such detail in a particular study, these aspects also need consideration when comparing the observed association across studies.

Numerous host and environmental factors influence the susceptibility to and manifestation of URI and asthma, and these need to be considered in studying their association. One practical point is the higher prevalence of URIs in children; therefore, utilizing children will increase the likelihood of observing URI-related asthma exacerbations in field studies. Less evident factors such as environmental exposures and activity levels might also impact the evaluation of the association of these two illnesses.

## Acknowledgments

The author thanks Drs. Terry Werick and Margaret Wecker for their reviews of the manuscript and Dr. Frederick Hayden for reviewing the virology section.

## References

1. NHLBI—National Institutes of Health. Global Initiatives for Asthma. Publication Number 95-3659, Washington, D.C., 1995.
2. Pattemore PK, Johnston SL, Bardin PG. Viruses as precipitants of asthma symptoms I. Epidemiology. Clin Exp Allergy 1992; 22:325–336.
3. Price WH. The isolation of a new virus associated with respiratory clinical disease in humans. Proc Natl Acad Sci USA 1956; 42:892–896.
4. Greve JM, Davis G, Meyer AM, Forte CP, Yost SC, Marlor CW, Kamarck ME, McClelland A. The major human rhinovirus receptor is ICAM-1. Cell 1989; 56: 839–847.
5. Staunton DE, Merluzzi VJ, Rothlein R, Barton R, Marlin SD, Springer TA. A cell adhesion molecule, ICAM-1, is the major surface receptor for rhinoviruses. Cell 1989; 56:849–853.
6. Arruda E, Crump CE, Rollins BS, Ohlin A, Hayden FG. Comparative susceptibles of human embryonic fibroblasts and HeLa cells for isolation of human rhinoviruses. J Clin Microbiol 1996; 34:1277–1279.
7. Olive DM, Al-Mufti S, Al-Mulla W, Khan MA, Pasca A, Stanway G, Al-Nakib W. Detection and differentiation of picornavirus in clinical samples following genomic amplification. J Gen Virol 1990; 71:2141–2147.
8. Johnston SL, Sanderson G, Pattemoe PK, Bardin PG, Bruce CB, Lambden PR, Smith S, Tyrrell DAJ, Holgate ST. Use of polymerase chain reaction for diagnosis of picor-

navirus infection in subjects with and without respiratory symptoms. J Clin Microbiol 1993; 31:111–117.

9.  Turner RB, Witek TJ, Riker DK. Comparison of symptom severity in natural and experimentally-induced colds. Am J Rhinol 1996; 10:167–172.

10. Rao SS, Hendley JO, Hayden FG, Gwaltney JM, Jr. Symptom expression in natural and experimental rhinovirus colds. Am J Rhinol 1995; 9:49–52.

11. Witek TJ, Cohen SD, Geist FC, Sorrentino JV, Riker DK. The clinical course of acute upper respiratory infection. Proceedings of XIV Congress of the European Rhinologic Society, Rome, 1992:104–105.

12. Chanock R, Finberg L. Recovery from infants with respiratory illness of a virus related to chimpanzee coryza agents. Epidemiologic aspects of infection in infants and young children. Am J Hyg 1957; 66:291–300.

13. Swierkosz EM, Flanders R, Melvin L, Miller JD, Kline MK. Evaluation of the Abbott TESTPACK RSV enzyme immonoassay for detection of respiratory syncytial virus in nasopharyngeal swab specimens. J Clin Microbiol 1989; 27:1151–1154.

14. Hall CB, Douglas RG Jr., Geiman IC. Possible transmission by fomites of respiratory syncytial virus. Infect Dis 1980; 141:98–102.

15. Lugo RA, Natiata MC. Pathogenesis and treatment of bronchiolitis. Clin Pharm 1993; 12:95–116.

16. Hayden FG, Gwaltney JH. Viral infections. In: Murray JF, Nadel JA, eds. Textbook of Respiratory Medicine. Philadelphia: WB Saunders, 1988: 748–802.

17. Shelhamer JH, Gill VJ, Quinn TC, Crawford SW, Kovacs JA, Masur H, Ognibene FP. The laboratory evaluation of opportunistic pulmonary infections. Ann Intern Med 1996; 124:585–599.

18. Johnston SL, Pattemore PK, Sanderson G, Smith S, Campbell MJ, Josephes LK, Cunningham A, Robinson SB, Myint SH, Ward ME, Tyrell DAJ, Holgate ST. The relationship between upper respiratory infections and hospital admissions for asthma: a time-trend analysis. Am J Respir Crit Care Med 1996; 154:654–660.

19. Sarkkinen HK, Halonen PE, Arstila PP, Salmi AA. Detection of respiratory syncytial, parainfluenza type 2, and adenovirus antigens by radioimmunoassay and enyzme immonoassay on nasopharyngeal specimens from children with acute respiratory disease. J Clin Microbiol 1981; 13:258–265.

20. Rowe WP, Huebner RJ, Gilmore LK, Parrott RH, Ward GT. Isolation of a cytopathogenic agent from human adenoids undergoing spontaneous degeneration in tissue culture. Proc Soc Exp Biol Med 1953; 84:570–573.

21. Macek V, Sorli J, Koprira S, Marin J. Persistant adenoviral infection and chronic airway obstruction in children. Am J Respir Crit Care Med 1994; 150:7–10.

22. Johnston SL, Pattemore PK, Sanderson G, Smith S, Lampe F, Josephs B, Symington P, O'Toole S, Myint H, Tyrell DA, Holgate ST. Community study of role of viral infections in exacerbations of asthma in 9–11 year old children. Br Med J 1995; 310:1225–1228.

23. Horn MEC, Brian EA, Gregg I, Inglis JM, Yealland SJ, Taylor P. Respiratory viral infection and wheezy bronchitis in childhood. Thorax 1979; 34:23–28.

24. Mitchell I, Inglis JM, Simpson H. Viral infection as a precipitant of wheeze in children: combined home and hospital study. Arch Dis Child 1978; 53:106–111.

25. Hudgel DW, Langston L, Selner JC, McIntosh K. Viral and bacterial infections in adults with chronic asthma. Am Rev Respir Dis 1979; 12:393–397.

26. Jennings LC, Barns G, Dawson KP. The association of viruses with acute asthma. NZ Med J 1987; 100:488–490.

27. McIntosh K, Ellis EF, Hoffman LS, Lybass TG, Eller JJ, Fuiginiti VA. The association of viral and bacterial respiratory infection with exacerbations of wheezing in young asthmatic children. J Pediatr 1973; 82:578–590.

28. Minor TE, Dick EC, DeMeo AN, Ouellette JJ, Cohen M, Reed CE. Viruses as precipitants of asthmatic attacks in children. J Am Med Assoc 1974; 227:292–298.

29. Mertsola J, Ziegler T, Ruuskanen O, Vanto T, Koivikko A, Halonen P. Recurrent wheezy bronchitis and viral respiratory infections. Arch Dis Child 1991; 66:124–129.

30. Podosin RL, Felton WL. The clinical picture of Far-East influenza occurring at the 4th National Boy Scout Jamboree. N Engl J Med 1958; 258:778–782.

31. Rebhan AW. An outbreak of Asian influenza in a girls camp. Can Med Assoc J 1957; 77:797–799.

32. Schuh S, Johnson DW, Callahan S, Canny G, Levinson H. Efficacy of frequently nebulized ipratropium bromide added to frequent high-dose albuterol therapy on severe childhood asthma. Pediatrics 1995; 126:639–645.

33. Sokhandan M, McFadden ER, Huang YT, Mazanec MB. The contribution of respiratory viruses to severe exacerbations of asthma in adults. Chest 1995; 107:1570–1575.

34. Jackson GG, Dowling HF, Spiesman IG, Boand AV. Transmission of the common cold to volunteers under controlled conditions. AMA Arch Intern Med 1958; 101:267–278.

35. Doyle WJ, McBride TP, Skoner DP, Maddern BR, Gwaltney JM, Jr, Uhrin M. A double-blind, placebo-controlled clinical trial of the effect of chlorpheniramine on the response of the nasal airway, middle ear and Eustachian tube to provocative rhinovirus challenge. Pediatr Infect Dis J 1988; 7:229–242.

36. Witek TJ, Canestrari DA, Hernandez JR, Miller RD, Yang JY, Riker DK. Nasal mucosal blood flow and nasal patency following oxymetazoline. Ann Allergy 1992; 68:165–168.

37. Druce HM, Bonner RF, Patow C et al. Response of nasal blood flow to neurohormones as measured by laser-Doppler velocimetry. J Appl Physiol Respir Environ Exercise Physiol 1984; 57:1276–1283.

38. Witek TJ. The nose as a target for adverse effects from the environment. Applying advances in physiologic measurements and mechanisms. Am J Indust Med 1993; 4:649–657.

39. Chanarin N, Miles J, Johnston SL, Sanderson G, Beasly R, Holgate ST. Virus infections are associated with acute severe asthma but not exacerbations of chronic persistent disease. Eur Respir J 1996; 9:1075.

40. Arruda E, Crump CE, Rollins BS, Ohlin A, Hayden FG. Comparative susceptibilities of human embryonic fibroblasts and HeLa cells for isolation of human rhinoviruses. J Clin Microbiol 1996; 34:1277–1279.

41. Arruda E, Pitkaranta A, Witek TJ, Doyle CA, Hayden FG. Etiology and clinical course of common colds during autumn months. Am J Respir Crit Care Med 1997.

42. Nicholson KG, Kent J, Ireland DC. Respiratory viruses and exacerbations of asthma in adults. Br Med J 1993; 307:982–986.

43. O'Connor GT, Weiss ST. Clinical and symptom measures. Am J Respir Crit Care Med 1994; 149:521–528.
44. Enright PL, Lebowitz MD, Cockcroft DW. Physiologic measures: pulmonary function tests. Am J Respir Crit Care Med 1994; 149:S9–S18.
45. O'Connor G, Sparrow D, Taylor D, Segal M, Weiss ST. Analysis of dose-response curves to methacholine: an approach suitable for population studies. Am Rev Respir Dis 1987; 136:1412–1417.
46. Monto AS, Ullman BM. Acute respiratory illness in an American community. JAMA 1974; 227:164–169.
47. Monto AS, Sullivan KM. Acute respiratory illness in the community: frequency of illness and the agents involved. Epidemiol Infect 1993; 110:145–160.
48. Monto AS, Ross H. Acute respiratory illness in the community: Effect of family composition, smoking, and chronic symptoms. Br J Prevent Social Med 1977; 31:101–108.
49. Gwaltney JM, Hendley JO, Simon G, Jordan WS. Rhinovirus infections in an industrial population. I. The occurrence of illness. N Engl J Med 1966; 275:1261–1268.
50. Henderson FW, Clyde WA, Collier AM, Denny FW, Senior RJ, Sheaffer CI, Conley WG, Christian RM. The etiologic and epidemiologic spectrum of bronchiolitis in pediatric practice. J Pediatr 1979; 95:183–190.
51. Monto AS, Bryan ER. Susceptibility to rhinovirus infection in chronic bronchitis. Am Rev Respir Dis 1978; 118:1101–1103.
52. Cunningham J, O'Connor GT, Dorkery DW, Speiger FE. Environmental tobacco smoke, wheezing, and asthma in children in 24 communities. Am J Respir Crit Care Med 1996; 153:218–224.
53. Nieman DC. Exercise, upper respiratory tract infection, and the immune system. Med Sci Sports Exerc 1994; 26:128–139.
54. Nieman DC. Upper respiratory tract infections and exercise. Thorax 1995; 50:1229–1231.

# 3

# Rates of Asthma Exacerbations During Viral Respiratory Infection

**JONATHAN M. CORNE and
SEBASTIAN L. JOHNSTON**

University of Southampton
Southampton, England

**RICHARD BEASLEY**

Wellington School of Medicine
Wellington, New Zealand

In his monograph "A Treatise of the Asthma" (1), published in 1698, Sir John Floyer wrote, "cannot remember the first Occasion of my Asthma; but have been told that it was a cold when I first went to school." Despite his experience and that of many asthmatics subsequently, the role of viral respiratory tract infection (VRTI) as precipitant of exacerbations of asthma has remained a subject of much debate. Indeed early investigators noted that viral infections lead to periods of anergy, as demonstrated by a reduction in delayed-type hypersensitivity responses, and concluded that viral infection, if anything, had a protective effect and would reduce the chances of an asthma exacerbation developing. In this chapter we will describe some of the early case reports that suggested that viral respiratory tract infections could lead to the development of exacerbations of asthma and then look at epidemiological and cohort studies that have investigated more fully their role. We will consider children and adults separately since the importance of VRTI in these two groups may differ.

## I. Early Case Reports

The first reports of VRTI leading to exacerbations of asthma were published by Podosin in 1958 (2). He described an outbreak of Far East influenza (influenza

A/Japan/305/57) occurring at a boy scout jamboree. Of 52,580 boy scouts aged 11–19 years present, 616 developed influenza, and the nature of the encampment allowed the natural history of their disease to be followed closely. The most consistent findings were fever, cough, sore throat, and symptoms of rhinitis and conjunctivitis. Of particular interest, however, is the fact that 27 children, all of whom had a history of asthma, developed acute asthma attacks as a complication of infection. Nineteen of the patients had no associated clinical or chest x-ray signs of parenchymal lung involvement, suggesting that they had developed an exacerbation of their asthma without any demonstrable pulmonary involvement of the influenza virus. Podosin also notes that 35 normal children (5.6%) developed wheezing following infection. These are not described in detail but may represent the development of increased bronchial hyperresponsiveness in some patients not previously diagnosed as having asthma.

A similar outbreak of influenza was described in the same year by Rebhan (3). This outbreak occurred at a centenary world guide camp held in Ontario at which 1600 people were present. Patterns of illness were similar to that described by Podosin and, again, seven girls with a previous history of asthma developed an exacerbation of their asthma as a complication of their infection.

Since these early observations a large number of studies have demonstrated the ability of viruses and other nonbacterial infective agents to cause episodes of wheezing. Roldaan and Masural (4), studying 32 mainly atopic children in a mountain resort, demonstrated that 29% of serologically proven VRTI and 67% of symptomatic VRTI infections led to exacerbations of asthma. Carlsen et al. (5) identified 979 children admitted to the hospital with diagnosed VRTI and showed that 13% of these infections were associated with exacerbations of asthma, with 47% of rhinovirus-type infections causing asthma exacerbations.

Although these studies suggest that VRTI can cause exacerbations of asthma, they do not define the proportion of exacerbations that are caused by viral infection, a figure that is important to know if we are to further our understanding of their role in exacerbations of asthma. A number of studies have addressed this question. These can be divided into indirect (time-series) studies, cross-sectional studies, and cohort studies involving both children and adults. As will become apparent, exacerbations of asthma have been studied far more extensively in children than in adults.

## II.   Indirect Evidence—Time-Series Studies

It has long been recognized that exacerbations of asthma have a marked seasonal variation, with a peak occurring during autumn (6). Various explanations of this have been advanced, including seasonal exposure to VRT infections, increases in aeroallergens (7), changes in weather systems (8), and changes in indoor air quality due to increased domestic heating (9). The possible role of VRTI was originally proposed following a study (10) of pediatric asthma admissions to a U.K. hospital in which the peak of admissions was noted to occur within the season in which the greatest number of respiratory tract viruses was isolated. Storr and Lenney (11) examined the admission rates for asthma at a children's hospital in Brighton over an 11-year period. They showed that admission rates showed a repeating yearly pattern with falling admission rates during the school holidays and two peaks of admissions during the school term, the first of which coincided with the return to school at the beginning of the term (the largest of which occurred at the beginning of the autumn term) and the second of which coincided with return following the half-term break. The authors concluded that this suggested a link between exacerbations of asthma and VRTI. It was proposed that the fall in admission rates during the school holidays occurred because there is less opportunity for spread of viruses when the children are away from school, and the peak immediately after the holidays was explained by new strains of virus being brought into the school community and spreading rapidly. A possible relationship between VRTI and episodes of asthma or bronchitis was sought by Ayres et al. (12). They examined general practitioner (GP) weekly returns for England and Wales over an 11-year period to determine the temporal association of episodes of acute asthma and bronchitis with viral isolation rates obtained from the Communicable Disease Surveillance Centre of the U.K. Public Health Laboratory Service. In children aged 0–4 years, peak consultation rates for wheezing illnesses (acute bronchiolitis and acute bronchitis) coincided with the peak for laboratory identifications of respiratory synoytial virus (RSV), suggesting a possible link. There were also positive correlations between GP-reported episodes of the common cold in children and acute asthma in children, although these did not reach statistical significance. A similar study has recently been reported from Singapore (13). Childhood emergency room attendances for asthma were compared over a 5-year period to virus isolation results from two large community hospitals. Although a significant positive correlation was found between daily frequency of RSV infection (lagged for 2 days) and asthma, this significance was lost when the data were analyzed using multiple regression and time-series analysis including confounding factors such as temperature and humidity.

In a later study, Dales et al. (14) examined seasonal patterns of emergency room visits and hospital admissions for asthma among children under 5 years of age in a reference population of 400,000 preschool children in Toronto, Canada. Admission rates and emergency presentation rates were examined over a 9-year period and were compared to those for nonrespiratory illnesses to allow for confounding factors such as bed closures and holiday periods. They showed a large peak in asthma admissions during the autumn period and were unable to demonstrate any significant correlation between this peak and levels of aeroallergens or levels of outdoor air pollutants measured during this period. In contrast, there was a significant correlation between rates of respiratory infections and both seasonal and week-to-week changes in admissions with asthma. They concluded that admissions for respiratory infections explained 20% of the variance in asthma admissions and 14% of the variance in asthma admissions after adjusting for climate, ambient air pollution, and aeroallergens.

A detailed analysis of seasonal changes in asthma exacerbations has been undertaken by Johnston et al. (15), who examined seasonal variations in hospital admissions for asthma over a 12-month period. The pattern of hospital admissions in the Wessex Regional Health Authority (previously one of 14 English Health Regions) and the Southampton District Health Authority (previously one of 9 districts within the Wessex region) were compared to viral infection rates recorded in a cohort of children aged 9–11 years with a history of wheeze or recurrent cough that had been investigated as part of another study (16) set within the Southampton District of the Wessex Regional Health Authority (Fig. 1). They confirmed the findings of Storr and Lenney showing that peaks of hospital admissions occurred within 2–4 weeks of the start of each school term. More significantly, however, they showed strong correlations between half-monthly rates of paediatric asthma admissions and viral detection rates from the Southampton cohort ($r = 0.67$, $p < 0.001$).

## III.  Studies in Adults

Fewer epidemiological studies have examined the link between URT viral infection and exacerbations of asthma in adults. In their study Ayres et al. (12) noticed a positive, though not statistically significant, correlation between rates of acute bronchitis and acute asthma. Since acute bronchitis is known to have an infective aetiology, it was suggested that, since there was a similar pattern of incidence, the etiology of acute asthma was also infective. Both showed a peak in autumn leading the authors to speculate that the infection was viral in nature.

Johnston et al. (15) extended their observations to demonstrate a correlation between virus-detection rates in their cohort of children and asthma admission rates among adults in the Wessex Regional Health Authority (Fig. 1). This correlation was less strong than for children ($r = 0.5$, $p = 0.013$) but nevertheless indicates that VRTI may be an important precipitant of asthma exacerbations in adults.

## IV.  Cross-Sectional Studies in Children

Studies based on time-series analysis have often relied on indirect or no virological data since virus isolations, if analyzed, apply to the population as a whole

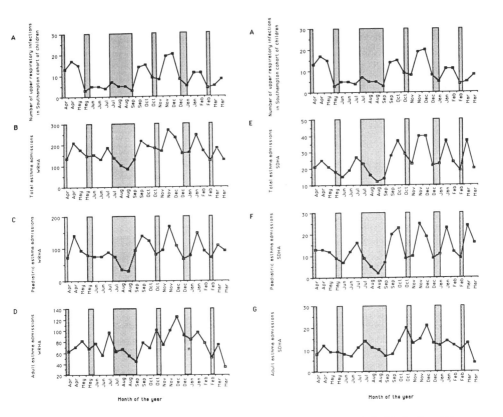

**Figure 1** A comparison of hospital admission rates for asthma and viral infection. (A) Number of upper respiratory tract infections identified in a cohort of 114 children aged 9–11 years with a history of wheeze or persistent cough and living in the city of Southampton in the Wessex Regional Health Authority (WRHA). These children were followed for 13 months and had nasal aspirates and venous blood taken every time they developed upper or lower respiratory tract symptoms. Upper respiratory tract viruses were identified by serology and rt-PCR. (B–D) Asthma admissions to the WRHA during the same period, showing total, pediatric, and adult admissions, respectively. (E–F) Asthma admissions in the city of Southampton showing total, pediatric, and adult admissions, respectively. The seasonal pattern of asthma admissions is similar to that of virus identification rates, suggesting that admissions to hospital with asthma may be precipitated by upper respiratory tract virus infection.

and are not specific to the patients presenting with exacerbations of asthma. Furthermore, viral identification rates are taken from a population of ill patients and so do not necessarily reflect the true prevalence of these viruses within the community. More exact information can be obtained by the direct investigation of patients presenting with acute exacerbations of asthma. This can take the form of prospective studies of cohorts or incidental studies in which patients presenting with a defined symptom complex and not previously recruited are examined to determine the frequency of infection.

A number of incidental studies have been reported that sought to identify infective agents in children presenting with episodes of asthma. Careful interpretation of these studies is necessary since they have varied considerably in the definition of an episode of asthma with some including any wheezing illness, some sampling children only with diagnosed asthma exacerbations, and some sampling children with wheezy bronchitis. We will categorize these studies according to the given definition of the episode since the denominator is important in comparing the results of different studies.

In order to overcome problems inherent in the definition of lower respiratory tract disease in children, a number of investigators have classified all types of lower respiratory symptoms together. Gregg (17) studied children who presented to his general practice with recurrent episodes of lower respiratory tract disease, which was defined as three or more episodes of cough accompanied by any generalized lower respiratory tract sign. No attempt was made to define further the nature of these episodes, but a number of factors including family history and atopic status suggested that a significant proportion of these children would be considered asthmatic. All children in the study were seen within 3 days of the onset of lower respiratory tract infection and isolation of viruses attempted from nose and throat swabs. Gregg demonstrated that VRTI was capable of causing lower respiratory tract disease, for example, rhinoviruses caused lower respiratory tract disease in 96% of the cases in which it was identified. This incidental study demonstrates the importance of VRTI as potential causes of exacerbations of asthma, but unfortunately the data were presented in a way that does not allow one to calculate the proportion of exacerbations caused by VRTI.

In another incidental study, Glezen et al. (18) surveyed children attending a pediatric group practice with episodes of lower respiratory tract disease and collected pharyngeal swabs on presentation to determine the rate of viral and *Mycoplasma* infection. Out of 3115 lower respiratory tract illnesses studied, evidence of VRTI or *Mycoplasma* infection was found in 28%. The authors extended their analysis by categorizing the episodes into croup, tracheobronchitis, bronchiolitis, and pneumonia. Of the episodes of bronchiolitis, defined as episodes of expiratory wheezing, VRTI or *Mycoplasma* infection was associated with 25.1% of episodes. In another community-based study, Horn et al. (19) examined URT virus infection rates in children presenting with ''wheezing bronchitis'' in a London general practice. Wheezy bronchitis was defined as an illness involving cough and the presence of wheeze and/or crackles. Five hundred and fifty-four such episodes were reported and nasal and throat swabs were taken within 5 days of the onset of symptoms for each of these. RT viruses were identified in 26.3% of reported episodes, the most common isolate being rhinoviruses (46.1% of viral isolations).

## V.  Hospital-Based Incidental Studies in Children

A large number of incidental studies have been performed in the hospital setting. These have focused on children admitted to the hospital with episodes variously defined as wheezing, wheezy bronchitis, or asthma, and in a number of studies the children have been followed to form a cohort.

In one early study Disney et al. (10) investigated 51 children admitted to hospital with acute attacks of asthma. In only 3 children (6%) were viruses isolated, and in only 2 out of the 26 tested (7.6%) was there serological evidence of recent viral infection, the conclusion being that viral infections were not important precipitants of acute asthma. Mitchell et al. (20) studied 267 children admitted to an Edinburgh hospital with wheezy bronchitis or exacerbations of asthma by taking throat and nasal swabs and nasopharyngeal aspirates on the day after admission. Viruses were isolated in 38 cases, giving an infection rate of only 14.2% although serological evidence suggested that a further 8 cases may have experienced recent infection, giving a total infection rate of 17.2%. As in other incidental studies in which they were sought, the most common virus identified was rhinovirus type, accounting for 34% of all possible infections.

In a combined inpatient and outpatient study, Carlsen et al. (21) studied a total of 256 attacks of asthma occurring in 169 children from 2 to 15 years of age. Nasopharyngeal secretions were collected together with sera either the morning after the patient was admitted or during their outpatient consultation. Viruses were identified in 73 cases, giving an identification rate of 29%, slightly higher than in previously published studies.

A much higher infection rate was found in a study by Jennings et al. (22), who investigated all children aged 0.5–12 years admitted to a New Zealand hospital with an acute respiratory illness. A virus or *Mycoplasma pneumoniae* was detected in 50% of all children and in 71% of children with a clinical diagnosis of bronchiolitis. No definition of bronchiolitis is given by the authors, but presuming it refers to children with a lower respiratory tract illness with wheeze, this is a very high viral isolation rate and one that is far higher than in other papers. The same authors, however, in another study (23) report on the association of VRTI infection with acute asthma in 204 children, of similar age profile, admitted to hospital over a one-year period. In this study viral infection was associated with 19% of acute asthma admissions. This suggests that the authors may have used a definition of bronchiolitis that was more specific than in other studies and led to a particularly high virus-identification rate in the bronchiolitis group. This explanation is also supported by the nature of the viruses identified, with 69% of viruses in the bronchiolitis group being RSV. Interestingly RSV was also the most common virus identified among the patients, with acute asthma accounting for 34.2% of viral infection and rhinoviruses accounting for 7.9%. As will be explained later, this may be due to methodological problems inherent in the identification of viruses such as rhinoviruses.

## VI.  Hospital-Based Incidental Studies in Adults

Only two published studies have attempted to determine the incidence of VRTI infection in adults admitted to hospital with exacerbations of asthma. In the first study of 63 asthmatics aged 15–77 years (24), blood was taken on admission and evidence of VRTI sought by serology. Evidence of recent viral infection was found in association with 19% of admissions for asthma, though the authors accepted that since only a small number of viruses were examined the actual incidence was probably higher.

In the second study Rossi et al. (25) studied all adult patients admitted to a university hospital with an acute attack of asthma, and virus identification was attempted by tissue culture and serology. Out of 142 episodes for which specimens were collected, VRTI or *Mycoplasma* infection was diagnosed in 41 (29%). This is a particularly high figure since the authors did not attempt to identify either rhinoviruses or coronavirus, which have been shown in most studies to far outnumber infection by other RT viruses. This high detection rate may reflect the use of enzyme immunoassay methods for virus detection or simply reflect severity of illness or speed of sampling.

## VII.  Cohort Studies in Children

A large number of cohort studies have been undertaken in children to determine the role of VRTI in exacerbations of asthma (Table 1). These studies have a number of advantages over the incidental studies outlined so far. First, such studies are, by their nature, prospective and allow for close monitoring of the participants so that samples can be taken as soon as symptoms develop. This avoids a delay between onset of symptoms and sampling of the patient, a problem that often occurs in incidental studies. Such a delay is likely to reduce the likelihood of isolating viruses, especially with conventional virological methods. Second, the population studied can be rigorously defined at the outset, allowing for much easier interpretation of results.

**Table 1**   Summary of Cohort and Cross-Sectional Studies Investigating the Role of Viruses in Exacerbating Asthma in Children

| First author | Year | Ref. | Type | Setting | Entry criteria | Episode type | No. of episodes studied | Viral detection rate (%) |
|---|---|---|---|---|---|---|---|---|
| Berkovich | 1970 | 26 | Cohort | Comm. | Asthma | Wheezing | 108 | 22.2 |
| Disney | 1971 | 10 | X Sect | Hosp. | Asthma | Asthma attacks | 51 | 9.8 |
| Glezen | 1971 | 18 | X Sect | Comm. | Lower RTI | Bronchiolitis with wheeze | 855 | 25.1 |
| McIntosh | 1973 | 27 | Cohort | Comm. | Asthma | RTI with wheezing | 139 | 41.7 |
| Minor | 1976 | 31 | X Sect | Comm. | Asthma | Asthma attacks | 71 | 23.9 |
| Mitchell | 1976 | 20 | X Sect | | Asthma/Wheezy bronchitis | Asthma/Wheezy bronchitis | 267 | 17.2 |
| Mitchell | 1978 | 28 | Cohort | Comm. | Asthma | Wheezing | 91 | 14.3 |
| Horn | 1979 | 27 | X Sect | Comm. | Wheezy bronchitis | Wheezy bronchitis | 72 | 48.6 |
| Roldaan | 1982 | 4 | Cohort | Comm. | Asthma | Exac. of asthma | 45 | 48.9 |
| Carlsen | 1984 | 21 | X Sect | Hosp. | Asthma | Acute bronchitis/Asthma | 256 | 29 |
| Jennings | 1985 | 22 | X Sect | Hosp. | Acute resp. illness | Acute resp. illness | 344 | 50 |
| Jennings | 1987 | 23 | X Sect | Hosp. | Asthma | Asthma attack | 204 | 18.6 |
| Mertsola | 1991 | 30 | Cohort | Comm. | Wheezy illness | Wheezing episode | 76 | 39.4 |
| Johnston* | 1995 | 16 | Cohort | Comm. | Wheeze or cough | LRT symptoms or fall in peak flow | 292 | 80 |

*Used PCR.

X Sect = cross-sectional study; Hosp = hospital-based study; Comm = community-based study; RTI = respiratory tract infection; LRT = lower respiratory tract; and resp = respiratory.

One of the first cohort studies was reported by Berkovich et al. (26). The cohort followed was part of a larger group of asthmatic children, aged 6 months to 16 years, who were participants in a study examining the effect of continuous treatment with antibiotics and were described as known asthmatics with recurrent disease. Throat and rectal swabs were taken for virus identification and blood taken for serology as soon as was possible after the development of a wheezy episode. Viral isolation rates from throat and rectal swabs were very low, with viruses identified in only 4 out of the 272 specimens detected (1.5%). However, out of the 84 volunteers from whom both acute and convalescent sera could be taken, there was evidence of recent viral infection in 27 of a total of 108 episodes of wheezing (25%), the most common virus being influenza type A followed by parainfluenza type 2.

McIntosh et al. (27) studied two cohorts of children hospitalized with asthma. Both cohorts consisted of severe asthmatics since they required prolonged hospital admission for intensive diagnostic study and assessment of treatment. In total, 32 children were studied, and nasopharyngeal and throat swabs and venous blood samples for serology were taken within 1–2 days of the development of a respiratory illness. There were 139 recorded episodes of wheezing, and RT viruses were associated with 58 of these (42%). The association between viral infection and wheezing was found to be stronger for certain respiratory viruses. Thus, RSV caused wheezing in all episodes of infection, whereas influenza A failed to cause wheezing despite being the cause of 11 incidents of infection. This latter observation is particularly interesting in view of the original case reports describing wheezing as a consequence of influenza A and may demonstrate important differences between strains of influenza virus.

Mitchell et al. (28) recruited 16 children attending a hospital respiratory clinic who were selected if they gave a history of three or more episodes of wheezing during the previous year. All volunteers kept diary cards of upper and lower respiratory symptoms as well as use of medication and were seen within 48 hours of the onset of respiratory illness. Nasal and throat swabs were taken for virological analysis. Of 127 reported episodes of wheezing, 91 samples were taken. Of these RT viruses were identified in 13 cases (14%), of which the most common were rhinoviruses (5.5% of episodes) and coxsackie (3.3% of episodes). Clinically, 56 episodes (61.5%) were thought to be associated with VRTI, which was interpreted as showing that clinical history was an unreliable guide to the presence of VRTI. However, a number of features suggest that it is more likely that the study methods resulted in an underestimate of the viral infection rate. These will be discussed in detail later, but it should be noted that only culture was used to detect the presence of virus and no additional serology was performed. Also, although the protocol required patients to be seen within 48 hours of the onset of illness, this was not always the case. Only 60 of the 91 episodes were reported as being seen within 48 hours, and in these the viral identification rate was higher (17%) than reported for the study as a whole. These figures are, however, consistent with the authors' previous identification rate of 17% in the hospital-based study described previously (20).

Horn et al. (29) collected a cohort of 22 children from those attending an asthma and bronchitis clinic held in a London general practice. Children were followed up for a period of up to 2 years, and nasal swabs, throat swabs, and sputum samples were collected within 5 days of the onset of respiratory symptoms. Seventy-two episodes of wheezy bronchitis were studied in which one or more viruses were identified in 35 (49%). Rhinovirus was the most common virus identified accounting for 20 of the 72 episodes (27.8%). Virus-isolation rates were higher in the more severe episodes, with viruses being identified in 17% of episodes classed as mild, 54% of episodes classed as moderate, and 63% of episodes classed as severe. The high isolation of viruses may partly be due to the addition of sputum samples since in 15% of episodes RT viruses were only found in the sputum and not in the nasal or throat swabs. Mertsola et al. (30) studied a cohort of 56 children who could be considered to suffer from severe wheezy illness in that they all had a history of two or more attacks of wheezy bronchitis involving one or more admissions to hospital. These children were followed up in the community and sampled during subsequent wheezing episodes. They found evidence of viral infection in 30 out of 76 (39.5%) episodes of wheezing, with the most commonly found virus type being coronavirus followed by rhinoviruses.

## VIII. Cohort Studies in Adults

A number of cohort studies have been undertaken in adults to determine the role of VRTI in the etiology of exacerbations of asthma (Table 2). In an early study

**Table 2**  Summary of Cohort and Cross-Sectional Studies Investigating the Role of Viruses in Exacerbating Asthma in Adults

| First author | Year | Ref. | Type | Setting | Entry criteria | Episode type | No. of episodes studied | Virus detect rate (%) |
|---|---|---|---|---|---|---|---|---|
| Huhti | 1974 | 24 | X Sect | Hosp. | Asthma | Asthma admission | 142 | 19 |
| Clark | 1979 | 32 | Cohort | Comm. | Asthma | Wheeze | 27 | 14.8 |
| Hudgel | 1979 | 33 | Cohort | Comm. | Asthma | Asthma exacerbation | 76 | 10.5 |
| Beasley | 1988 | 34 | Cohort | Comm. | Asthma | Asthma exacerbation | 178 | 10.0 |
| Rossi | 1994 | 25 | X Sect | Hosp. | Asthma | Asthma admission | 142 | 29 |
| Nicholson | 1993 | 36 | Cohort | Comm. | Asthma | Drop in peak flow | 84 | 44 |

X Sect = cross-sectional study; Hosp = hospital-based study; Comm = community-based study.

Minor et al. (31) investigated a cohort consisting of both children and adults. They noted that recovery of viruses was far more common during exacerbations of asthma in children than in adults, but unfortunately it is not possible to determine from the paper exact figures as to the relative rates of infection. Clarke (32) followed a cohort of 51 adult asthmatics, recruited from a hospital outpatient clinic, for 18 months. Volunteers were seen as soon as possible following the development of wheeze, and sputum was taken for bacteriology and blood for serology. A total of 111 exacerbations were studied. Nasopharyngeal swabs were taken during 27 of these exacerbations and RT viruses isolated in 4 of these (14.8%). Paired serological samples were taken during and following 102 exacerbations, and a rise in viral antibody titer found in 4 cases (3.6%), giving an overall viral infection rate of 10.8%. A similar identification rate was found by Hudgel et al. (33) in a study of 19 patients from a hospital clinic. Viral identification was undertaken by culture of nasopharyngeal washings and by serology. Viruses were identified in 8 out of the 76 episodes of wheezing in which a full analysis was undertaken giving a viral infection rate of 11% compared to an infection rate in remission of 3.3%. Although this is a low rate of infection, there was a statistically significant difference between the infection rate during exacerbations and when the volunteers were well, suggesting that an association, even if minor, did exist. In another cohort study Beasley et al. (34) recruited 31 patients aged 15–56 years with atopic asthma. Volunteers kept a diary card of symptoms and reported when they developed symptoms of respiratory tract infection or worsening of asthma. Nasopharyngeal aspiration for viral culture and venesection for serology was performed at each visit. Viruses were identified during 18 of the 178 reported episodes of asthma (10.1%). Viral identification was considerably higher during exacerbations classed as severe (35.7%) than in those classed as mild and moderate (5.3%).

## IX.  Studies Utilizing PCR—Children

Application of the polymerase chain reaction (PCR) has lead to an increase in the sensitivity of detection of RT viruses (35). This is because the most common RT viruses, rhinoviruses and coronavirus, which together account for more than 50% of episodes of the common cold, are very difficult to detect using the conventional virological techniques of tissue culture and serology. PCR relies on the exponential amplification of areas of the viral genome that are specific to that virus. The reaction is designed to incorporate enough cycles to allow amplification to such an extent that products can be detected by standard gel electrophoresis or by probing with specific nucleotide probes.

One study has so far been published that has used this technology to give an accurate determination of the role of VRTI in exacerbations of asthma in children (16). This important study probably gives the most accurate determination yet of the importance of VRTI in childhood asthma. One hundred and fourteen children, aged 9–11 years, with a history of wheeze or persistent cough were recruited and followed for 13 months. All children kept diary card records of upper and lower respiratory tract symptoms as well as twice-daily peak flow recordings. Parents contacted the investigators as soon as the child developed upper or lower respiratory tract symptoms, or if they felt the child was about to develop a cold, or if the child had an exacerbation of asthma. They also contacted the investigators should the child's peak flow fall by 50 liters/min. Within 48 hours of each report nasal aspiration was performed and blood taken. Rhinoviruses and coronavirus were identified using PCR and the other viruses by serology, tissue culture, and immunofluorescence. RT viruses were detected in 80% of reported falls in peak flow, 80% of episodes of wheeze, and 81% of all episodes of lower respiratory tract symptoms. Rhinovirus was the predominant organism identified and was responsible for 60.7% of all virus isolations (Fig. 2). This compared with a rhinovirus type isolation rate of 12% when the children were asymptomatic, giving a statistically significant difference ($p = 0.001$).

This study gives a far higher association rate of exacerbations of asthma and VRTI than any previously published study. Much of this is due to the ability of PCR technology to detect rhinoviruses, and the high pick of rate for rhinoviruses confirms this. Also important, however, are other methodological factors. The study was cohort in nature, its design ensured that children were sampled early on in the development of symptoms, and specimens were handled in a manner that maximized the chances of viral identification.

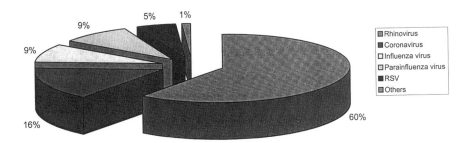

**Figure 2**  Upper respiratory tract viruses identified in a cohort of 114 children aged 9 to 11 years with a history of wheeze or persistent cough. The children were followed for 13 months and nasal aspirates were taken when they developed upper or lower respiratory tract symptoms. The figures refer to the percentage of the total number of viruses identified.

## X.  Studies Utilizing PCR—Adults

One study has so far been published that has used PCR to determine the importance of RT viruses as precipitants of asthma in adults (36). In this study 138 adult asthmatics were followed for a period of up to 2 years. Volunteers reported as soon as they developed upper or lower respiratory tract symptoms, at which point they were asked to keep diary card records of symptoms and to continue with twice-daily peak flow recordings. Nasal swabs were taken for identification of rhinoviruses by PCR and paired sera sample taken for serology for the other upper respiratory tract viruses. Of 315 symptomatic episodes, 84 were associated with a drop in mean peak flow of $> 50$ liters/min for the first 7 days after the episode. RT viruses were identified in 27 of these episodes (44%), though in 60 episodes (71%) volunteers had symptoms of the common cold preceding the asthma attack. Rhinovirus type was again the most common pathogen identified.

## XI.  Summary of Studies

In this chapter we have critically reviewed some of the most important published studies that have examined the association of VRTI and exacerbations of asthma. Most studies have used conventional methods for virus detection. In summarizing these we can first compare incidental and cohort studies. Cohort studies have demonstrated a much greater association between the VRTI and exacerbations of asthma. This is probably because use of a cohort allows participants to be followed closely and be sampled early in their illness, therefore increasing the chances of sampling during a period of virus shedding. This may also be a reason why hospital studies have generally given lower rates for virus identification. Although patients are more severely ill and therefore may be expected to have a higher virus load, by the time they are admitted they have often had the illness for a few days.

Another important comparison is between studies in adults and children. It is interesting in itself that far fewer studies have been undertaken in adults— a fact that may reflect the perception of clinicians that RT viruses are less important as precipitants of asthma in adults. To a certain extent this is justified by the studies so far described. The indirect studies have shown a far weaker correlation between peaks of viral infection and peaks of adult hospital admissions. However, this could partly be explained by the fact that the comparison was with virus detection rates in children, which may differ from those in adults. Cohort and incidental studies have also suggested that RT viruses are less important as precipitants of asthma attacks in adults. A weighted average of both incidental and cohort studies in children (37) carried out before the advent of PCR suggested that viruses were associated with 25% of wheezy episodes, whereas cohort studies alone suggested an association of RT viruses with 31.9% of wheezy episodes. In contrast, in adults the weighted average of the three incidental studies performed suggested that 13.3% of exacerbations of asthma can be associated with VRTI. Of particular interest is the study of Minor et al. (38), which investigated a cohort consisting of both adults and children and noted that viruses were isolated more frequently from children than from adults. This would suggest that the differences may not due to methodological problems. It may reflect differences in the nature of populations studied or the diagnostic category used. Many children without the features of asthma in between exacerbations wheeze in response to viral infection, and it is debatable whether these children are getting true exacerbations of asthma. Their inclusion in a cohort will result in a higher virus-detection rate since, by definition, these subjects will all have a viral infection. Adult asthma appears distinct from the syndrome of ''virus-induced wheeze'' observed in children, in that almost all subjects do have features of asthma in between exacerbations. The lower virus detection rates observed in adults may reflect the absence of a group with virus-induced wheeze. Virus infections become less frequent with increasing age, and it is therefore likely that the proportion of exacerbations induced by factors other than viruses (e.g., allergens) will also increase with age. The relative roles of allergen exposure and viral infection in inducing asthma exacerbations in various age groups have not so far been adequately studied.

Although limited in number, studies utilizing PCR have given much higher rates of virus identification than studies using conventional virological methods. This is largely due to improved detection of rhinoviruses, a virus type difficult to identify with conventional techniques but which is the major virus type associated with exacerbations of asthma. Indeed, previous studies showing higher rates of virus infection have generally been those that have been more successful in identifying rhinoviruses.

Studies using PCR give a more accurate reflection of the importance of RT viruses as causes of exacerbations of asthma than those using conventional virology. However, the sensitivity of this technique means that care must be taken in the design of these studies. In our experience PCR is so sensitive that by increasing the number of cycles minute amounts of viral genome can be detected in many asymptomatic samples of nasal aspirate. Thus, studies *must* be adequately controlled with either an asymptomatic control group or volunteers being sampled during asymptomatic periods and the rate of virus detection in these control groups being assessed critically when interpreting results.

## XII.  Future Studies

PCR techniques have now been developed for most of the RT viruses, and application of these should allow more accurate identification of their role in exacerbations of asthma. Studies of the importance of RT viruses in wheezy infants and a comparison of the characteristics of those with confirmed virus induced wheeze in infancy, childhood, and adulthood may throw some light on possible differences in the etiology of wheeze in these age groups. Such technology can also be used to determine the importance of RT viruses in other respiratory diseases. The role of RT viruses in cystic fibrosis has already been investigated, and other areas in which such research would be beneficial include the role of RT viruses in exacerbations of chronic obstructive pulmonary disease and interstitial lung disease such as pulmonary fibrosis.

## XIII.  Conclusions

Early case reports suggested a role for RT viruses as causes of asthma exacerbations, and this was supported by a number of epidemiological investigations. Limitations in virological techniques precluded definitive demonstration of such a link in either cohort or cross-sectional studies. The development of a PCR for rhinoviruses has allowed more accurate documentation of the role of rhinoviruses and suggested that these viruses are responsible for more than 80% of asthma exacerbations in children and around 50% in adults. The development of PCR for the other RT viruses will allow more accurate documentation of the role of RT viruses in exacerbations of asthma and also exacerbations of other respiratory diseases.

### References

1.  Floyer J. A Treatise of the Asthma. London: R Wilkin, 1698.
2.  Podosin RL, Felton WL. The clinical picture of far east influenza occuring at the fourth national boy scout jamboree. N Engl J Med 1958; 258:778–782.
3.  Rebhan AW. An outbreak of Asian influenza in a girls camp. Can Med Assoc J 1957; 77:797–799.
4.  Roldaan AC, Masural N. Viral respiratory infections in asthmatic children staying in a mountain resort. Eur J Respir Dis 1982; 63:140–150.
5.  Carlsen K-H, Orstavik I, Halvorsen K. Viral infections of the respiratory tract in hospitalized children. Acta Paediatr Scan 1983; 72:53–58.
6.  Adams F. The Genuine Works of Hippocrates. Baltimore: The Williams and Wilkins Co, 1939.
7.  Salvaggio S, Hasselblad V, Seabury C, Heiderscheit L. New Orleans asthma. II. Relationship of climatologic and seasonal factors to outbreak. J Allergy 1970; 45: 257–265.
8.  Goldstein I. Weather patterns and asthma epidemics in New York City and New Orleans. Int J Biometeorol 1980; 24:329–339.

9. Bates D, Baker-Anderson M, Sizto R. Asthma attack periodicity: a study of hospital emergency visits in Vancouver. Environ Res 1990; 51:51–70.

10. Disney M, Matthews R, Williams J. The role of infection in the morbidity of asthmatic children admitted to hospital. Clin Allergy 1971; 1:399–406.

11. Storr J, Lenney W. School holidays and admissions with asthma. Arch Dis Child 1989; 64:103–107.

12. Ayres JG, Noah ND, Fleming DM. Incidence of episodes of acute asthma and acute bronchitis in general practice 1976–87. Br J Gen Pract 1993; 43:361–4.

13. Chew F, Doraisingham S, Goh D, Kumaransinghe G, Ooi B, Lim Y, Soh S, Lee B. Patterns of respiratory virus infections and its association with acute childhood asthma (abstr). J Allergy Clin Immunol 1996; 97:307.

14. Dales R, Schweitzer I, Toogood J, Drouin M, Yang W, Dolovich J, Boulet J. Respiratory infections and the autumn increase in asthma morbidity. Eur Respir J 1996; 9: 72–77.

15. Johnston S, Pattemore P, Sanderson G, Smith S, Campbell M, Josephs L, Cunningham A, Robinson B, Myint S, Ward M, Tyrrell D, Holgate S. The relationship between upper respiratory infections and hospital admissions for asthma: A time trend analysis. Am J Respir Crit Care Med 1996; 154:654–660.

16. Johnston S, Pattemore P, Sanderson G, Smith S, Lampe F, Josephs L, Symington P, O'Toole S, Myint S, Tyrell D, Holgate S. Community study of role of viral infections in exacerbations of asthma in 9–11 year old children. Br Med J 1995; 310: 1225–1229.

17. Gregg I. A study of recurrent bronchitis in childhood. Respiration 1970; 27:133–138.

18. Glezen W, Loda F, Clyde W, Senior R, Sheaffer C, Conley W, Denny F. Epidemiologic patterns of acute lower respiratory disease of children in a pediatric group practice. J Pediatr 1971; 78:397–406.

19. Horn M, Brain E, Gregg I. Respiratory viral infection in childhood. A survey in general practice, Roehampton 1967–1972. J Hygeine 1975; 74:157–168.

20. Mitchell I, Inglis H, Simpson H. Viral infection in wheezy bronchitis and asthma in children. Arch Dis Child 1976; 51:707–711.

21. Carlsen KH, Orstavik I, Leegaard J, Hoeg H. Respiratory virus infections and aeroallergens in acute bronchial asthma. Arch Dis Child 1984; 59:310–315.

22. Jennings LC, Dawson KP, Abbott GD, Allen J. Acute respiratory tract infections if children in hospital: a viral and mycoplasma pneumoniae profile. NZ Med J 1985; 98:582–585.

23. Jennings L, Barns G, Dawson K. The association of viruses with acute asthma. NZ Med J 1987; 100:488–490.

24. Huhti E, Mokka T, Nikoskelainen J, Halonen P. Association of viral and mycoplasma infections with exacerbations of asthma. Ann Allergy 1974; 33:145–149.

25. Rossi O, Kinnula V, Tuokko H, Huhti E. Respiratory viral and *Mycoplasma* infections in patients hospitalized for acute asthma. Monaldi Arch Chest Dis 1994; 49: 107–111.

26. Berkovich S, Millian S, Snyder R. The association of viral and mycoplasma infections with recurrence of wheezing in the asthmatic child. Ann Allergy 1970; 28:43–49.

27.  McIntosh K, Ellis EF, Hoffman LS, Lybass TG, Eller JJ, Fulginiti VA. The association of viral and bacterial respiratory infections with exacerbations of wheezing in young asthmatic children. J Paediatr 1973; 82:578–90.

28.  Mitchell I, Inglis J, Simpson H. Viral infection as a precipitant of wheeze in children. Combined home and hospital study. Arch Dis Child 1978; 53:106–111.

29.  Horn MEC, Reed SA, Taylor P. Role of viruses and bacteria in acute wheezy bronchitis in childhood: a study of sputum. Arch Dis Child 1979; 54:587–592.

30.  Mertsola J, Ziegler T, Ruuskanen O, Vanto T, Koivikko A, Halonen P. Recurrent wheezy bronchitis and viral respiratory infections. Arch Dis Child 1991; 66:124–129.

31.  Minor TE, Dick EC, Baker JW, Ouellette JJ, Cohen M, Reed CE. Rhinovirus and influenza type A infections as precipitants of asthma. Am Rev Respir Dis 1976; 113:149–153.

32.  Clarke CW. Relationship of bacterial and viral infections to exacerbations of asthma. Thorax 1979; 34:344–347.

33.  Hudgel DW, Langston L, Selner J, McIntosh K. Viral and bacterial infections in adults with chronic asthma. Am Rev Respir Dis 1979; 120:393–397.

34.  Beasley RB, Coleman ED, Hermon Y, Holst PE, O'Donnell TV, Tobias M. Viral respiratory tract infection and exacerbations of asthma in adult patients. Thorax 1988; 43:679–683.

35.  Johnston S, Sanderson G, Pattemore P, Smith S, Bardin P, Bruce C, Lambden P, Tyrrell D, Holgate S. Use of polymerase chain reaction for diagnosis of picornavirus infection in subjects with and without respiratory symptoms. J Clin Microbiol 1993; 31:111–117.

36.  Nicholson KG, Kent J, Ireland DC. Respiratory viruses and exacerbations of asthma in adults. Br Med J 1993; 307:982–6.

37.  Pattemore PK, Johnston SL, Bardin PG. Viruses as precipitants of asthma symptoms. I. Epidemiology. Clin Exp Allergy 1992; 22:325–36.

38.  Minor TE, Dick EC, De Meo AN, Ouellette JJ, Cohen M, Reed CE. Viruses as precipitants of asthmatic attacks in children. J Am Med Assoc 1974; 227:292–8.

# 4

## Risk Factors for Wheezing with Viral Upper Respiratory Tract Infections in Children

**MICHAEL KABESCH and ERIKA VON MUTIUS**

University Children's Hospital
Munich, Germany

## I. Introduction

Approximately one-half of all consultations in pediatric practice for children under the age of 5 years is due to respiratory illnesses, and about 20% of childhood hospital admissions are attributable to respiratory diseases. Infections of the respiratory tract, largely observed as common colds, are the most frequent cause of illness in humans. Children in particular go through a series of these viral infections within their first few years of life. Respiratory syncytial virus (RSV), human rhinovirus, coronavirus, parainfluenza virus types 1–3, adenovirus, and influenza virus types A and B have all been associated with infections of the respiratory tract in children (1–11). In general, any respiratory virus can cause any picture of acute respiratory infection, but certain viruses tend to associate with a particular group of diseases (12). This tendency probably reflects the fact that viruses seem to have a particular affinity to certain types of cells and certain anatomic levels of the airways, although they affect quite a wide area of the airway epithelium. For example, clinical colds are more strongly associated with rhinoviruses and coronaviruses, which particularly affect the nasal epithelium, whereas croup is more often related to parainfluenza virus, which also attacks the larynx and trachea. In turn, adenovirus is often involved in eliciting sore throat, but it can also cause severe pneumonia and bronchiolitis in some subjects.

Wheeze is a very common respiratory symptom in early childhood. About half of a random sample of children enrolled as newborns in a prospective, longitudinal, population-based survey—the Tucson Children's Respiratory Study in the United States—wheezed at some time from birth up to the age of 6 years (13). Similar figures have been reported from a smaller Australian birth cohort study in which 42% of infants developed wheezing in the first 2 years of life (14). In European population studies estimates have been slightly lower, ranging from 15 to 32% of children who wheezed at some time during the first 5 years of life (15).

A number of studies have shown that childhood wheeze is often associated with viral respiratory tract infections (16–19). Subjects on their first visit to a clinic because of wheezing often present with rhinorrhea, nasal congestion, mild fever, cough, and other features of viral upper respiratory tract infection. A significant proportion of these children will develop recurrent episodes of wheeze, and some will become atopic and develop airway hyperresponsiveness and asthma following the initial viral illness. The factors that determine the prognosis and further progression or remission of the disease relate to both intrinsic and extrinsic characteristics. Intrinsic host factors will determine a subject's ability to limit the clinical response to a viral infection to no symptoms or only local signs of infection, such as rhinorrhea and sneezing, or to extend the response to the lower respiratory tract and other organ systems. Extrinsic factors, which may be attributable to different virus species or to environmental conditions, will further determine a subject's outcome.

Section II of this chapter will discuss the different phenotypes of wheezing illness in infancy and childhood, and the second part the incidence and type of viral infections detected in wheezing lower respiratory tract illnesses (LRIs) in children. Finally, several risk factors for these wheezing conditions will be discussed.

## II. Wheezing in Infancy and Childhood

In a large prospective birth cohort study in the United States, the Tucson Children's Respiratory Study, Martinez and coworkers investigated pulmonary function in a subgroup of infants shortly after birth before any wheezing LRI had occurred (20). The risk for developing a wheezing illness in the first year of life was 3.7 times higher among infants whose premorbid total respiratory conductance ranged in the lowest tertile as compared to the rest of the group. Decrements in lung function were seen in both, boys and girls. However, gender differences were found for the respective indices of pulmonary function: in boys Tme/TE was significantly reduced, whereas functional residual capacity was significantly diminished in girls. These children were further followed up to their third and sixth birthdays (13,21). Those infants who started to wheeze during the first 3 years of life had lower initial levels of lung function than children with no LRI or with nonwheezing LRIs.

The shape of the tidal-breathing expiratory-flow-time curve as assessed by calculating the percentage of expiratory time to reach peak tidal expiratory flow ($T_{me}$/TE) has been shown to correlate well with specific airway conductance, $FEV_1$ and the $FEV_1$/FVC ratio (22). The conductance, in turn, is a function of the fourth power of the airway radius and depends on the conductance of the lower and upper airways and on characteristics of the lung tissue and the chest wall. Therefore, not only differences in the size and length of airways but also differences in the elastic recoil properties of the lung and the chest wall may exist between infants who subsequently develop wheezing with a viral lower respiratory tract illness and those who do not wheeze with a similar illness. In the Tucson study, airway conductance seemed to be the critical factor in boys, whereas a significantly smaller lung size may predispose girls to wheezing lower respiratory tract illnesses. These discrepancies between genders may confirm previous observations that boys have smaller airways relative to lung size than girls (23).

A recent study from western Australia by Young and colleagues (14) confirmed these findings. Two hundred and fifty-three infants underwent lung function testing at a mean age of 5 weeks and were followed during the first 2 years of life with lung function measurements at 1 month of age. Maximum flow at functional residual capacity ($V_{max}$FRC) and resistance were measured. In addition, airway hyperresponsiveness was assessed by histamine challenge. Seven percent of these children developed bronchiolitis in the first 2 years of life. No difference was found for family history of atopy, the number of older siblings, the number breast fed, the duration of breast feeding, or socioeconomic status of the families between groups. However, $V_{max}$FRC values in the lowest tertile at the age of one month were related to the subsequent development of bronchiolitis in the first year of life. No significant difference in histamine responsiveness between groups was seen. The results of both the American and the Australian studies thus indicate that diminished lung function is a predisposing factor for the development of recurrent wheezing illnesses in infancy, whereas airway hyperresponsiveness is not, as results of other studies have confirmed (24).

Interestingly, in the Tucson Children's Study many children with postnatally diminished lung function grew out of their wheezing symptoms around the age of 3 years, while reductions in pulmonary function were still documented at the age of 6 years (13). This benign course of wheezing illness was not associated with any feature known to be associated with childhood asthma such as atopy or parental history of atopy. In turn, at the age of 6 years a second group of wheezing children was identified, who also started wheezing early in life but went on with recurrent wheezing episodes up to the age of 6 years. These children, whose lung function had been within normal limits at birth, showed decrements in pulmonary function at school age, suggesting a more severe form of the disease. This condition was furthermore related to increased total IgE levels, skin test reactivity to a panel of aeroallergens, the presence of eczema in the child, bronchial hyperresponsiveness to methacholine, and a family history of atopic diseases. This subgroup might be comparable to subjects with a doctor diagnosis of asthma in other studies. Finally, a third subgroup of children who started wheezing late after their third birthday but continued to wheeze at school age was identified. This subgroup was associated with atopy, parental history of atopy, and peak flow variability, but not bronchial hyperresponsiveness to methacholine (25).

These findings are of particular interest because they suggest that different phenotypes of wheezing illnesses develop during childhood, which are related to different intrinsic characteristics and possibly to different external risk factors. However, few longitudinal studies have been performed, which may have allowed the identification of these subgroups and their respective risk factors in more detail. Most studies have used cross-sectional study designs in which the correct classification of subjects is limited because of potential severe recall bias. Nevertheless, all of these wheezing conditions are known to be triggered by viral infections of the upper respiratory tract.

### III.  Incidence and Type of Viral Infections in Wheezing Lower Respiratory Tract Illnesses

Up to 70% of wheezing episodes in the first year of life have been found to be associated with evidence of viral respiratory infections (26). These epidemiological observations have been confirmed by studies detecting viruses in nasal washes of infants under the age of 2 years (27). Duff and coworkers (27) demonstrated that in wheezing patients ($n = 20$) 70% of the cultures were positive for virus as compared to 20% of a nonwheezing control group ($n = 13$). The majority of these cultures were positive for RSV, followed by rhinovirus and influenza B.

In earlier studies enrolling older wheezing children, virus-isolation rates were relatively low and varied significantly between studies (9.8–48.6%) depending on different approaches in sampling and processing different materials (1–10). These rates were, however, higher in cases than in controls. Furthermore, identification rates of viruses during exacerbations of asthma were similar to those generally found during respiratory infections without wheeze. Moreover, the rate of virus identification decreased substantially after the acute stage of respiratory illness, suggesting that virus infections are indeed causally involved in the triggering or development of wheezing LRIs. The wheezing and other observed changes during viral infections such as increases in asthma medication and symptom scores (16,18) and decreases in daily $FEV_1$ (28) start early, in mean 43 hours after the first symptoms of respiratory infection, and last from several days up to 2 weeks (29). Several studies (3,18,28) have also shown that more severe exacerbations of asthma correlate with a higher viral detection rate.

There are considerable difficulties involved in isolating respiratory viruses (11). The detection rate depends on the prevalence of certain viruses, which varies from year to year and season to season, the age of the enrolled subjects, and the time elapsed between notification and investigation of a symptomatic episode. Further technical problems arise with obtaining satisfactory specimen, with transport, storage, and eventually the culture of the material. These difficulties result in very low false-positive rates for identification of respiratory viruses but in significant false-negative rates, particularly for rhinoviruses.

Altogether RSV, rhinovirus, and parainfluenza virus were the most frequent isolates in studies investigating viral respiratory tract infections in wheezy children (1,3–6,8). All studies found RSV and parainfluenza viruses, and all but one identified rhinoviruses and adenoviruses. As might be expected from the difficulties in isolating rhinoviruses, these organisms showed the most variable detection rates. In studies closely following children either in the hospital (16) or in an Alpine asthma resort (28), where children were followed over months, coronaviruses and influenza viruses were also found in a significant proportion of wheezing episodes. *Mycoplasma pneumoniae* was only identified in studies using appropriate methods (11). In contrast, several studies failed to demonstrate an association between episodes of wheeze, symptoms of respiratory tract infections, and the isolation of bacteria (3,16,19).

A recent study using PCR techniques in addition to conventional methods and assuring prompt sampling of specimens yielded much higher virus identification rates. Johnston and colleagues (30) studied the relation between exacerbations of asthma and upper and lower respiratory viral infections in 108 asthmatic children aged 9–11 years. Over a 13-month period viruses were detected in 80% of nasal aspirates taken within 4 days after parents reported episodes of wheezing. Picornaviruses and among these rhinoviruses were found in most (about 50%) of the episodes. In turn, the identification rate of rhinoviruses in samples taken during asymptomatic control periods amounted to 12%. It thus seems very unlikely that these high virus-isolation rates reflect only a continuing colonization of the airways that is not related to the exacerbation of the disease.

## IV.   Risk Factors for Wheeze with Viral Respiratory Tract Infections

Viral infections result in increased mucus secretion, submucosal edema, and airway inflammation (31), all obstructing the airway lumen and increasing airway resistance. Although knowledge about virus structure, replication, and host responses is increasing rapidly, the mechanisms by which wheezing occurs remain to be elucidated. Two major hypotheses have been proposed to explain the relationship between respiratory tract infections and subsequent respiratory abnormalities (32). One hypothesis states that viral infections early in life damage the growing lung or alter host immune regulation. The second hypothesis holds that respiratory infections are more severe in infants and children with some underlying predisposition. In this case, the symptomatic viral infection is merely an indicator of an otherwise silent condition, whereas viral infections were causal risk factors if the first hypothesis holds true. These two arguments are not mutually exclusive. It is conceivable that severe viral lower respiratory infections occur primarily in infants and children with an inherent predisposition and that both the infection and the predisposition contribute to the development of wheezing illness or other long-term respiratory abnormality.

There is still an ongoing debate about a potential causal role of virus infections, mainly RSV, for the subsequent development of childhood wheezing illness, asthma, and atopy. RSV infection is very common in the first year of life. According to Long and colleagues (32), 80% or more of all infants are infected with RSV in the first year of life. Lower respiratory tract disease is evident in about 40% of these children. One percent of all infants are hospitalized for RSV disease, and 0.1% require intensive care. Thus, a significant proportion of children undergo inapparent RSV infections in the first years of life, suggesting that there is at least one host factor for the development of bronchiolitis.

Several researchers have followed children with proven RSV bronchiolitis to study their outcome after several years. Most authors (33–35) reported decrements in pulmonary function and increased prevalences of airway hyperresponsiveness in cases as compared to controls. These findings are, however, also consistent with the notion of an underlying respiratory abnormality rather than a subsequent damage of the airways through the RSV infection. In a study by Pullen and Hey (34), who followed 130 infants admitted to hospital at a mean age of 14 weeks with proven RSV bronchiolitis and compared them with matched controls, 6.2% of the RSV group were wheezing at the age of 10 years as compared to 4.5% of the control group. A slightly increased prevalence of repeated mild episodes of wheeze was found during the first 4 years of age (38% vs. 15%), but no increased rate of atopic sensitization was seen in the cases as compared to the controls. Others confirmed these findings (33,35). In a predisposed host an infection by RSV may, however, not only unmask latent asthma but also elicit a $TH_2$ response (36,37), transiently enhance IgE production (38,39), and thereby significantly add to the manifestation of the disease at an early age.

When considering the second hypothesis, several risk factors associated with an underlying predisposition to wheeze may be relevant. If wheeze is a nonspecific symptom of airway narrowing, then either underlying abnormalities of lung and airway structure, which result in smaller airway diameters, or a propensity to obstruct the airway lumen by mechanisms such as airway hyperresponsiveness to a variety of stimuli may be important. Risk factors for the occurrence of wheezing LRIs may thus relate to a multitude of underlying intrinsic and environmental conditions such as risks associated with airway damage and resulting reduction of airway size, risks for the development of childhood asthma, risks to acquire viral infections at different ages and stages of lung maturation, and finally a combination of all the above.

### A. Gender

Boys are more often affected by asthma than girls, and they also have a higher incidence of viral respiratory infections than females once they are asthmatic (4,9,40,41). Young boys may be predisposed to wheeze because of smaller airways relative to their lung size (24,42). In addition, a variety of other gender-related differences in the mechanical properties of the lung in children has been described. These include greater respiratory resistances for boys than girls, larger lung volumes for boys than girls of comparable height, and greater resting airway tone in boys (43). Thus, viral infections of the respiratory tract may more often become symptomatic in boys because of gender-related characteristics of airway size and lung structure. This male "disadvantage" regarding asthma disappears during puberty. After the age of 20 years, the asthma incidence is greater in females than in males (44), and morbidity rates in women are higher than in men after the age of 40 years (45).

### B. Prematurity and Birthweight

In 1967, the term bronchopulmonary dysplasia (BPD) was introduced to describe the chronic lung disease that occurs in some infants who require increased levels of oxygen and mechanical ventilation after birth. BPD is a leading cause of morbidity and mortality in infants surviving respiratory distress syndrome and reportedly develops in 15–38% of all infants weighing less than 1500 g who require mechanical ventilation (46,47). Airway reactivity has been implicated as a causal mechanism for the development of this obstructive airway disease (48).

Several studies have shown that infants who survive neonatal respiratory distress syndrome are at higher risk for reduced lung function and the development of wheezing lower respiratory tract illnesses in the first year of life (49–53). Elder and colleagues (54) prospectively followed a cohort of 525 very preterm infants with a gestational age of less than 33 weeks up to their first birthday. When compared to a control group of 657 term-born infants, the preterm-born children showed a significantly higher incidence of recurrent wheezing (14.5% vs. 3%). An even stronger effect was seen when the children had required mechanical ventilation after birth. These findings were confirmed by the results of a study by Lucas and coworkers (55), who followed 777 preterm born infants weighing less than 1850 g up to the age of 18 months. The crude prevalence of wheezing was found to be 18% in children who did not require respiratory support, whereas among infants who had been ventilated for at least 10 days 38% developed wheezing during this time period.

Most of these children improve rapidly over the first years of life (50,56). However, in a significant proportion recurrent wheezing persists into childhood and adolescence and decrements in pulmonary function are still seen (57,58). Northway and colleagues (47) reported that wheezing occurred more frequently in young adults (age 18 years) with BPD in infancy than in age-matched controls of similar birthweight but no BPD or age-matched normal controls. Furthermore, airway obstruction present in 68% of the subjects in the bronchopulmonary dysplasia group was manifest by significant decreases of several indices of pulmonary function such as $FEV_1$, PEFR, $FEF_{25-75}$, and $V_{max50}$ as compared to both control groups. Similarly, Bader and colleagues (59) reported that long-term survivors of BPD have evidence of airway obstruction and airway hyperresponsiveness to an exercise challenge test at a mean age of 10 years as compared to an age-matched normal control group. In a cross-sectional survey of 5573 British children (60), the relationship between birthweight and gestational age as recalled by parents and the occurrence of respiratory symptoms and pulmonary function at the age of 5–11 years was studied. Differing effects for birthweight and gestational age were found. Length of gestation, but not birthweight, was associated with the development of respiratory symptoms, whereas birthweight but not gestational age was related to decrements in FEV and $FEV_1$ at school age.

Other studies (61,62) also found that low birthweight is associated with impairment of lung function at school age regardless of respiratory illness during the neonatal period. These findings thus suggest that low birthweight is an indicator of intrauterine growth retardation, which may relate to impaired lung growth and decrements in lung function throughout childhood. In turn, gestational age may be a surrogate for the maturity of the respiratory system at birth and may be conceived as a significant independent risk factor for the development of wheezing respiratory illness in childhood.

We have previously shown that prematurely born girls had significantly more often been diagnosed as asthmatics and had significantly more respiratory symptoms such as recurrent wheezing or shortness of breath and frequent cough with exercise than term girls, especially if they had required mechanical ventilation after birth (63). Significant decrements could also be demonstrated for different parameters of lung function in these children. No difference, however, was found for atopic sensitization between groups. Thus, wheeze and cough of prematurely born children may rather be attributable to decrements in lung function present at birth reflecting impaired lung development in utero with subsequent abnormalities of the airways or the lung parenchyma. Alternatively, an increased thickness of the bronchial smooth muscle and increasing numbers of goblet cells in premature airways (64) may explain the reduced flows. Neonatal respiratory therapy can further affect the alveolar development, as Hislop and colleagues (65) have convincingly shown in morphometric and biochemical studies of infant autopsies. Finally, the increased risk of developing lower respiratory tract illnesses in infancy and later in childhood may further add to the lung function decrements. There is, however, no evidence that atopy is causally related to these conditions.

As with transient early wheezing the main triggers of obstructive episodes in preterm-born children are viral infections of the upper respiratory tract. It is unknown whether prematurely born children have a higher likelihood of acquiring these viral infections or whether their lung abnormalities predispose to earlier manifestation of symptoms of the lower respiratory tract.

### C. Environmental Tobacco Smoke Exposure

The effects of exposure to environmental tobacco smoke (ETS) on the respiratory tract of children have been extensively investigated. Tobacco smoke is a complex mixture of gases and particles. Levels of respirable particulates, nicotine, polycyclic aromatic hydrocarbons, CO, $NO_2$, and many other substances in indoor environments increase with the number of smokers and the intensity of their smoking and decrease with air-exchange rate (66). Among other constituents of sidestream tobacco smoke, concentrations of respirable particulates have been shown to exceed the 24-hour National Ambient Air Quality Standard of 260 $\mu g/m^3$ for total suspended particulates in homes with two or more heavy smokers (67).

Environmental tobacco smoke exposure has repeatedly and consistently been shown to increase the risk of developing lower respiratory tract illnesses in infancy and childhood (68). A review on adverse health effects of ETS exposure has been provided to the U.S. Environmental Protection Agency (69). The report concludes that passive smoke exposure is causally associated with an increased risk of lower respiratory tract infections such as bronchitis and pneumonia mainly in infants and young children; a small but significant and dose-dependent reduction in pulmonary function; and additional episodes and increased severity of symptoms in children with asthma. Furthermore, ETS exposure was considered to be a risk factor for the development of new cases of asthma in children not previously displaying symptoms.

Most studies documented a dose-response relationship between the number of cigarettes smoked and the risk of developing lower respiratory tract illnesses. This finding is consistent with a stronger effect of maternal than paternal smoking found in most studies, suggesting a higher exposure through the mother than the father or alternatively persisting effects of passive smoke exposure through the mother in utero. Since most mothers who smoked during pregnancy continue to smoke thereafter, adverse health effects from intrauterine exposure are difficult to disentangle from environmental exposure after birth.

The consequences of maternal cigarette smoking during pregnancy on infants' pulmonary function was studied in 80 infants shortly after birth (mean 4.2 weeks) in Boston (70). Maternal smoking habits were assessed prior to birth via questionnaires that had been validated by measuring urine cotinine concentrations. In infants of smoking mothers, forced expiratory flow levels were significantly reduced as compared to nonexposed children. Since lung function testing had been performed shortly after birth and passive smoke exposure during this short time interval had been controlled in multivariate analysis, the results of this study indicate that maternal smoking impairs airway development in utero, causing smaller airway calibers at birth. In further studies by the same group (71), the detrimental effects of maternal smoking during pregnancy on infant respiratory function have been shown to persist at least over the first 18 months of life. The reductions were greater for measures of flow than for volume and for female than for male infants and were related to the development of wheezing lower respiratory tract illnesses during the first year of life (71,72).

The relationship between maternal smoking and lower respiratory tract illness was further studied in a large birth cohort study in Tucson, Arizona (73). ETS exposure was assessed via questionnaires and umbilical cord cotinine measurements; wheezing and nonwheezing LRIs were confirmed by physicians. The odds of developing an LRI in the first year of life were significantly higher in children whose mothers smoked heavily, i.e., more than 20 cigarettes a day (OR = 1.82; 95% CI 1.13–2.94) than in those infants whose mothers smoked lightly or not at all. The proportion of symptomatic children was higher if the mother had smoked heavily during pregnancy and thereafter as compared to heavy maternal smoking after birth only (46.2% vs. 36.4%; $p < 0.03$). Interestingly, the odds for having wheezing LRIs in the first year of life further increased if the child stayed at home rather than attending day care (OR = 2.8; 95% CI 1.43–5.5), pointing toward the importance of modifying factors affecting the effective level of passive smoke exposure in a given child. However, smoking caregivers in day-care centers have also been shown to increase the risk of LRIs in the first 3 years of life (74). Maternal smoking was related not only to the development of wheezing and nonwheezing LRIs, but also to an earlier manifestation of these illnesses (73).

The strong link between maternal smoking during pregnancy and decrements in infant pulmonary function with subsequent occurrence of wheezing LRIs in the first years of life may indicate that mainly the risk of developing benign transient wheeze in early infancy and not the risk of acquiring childhood asthma is increased by ETS exposure. However, in the large prospective birth cohort study in Tucson, Arizona, the occurrence of both transient early wheezing and persistent wheezing up to the age of 6 years was related to passive smoke exposure. Children of mothers with 12 or fewer years of education and who smoked 10 or more cigarettes per day were 2.5 times more likely to develop asthma (OR = 2.5; 95% CI 1.42–4.59; $p$ = 0.002) than children of mothers with the same educational level who did not smoke or smoked fewer than 10 cigarettes a day (75). No relationship was found in children of mothers with a higher education. In a British birth cohort study following 9670 children up to the age of 10 years, a 14% increase in childhood wheezy bronchitis was noted when mothers smoked more than 4 cigarettes per day (76). This rate increased to 49% when maternal smoking exceeded 14 cigarettes daily. No association was found with asthma, but no clear distinction between wheezy bronchitis and asthma was made in this study. Interestingly, in a recent case-control study performed in South Africa in 7- to 9-year-old children (77), maternal smoking during pregnancy was found to increase the child's risk of developing asthma and wheeze almost two-fold (OR = 1.9, 95% CI 1.2–2.8). Yet, each additional smoking household member added significantly to this risk (OR = 1.15; 95% CI 1.0–1.3), suggesting that the odds for asthma do not only increase with ETS exposure in utero (though the effect is stronger), but also after birth by passive inhalation of sidestream cigarette smoke.

Studies including objective measures of features closely associated with asthma may help in further understanding the effects of ETS exposure. Forastiere and associates studied the effect of passive smoking on the degree of bronchial responsiveness to a methacholine challenge in a cross-sectional survey of 1215 children aged 7–11 years in Italy (78). Higher odds ratios were found among girls in whom a dose-response relationship with the number of cigarettes smoked by the mother could be established. No increased risk was seen in boys. An effect modification was detected for father's education and household crowding: maternal and paternal smoking were strong predictors of bronchial hyperrespon-siveness (BHR) in families in which the head was less educated and in over-crowded houses. Likewise, a strong association between parental smoking and BHR to carbachol was found in another Italian survey (79). Yet, in this survey boys were more strongly affected than girls, and the association was strongest for children with asthma. In Frischer's studies, diurnal variability of peak flow rates was associated with maternal smoking in nonasthmatic and asthmatic non-atopic Austrian children (80). In the atopic group, there was evidence that mothers changed their smoking habits subsequent to the development of disease in their children, thus biasing the study results towards null. Several other studies, how-ever, were unable to reproduce these findings: maternal smoking was not found to be associated with BHR to methacholine challenge (81,82) or to hyperventila-tion of cold, dry air (83).

Conflicting results have furthermore been reported from studies investigat-ing the effects of passive smoke exposure on the development of atopic sensitiza-tion in children. Whereas two investigators found enhanced allergic sensitization

(83,84), increased serum IgE levels (85), and an increased prevalence of eosino-philia (85) in 9-year-old children of smoking parents, others failed to show any correlation between allergic sensitization and ETS exposure (86–88).

In contrast several reports conclude that ETS exposure is significantly associated with increased prevalence of otitis media in infants and schoolchildren. Ey and colleagues studied more than 1000 newborns, who were followed from birth up to their first birthday as part of the Tucson Children's Study (89). Their medical records were reviewed for a diagnosis of otitis and recurrent otitis media. Heavy maternal smoking of more than 20 cigarettes a day was significantly associated with the development of recurrent otitis media in the first year of life. If the infant weighted less than the mean at birth (3.5 kg), the risk increased threefold. In a British study including almost 900 schoolchildren aged 6–7 years, middle ear pressure and compliance were measured in both ears by impedance tympanometry. ETS exposure was assessed by salivary cotinine measurements. About one-third of the cases with middle ear effusion were statistically attributable to exposure to tobacco smoke.

In summary, most studies reporting an association between ETS exposure and the acquisition of asthma or BHR were found for heavy ETS exposure, which may particularly occur in families of lower socioeconomic status. Some studies found stronger effects on wheezy bronchitis than asthma possibly reflecting underdiagnosis of asthma, reporting bias or smoking cessation by parents whose child was labeled asthmatic. Alternatively, effects of passive smoke exposure may be stronger for viral-induced asthmatic symptoms. This notion is supported by the finding of an increased prevalence of infectious dieseases of the upper and lower respiratory tract such as recurrent otitis media, middle ear effusion, bronchitis, and pneumonia in infants, toddlers, and schoolchildren exposed to environmental tobacco smoke.

### D.  Childhood Asthma and Bronchial Hyperresponsiveness

There is some evidence that asthmatics may be more susceptible to viral infections than healthy children. Minor and colleagues (90) observed that asthmatic children experienced significantly more viral respiratory tract infections than did their nonasthmatic siblings. Similarly, Bardin and coworkers (91) reported that atopic subjects who were experimentally infected with rhinovirus experienced more severe symptoms than nonatopic controls. Rhinoviruses use receptors on the cell surface for cellular attachment. The best known and most common receptor is ICAM-1 (92). Epithelial cells of asthmatics have been found to express more ICAM-1 as compared to normal subjects or subjects with chronic bronchitis (93). Thus, rhinoviruses may attack epithelial cells more easily and more effectively in these subjects, resulting in an enhanced clinical manifestation of symptoms or more severe complaints.

Unlike in infants and preschool children, (BHR) is strongly associated with asthma and active wheezing in school-age children. In clinical studies the presence and degree of BHR correlated well with the physician's diagnosis and the severity of the disease. In population-based surveys, however, only partial overlap between the lifetime prevalence of asthma, the period prevalence of respiratory symptoms, and the point prevalence of BHR to histamine (94), methacholine (95), or cold, dry air (96) was found. Pattemore and colleagues showed that even of those children who wheezed within the previous month, more than 40% had normal bronchial responsiveness to methacholine (93). Conversely, bronchial responsiveness to pharmacological and physical stimuli was found in a significant proportion of asymptomatic, normal children (94–96).

One possible explanation for this discrepancy is that BHR is probably as episodic and variable over time as are clinical symptoms of asthma (97,98). BHR can transiently be enhanced by many different factors such as exposure to allergens and viral respiratory tract infections (99,100) and may thus reflect the activity and severity of the disease at a given point in time. Different methods of assessing bronchial responsiveness are furthermore likely to reflect only a limited aspect of the disease. Responses to a physical provocation are mediated by factors other than those inducing the bronchial muscular contraction by pharmacological agents. Moreover, BHR may persist independently from asthma. In a longitudinal follow-up of an asymptomatic, bronchial hyperresponsive population, no significant loss of BHR over time was found (101). The finding of increased nonspecific BHR in asymptomatic relatives of subjects with asthma (102,103) supports this hypothesis.

It has long been recognized that airway hyperresponsiveness and asthma are associated with immunological processes that induce an increased production of total serum IgE. Burrows and coworkers (104) showed that the prevalence of physician-diagnosed asthma after the age of 6 years was closely related to serum IgE levels in the population and that no asthma was present in the subjects with the lowest IgE levels. Sears and colleagues (105) reported that airway responsiveness was closely linked to serum IgE even in children who have been asymptomatic throughout their lives. Many studies have furthermore consistently shown that atopy, i.e., the production of specific IgE antibodies to environmental allergens, is strongly associated with airway hyperresponsiveness and childhood asthma. In cross-sectional and clinical studies atopic sensitization was related to an increased prevalence of asthma, airway hyperresponsiveness, and a greater severity of respiratory symptoms as compared with the absence of atopy (106–108). Moreover, the strength of atopic sensitization as assessed by increasing numbers of positive skin prick test results (109) or increasing wheal sizes (110) was linearly related to the severity of childhood asthma and airway hyperresponsiveness. Thus, factors enhancing the production of specific IgE antibodies or the lack of protective mechanisms to induce tolerance toward environmental allergens early in life may also increase the risk for airway hyperresponsiveness and asthma.

In many studies an inverse relation between asthma and the overall incidence of respiratory infections has been reported. Anderson observed in his studies in Papua New Guinea that respiratory infections were more common among young children in the highlands, where asthma was exceedingly low, than in the coastal regions of the country, where asthma occurred more frequently (111). Flynn studied two groups of children of the Fiji Islands: the indigenous Fijians, who showed a high hospital admission rate for pneumonia, and the Fiji Indians, whose asthma admission rate was three times higher than in the Fijians (112,113). Consistent with the hospitalization rates, Indian children had a threefold higher prevalence of asthma and airway hyperresponsiveness than Fijians, whereas respiratory infection was more than twice as common in Fijian than in Indian children. In the East European countries a higher prevalence of respiratory infections was found, whereas atopic sensitization, hay fever, asthma, and BHR were all significantly lower as compared to Sweden or West Germany (114,115).

The results of three recent studies further substantiate the potential protective effect of infections early in life on the development of atopy. Shaheen and coworkers studied young adults who were first surveyed at the age of 0–6 years in Guinea-Bissau, West Africa (116). Among the participants who had had measles during childhood, the prevalence of atopic sensitization defined as skin prick test positivity to aeroallergens was about half the rate of those who had been vaccinated and did not have measles (12.8% vs. 25.6%). A recent report from Southern Italy demonstrated that military students who were seropositive for hepatitis A also had a significantly lower prevalence of atopic sensitization to common aeroallergens and atopic diseases as compared to their peers who had no antibodies to hepatitis A (117). In the prospective Tucson Cohort Study, children who had nonwheezing LRIs in the first 3 years of life had subsequently reduced skin test reactivity and depressed levels of IgE at the age of 6 years (118).

Recent immunological findings show biological plausibility for those hypotheses inferred from epidemiological studies. They indicate that two mutually exclusive T-helper-cell phenotypes develop from a common ancestor cell. Different patterns of cytokine release are produced by these different T-helper cells. $TH_2$-like T cells produce interleukin 4 (IL-4) and 5 (IL-5) and may particularly be implicated in allergic disease, whereas $TH_1$-like T cells produce interleukin 2 (IL-2) and interferon gamma (119). IL-4 is one of the necessary signals that induce B-cell clones to switch from the production of IgM to IgE. Interferon gamma, on the other hand, is produced in the course of viral infectious diseases and inhibits the proliferation of $TH_2$ clones and the production of IgE by B cells (120,121). Thus, a predominant activation of $TH_1$-like T-helper cells in the course of recurrent viral or bacterial infections may prevent the proliferation of $TH_2$ clones and the development of allergic disease (119).

Therefore, a subject's overall burden of continuing infections early in life and throughout childhood may direct the immune response toward a predominant $TH_1$-like response suppressing the $TH_2$ pathway. A suppressed $TH_2$ response may then reduce the risk to develop atopy and asthma. In contrast, infections by some respiratory viruses such as RSV at certain stages of lung maturation and in predisposed hosts may transiently induce a $TH_2$ response (36,37) with increased IgE production (38,39), thereby unmasking the manifestation of asthma.

### E. Day-Care Attendance

Several studies have shown that a child's risk of acquiring infectious illnesses is increased if the child is looked after in day-care centers or to a lesser extent in family day care as compared to children reared at home (122). The strongest relation has been found for otitis media and recurrent otitis media. Two Scandinavian studies (123,124) used tympanometry to examine middle ear problems in 1–2 and 3-year-old children, respectively. Both groups found approximately twice as many abnormal tympanograms in those children attending day-care centers than in children reared at home. Interestingly, in one of these studies (123) the findings for children in family day care were similar to those of children in home care in the summer or fall, whereas in the winter months both children in day-care centers and in family day care had more abnormal findings than children reared at home.

The association between day-care attendance and respiratory infections seems weaker, although most studies found evidence of increased rates of respiratory illness in children attending day-care centers (122). Rasmussen and Sundelin (125) reported that the rates of physician visits for acute respiratory infections were 1.4–1.8 times higher in children attending day-care centers or family day care than in children raised at home. In a prospective birth cohort study in Pittsburgh, 153 children were enrolled at birth and observed for 12–18 months (126). Children in group care and day care were more likely than children reared at home to experience at least six respiratory infections, more than 60 days of illness, and more than four severe illnesses ($p < 0.01$). Furthermore, hospitalization for lower respiratory tract illness has been found to be related to regular attendance of a day-care center (127).

### F. Lack of Breast Feeding

The occurrence of infectious diseases of the respiratory and gastrointestinal tracts may be prevented by nursing the babies. Several studies have shown a beneficial effect of breast feeding on the incidence of infectious respiratory illnesses

(26,128–131). This protective effect was, however, mainly present in the first weeks or months of life and most pronounced when other risk factors were also apparent. Wright and colleagues (26) reported that in a prospective birth cohort study in Tucson, breast feeding was associated with a decreased incidence of wheezing illnesses in the first 4 months of age. The risk associated with lack of breast feeding increased if other people were sharing the child's bedroom (OR = 3.3; 95% CI 1.8–6.0). Similarly, Nafstad and coworkers (132) reported a protective effect of long-term breast feeding on the risk of developing lower respiratory tract infections during the first year of life. The effect was strongest in children exposed to environmental tobacco smoke.

### G. Air Pollution

Few studies have investigated the effects of air pollution on the development of infectious respiratory diseases in children. Braun-Fahrländer and colleagues (133) reported a correlation of total suspended particulates (TSP) and $NO_2$ with the incidence and duration of upper respiratory symptom episodes among preschool children in Switzerland. Others found a correlation between these two pollutants and croup among German children of the same age (134). Furthermore, a significant association between the prevalence of upper respiratory infections and the residence in a Finnish community that was moderately polluted by $SO_2$ has been reported (135). Results from studies in East Germany where air pollution levels had been high suggest that high concentrations of $SO_2$ and moderate levels of particulate matters and $NO_x$ are associated with an increased risk of developing upper respiratory symptoms in childhood (136). The highest risk was found when the concentrations of all three pollutants ranged in their upper quartiles. Similarly, an adverse effect on the prevalence of symptoms of colds was found when children were exposed to heavy car traffic in Munich, West Germany (137).

### V. Summary

Wheezing with upper respiratory tract infections is a very common childhood condition. A multitude of viral agents have been associated with these episodes, although the methods to detect viral infections were cumbersome until recent advances introducing PCR techniques were achieved. These new methods may in the future allow us to better understand the role of viruses in triggering and eliciting wheezing episodes in children predisposed either by anatomical abnormalities of airway size and lung parenchyma or by reactive airway disease. Particularly, the reasons why in some subjects a viral infection remains inapparent, whereas others react with upper or even lower respiratory symptoms such as a runny nose, cough, and wheeze, needs further attention. It still remains a matter of debate whether asthmatic subjects are more susceptible to viral infections than their healthy siblings (90) and peers, and how this susceptibility may be mediated. However, several distinct risk factors that increase the risk of wheezing with viral infections: have been identified: prematurity and maternal smoking. Both are amenable to preventive measures and may be endorsed by encouraging a mother to nurse her baby for the first 6 months of life.

## References

1. Horn ME, Brain EA, Gregg I, Inglis JM, Yealland SJ, Taylor P. Respiratory viral infection and wheezy bronchitis in childhood. Thorax 1979; 34:23–28.
2. Jennings LC, Barns G, Dawson KP. The association of viruses with acute asthma. NZ Med J 1987; 12(100):488–490.
3. Horn ME, Reed SE, Taylor P. Role of viruses and bacteria in acute wheezy bronchitis in childhood: a study of sputum. Arch Dis Child 1979; 54:587–592.
4. Henderson FW, Clyde WA Jr, Collier AM, Denny FW, Senior RJ, Sheaffer CI, Conley WG 3d, Christian-RM. The etiologic and epidemiologic spectrum of bronchiolitis in pediatric practice. J Pediatr 1979; 95:183–190.
5. Mitchell-I'Inglis H, Inglis H, Simpson H. Viral infection in wheezy bronchitis and asthma in children. Arch Dis Child 1976; 51:707–711.
6. Carlsen KH, Orstavik I, Leegaard J, Hoeg H. Respiratory virus infections and aeroallergens in acute bronchial asthma. Arch Dis Child 1984; 59:310–315.
7. Horn ME, Brain E, Gregg I, Yealland SJ, Inglis JM. Respiratory viral infection in childhood. A survey in general practice, Roehampton 1967–1972. J Hyg Lond 1975; 74:157–168.
8. Disney ME, Matthews R, Williams JD. The role of infection in the morbidity of asthmatic children admitted to hospital. Clin Allergy 1971; 1:399–406.
9. Glezen WP, Loda FA, Clyde WA Jr, Senior RJ, Sheaffer CI, Conley WG, Denny FW. Epidemiologic patterns of acute lower respiratory disease of children in a pediatric group practice. J Pediatr 1971; 78:397–406.
10. Tyrerell DAJ. A collaborative study of the aetiology of acute respiratory infections in Britain 1961-4. A report of the Medical Research Council Working Party on acute respiratory virus infections. Br Med J 1965; 2:319–326.
11. Pattemore PK, Johnston SL, Bardin PG. Viruses as precipitants of asthma symptoms. I. Epidemiology. Clin Exp Allergy 1992; 22:325–336.
12. Busse WW. Viral infections in humans. Am J Respir Crit Care Med 1995; 151: 1675–1677.
13. Martinez FD, Wright AL, Taussig LM, Holberg CJ, Halonen M, Morgan WJ. Asthma and wheezing in the first six years of life. N Engl J Med 1995; 332: 133–8.
14. Young S, O'Keeffe PT, Arnott J, Landau LI. Lung function, airway responsiveness, and respiratory symptoms before and after bronchiolitis. Arch Dis Child 1995; 72: 16–24.
15. Wilson NM. The significance of early wheezing. Clin Exp Allergy 1994; 24:522–529.

16. McIntosh K, Ellis EF, Hoffman LS, Lybass TG, Eller JJ, Fulginiti VA. The association of viral and bacterial respiratory infections with exacerbations of wheezing in young asthmatic children. J Pediatr 1973; 82:578–590.

17. Minor TE, Dick EC, Baker JW, Ouellette JJ, Cohen M, Reed CE. Rhinovirus and influenza type A infections as precipitants of asthma. Am Rev Respir Dis 1976; 113:149–153.

18. Minor TE, Dick EC, DeMeo AN, Ouellette JJ, Cohen M, Reed CE. Viruses as precipitants of asthmatic attacks in children. JAMA 1974; 227:292–298.

19. Hudgel DW, Langston L Jr, Selner JC, McIntosh K. Viral and bacterial infections in adults with chronic asthma. Am Rev Respir Dis 1979; 120:393–397.

20. Martinez FD, Morgan WJ, Wright AL, Holberg CJ, Taussig LM. Diminished lung function as a predisposing factor for wheezing respiratory illness in infants. N Engl J Med 1988; 319:1112–1117.

21. Martinez FD, Morgan WJ, Wright AL, Holberg C, Taussig LM. Initial airway function is a risk factor for recurrent wheezing respiratory illnesses during the first three years of life. Group Health Medical Associates. Am Rev Respir Dis 1991; 143: 312–316.

22. Morris MJ, Lane DJ. Tidal expiratory flow patterns in airflow obstruction. Thorax 1981; 36:135–142.

23. Tepper RS, Morgan WJ, Cota K, Wright A, Taussig LM, GHMA Pediatricians. Physiologic growth and development of the lung during the first year of life. Am Rev Respir Dis 1986; 134:513–519.

24. Clarke JR, Reese A, Silverman M. Bronchial responsiveness and lung function in infants with lower respiratory tract illness over the first 6 months of life. Arch Dis Child 1992; 67:1454–1458.

25. Stein RT, Holberg CJ, Morgan WJ, Lombardi E, Wright AL, Martinez FD. Determinants of peak flow variability and methacholine responsiveness in children: a prospective study. Am J Respir Crit Care Med 1996; 153:A428.

26. Wright AL, Holberg CJ, Martinez FD, Morgan WJ, Taussig LM, GHMA. Breast feeding and lower respiratory tract illness in the first year of life. Br Med J 1989; 299:946–949.

27. Duff AL, Pomeranz ES, Gelber LE, Price GW, Farris H, Hayden FG, Platts-Mills TA, Heymann PW. Risk factors for acute wheezing in infants and children: viruses, passive smoke, and IgE antibodies to inhalant allergens. Pediatrics 1993; 92:535–540.

28. Roldaan AC, Masural N. Viral respiratory infections in asthmatic children staying in a mountain resort. Eur J Respir Dis 1982; 63:140–50.

29. Mertsola J, Ziegler T, Ruuskanen O, Vanto T, Kiovikko A, Halonen P. Recurrent wheezy bronchitis and viral respiratory infections. Arch Dis Child 1991; 66:124–129.

30. Johnston SL, Pattemore PK, Sanderson G, Smith S, Lampe F, Josephs L, Symington P, O'Toole S, Myint SH, Tyrrell DA, et al. Community study of role of viral infections in exacerbations of asthma in 9–11 year old children. Br Med J 1995; 310:1225–1129.

31. Price JF. Acute and long-term effects of viral bronchiolitis in infancy. Lung 1990; 168(suppl):414–421.

32. Long CE, McBride JT, Hall CB. Sequelae of respiratory syncytial virus infections. A role for intervention studies. Am J Respir Crit Care Med 1995; 151:1678–1681.
33. Sims D, Downham M, Gardner P, Webb J, Weightman D. Study of 8 year old children with a history of RSV bronchiolitis in infancy. Br Med J 1978; 1:11–14.
34. Pullen CR, Hey EN. Wheezing, asthma and pulmonary dysfunction 10 years after infection with respiratory syncytial virus in infancy. Br Med J 1982; 284:1665–1669.
35. Hall CB, Hall WB, gala CL, Magill FB, Leddy JP. Long term prospective study in children after respiratory syncytial virus infection. J Pediatr 1984; 105:358–364.
36. Roman M, Calhoun WJ, Hinton KL, Avendano LF, Simon V, Escobar AM, Gaggero A, Diaz PV. Respiratory syncitial virus infection in infants is associated with predominant TH2-like response. Am J Respir Crit Care Med 1997; 156:190–195.
37. Matzuzaki Z, Okamoto Y, Sarashina N, Ito E, Togawa K, saito I. Induction of intercellular adhesion molecule-1 in human nasal epithelial cells during respiratory syncytial virus infection. Immunology 1996; 88:565–568.
38. Welliver RC, Wong DT, Sun M, Middleton E, Vaughan RS, Ogra PL. The development of respiratory syncytial virus-specific IgE and the release of histamine in nasopharyngeal secretions after infection. N Engl J Med 1981; 305:841–846.
39. Welliver RC, Kaul TN, Ogra PL. The appearance of cell-bound IgE in respiratory-tract epithelium after respiratory-syncytial virus infection. N Engl J Med 1980; 303:1198–1202.
40. Report to the Medical Research Council Subcommittee on Respiratory Syncytial Virus Vaccines. Respiratory syncytial virus infection: admissions to hospital in industrial, urban, and rural areas. Br Med J 1978; 2:796–798.
41. Welliver RC, Wong DT, Sun M, McCarthy N. Parainfluenza virus bronchiolitis. Epidemiology and pathogenesis. Am J Dis Child 1986; 140:34–40.
42. Hanrahan J, Tager I, Castile R, Segal M, Weiss S, Speizer FE. Pulmonary function measures in healthy infants. Am Rev Respir Dis 1990; 140:1127–1135.
43. Landau LI, Morgan W, McCoy KS, Taussig LM. Gender related differences in airway tone in children. Ped Pulmonol 1993; 16:31–35.
44. Dodge RR, Burrows B. The prevalence and incidence of asthma-like symptoms in a general population sample. Am Rev Respir Dis 1980; 122:557–575.
45. Skobeloff EM, Spivey WH, St Clair SS, Schoffstall JM. The influence of age and sex on asthma admissions. JAMA 1992; 288:3437–3440.
46. O'Brodovich HM, Mellins RB. Bronchopulmonary dysplasia: Unresolved neonatal acute lung injury. Am Rev Respir Dis 1985; 132:694–699.
47. Northway WH, Moss RB, Carlisle KB, Parker BR, Popp RL, Pitlick PT, Eichler I, Lamm RL, Brown BW. Late pulmonary sequelae of bronchopulmonary dysplasia. N Engl J Med 1990; 323:1793–1799.
48. Motoyama EK, Fort MD, Klesh KW, Mutich RL, Guthrie RD. Early onset of airway reactivity in premature infants with bronchopulmonary dysplasia. Am Rev Respir Dis 1987; 136:50–57.
49. Bryan MH, Hardie MJ, Reilly BJ, Sawyer RR. Pulmonary function studies during the first year of life in infants recovering from respiratory distress syndrome. Pediatrics 1973; 52:169–178.
50. Wong YC, Beardsmore CS, Silverman M. Pulmonary sequelae in neonatal respira-

tory distress in very low birth weight infants: a clinical and a physiological study. Arch Dis Child 1982; 57:418–424.
51. Lindroth M, Mortensson W. Long-term follow-up of ventilator treated low birth weight infants. Acta Paediatr Scand 1986; 75:819–826.
52. Arad I, Bar-Yishay E, Eyal F, Gross S, Godfrey S. Lung function in infancy and childhood following neonatal intensive care. Pediatr Pulmonol 1987; 3:29–33.
53. Kitchen WH, Olinsky A, Doyle LW, Ford GW, Murton LJ, Slonim L, Callanan C. Respiratory health and lung function in 8-year-old children of very low birth weight: a cohort study. Pediatrics 1992; 89:1151–1158.
54. Elder DE, Hagan R, Evans SF, Benninger HR, French NP. Recurrent wheezing in very preterm infants. Arch Dis Child Fetal Neonatal Ed 1996; 74:F165–171.
55. Lucas A, Brooke OG, Cole TJ, Morley R, Bamford MF. Food and drug reactions, wheezing, and eczema in preterm infants. Arch Dis Child 1990; 65:411–415.
56. Gerhardt T, Hehre D, Feller R, Reifenberg L, Bancalari E. Serial determination of pulmonary function in infants with chronic lung disease. J Pediatr 1987; 110:448–456.
57. Schwartz J, Gold D, Dockery DW, Weiss ST, Speizer FE. Predictors of asthma and persistent wheeze in a national sample of children in the United States. Am Rev Respir Dis 1990; 142:555–562.
58. Seidman DS, Laor A, Gale R, Stevenson DK, Danon YL. Is low birth weight a risk factor for asthma during adolescence? Arch Dis Child 1991; 66:584–587.
59. Bader D, Ramos AD, Lew CD, Platzker ACG, Stabile MW, Keens TG. Childhood sequelae of infant lung disease: exercise and pulmonary function abnormalities after bronchopulmonary dysplasia. J Pediatr 1987; 110:693–699.
60. Rona RJ, Gulliford MC, Chinn SBMJ. Effects of prematurity and intrauterine growth on respiratory health and lung function in childhood. 1993; 306:817–820.
61. Chan KN, Noble-Jamieson CM, Elliman A, Bryan EM, Silverman M. Lung function in children of low birth weight. Arch Dis Child 1989; 64:1284–1293.
62. Galdès-Sebaldt M, Sheller JR, Grogaard J, Stahlman M. Prematurity is associated with abnormal airway function in childhood. Pediatr Pulmonol 1989; 7:259–264.
63. Khoury MJ, Marks JS, McCarthy BJ, Zaro SM. Factors affecting the sex differential in neonatal mortality: the role of respiratory distress syndrome. Am J Obstet Gynecol 1985; 151:777–782.
64. Hislop AA, Haworth SG. Airway size and structure in the normal fetal and infant lung and the effect of premature delivery and artificial ventilation. Am Rev Respir Dis 1989; 140:1717–1726.
65. Hislop AA, Wigglesworth JS, Desai R, Aber V. The effects of preterm delivery and mechanical ventilation on human lung growth. Early Hum Dev 1987; 15:147–164.
66. Samet JM, Marbury MC, Spengler JD. Health effects and sources of indoor air pollution. Part I. Am Rev Respir Dis 1987; 136:1486–1508.
67. Spengler JD, Dockery DW, Turner WA, Wolfson JM, Ferris BG Jr. Long-term measurements of respirable sulfates and particles inside and outside homes. Atmos Environ 1981; 15:23–30.
68. National Research Council. Environmental Tobacco Smoke: Measuring Exposures and Assessing Health Effects. Washington, DC: National Academy Press, 1986.

69. Neuspiel DR, Rush D, Butler NR, Golding J, Bijur PE, Kurzon M. Parental smoking and post-infancy wheezing in children: a prospective cohort study. Am J Publ Health 1989; 79:168–171.

70. Hanrahan JP, Tager IB, Segal MR, Tosteson TD, Castile RG, Van Vunakis H, Weiss ST, Speizer FE. The effect of maternal smoking during pregnancy on early infant lung function. Am Rev Respir Dis 1992; 145:1129–1135.

71. Tager IB, Ngo L, Hanrahan JP. Maternal smoking during pregnancy. Effects on lung function during the first 18 months of life. Am J Respir Crit Care Med 1995; 152:977–983.

72. Tager IB, Hanrahan JP, Tosteson TD, Castile RG, Brown RW, Weiss ST, Speizer FE. Lung function, pre and post natal smoke exposure, and wheezing in the first year of life. Am Rev Respir Dis 1993; 147:811–817.

73. Wright AL, Holberg C, Martinez FD, Taussig LM. Relationship of parental smoking to wheezing and nonwheezing lower respiratory tract illnesses in infancy. Group Health Medical Associates. J Pediatr 1991; 118:207–214.

74. Holberg CJ, Wright AL, Martinez FD, Morgan WJ, Taussig LM, GHM Associates. Child day care, smoking by caregivers, and lower respiratory tract illness in the first 3 years of life. Pediatrics 1993; 91:885–892.

75. Martinez FD, Cline M, Burrows B. Increased incidence of asthma in children of smoking mothers. Pediatrics 1992; 89:21–26.

76. Neuspiel DR, Rush D, Butler NR, Golding J, Bijur PE, Kurzon M. Parental smoking and post-infancy wheezing in children: a prospective cohort study. Am J Public Health 1989; 79:168–171.

77. Ehrlich RI, Du Toit D, Jordaan E, Zwarenstein M, Potter P, Volmink JA, Weinberg E. Risk factors for childhood asthma and wheezing. Importance of maternal and household smoking. Am J Respir Crit Care Med 1996; 154:681–688.

78. Forastiere F, Agabiti N, Corbo GM, Pistelli R, Dell'Orco V, Ciappi G, Perucci CA. Passive smoking as a determinant of bronchial responsiveness in children. Am J Respir Crit Care Med 1994; 149:365–370.

79. Martinez FD, Antognoni G, Macri F, Bonci E, Midulla F, De Castro G, Ronchetti R. Parental smoking enhances bronchial responsiveness in nine-year-old children. Am Rev Respir Dis 1988; 138:518–523.

80. Frischer T, Kuehr J, Meinert R, Karmaus W, Urbanek R. Influence of maternal smoking on variability of peak expiratory flow rate in school children. Chest 1993; 104:1133–1137.

81. Peat JK, Salome CM, Woolcock AJ. Bronchial hyperresponsiveness in Australian adults and children. Eur Respir J 1992; 5:921–929.

82. Soyseth V, Kongerud J, Boe J. Postnatal maternal smoking increases the prevalence of asthma but not of bronchial hyperresponsiveness or atopy in their children. Chest 1995; 107:389–394.

83. Weiss ST, Tager IB, Munoz A, Speizer FE. The relationship of respiratory infections in early childhood to the occurrence of increased levels of bronchial responsiveness and atopy. Am Rev Respir Dis 1985; 131:573–578.

84. Ronchetti R, Bonci E, Cutrera R, De Castro G, Indinnimeo L, Midulla F, Tancredi G, Martinez FD. Enhanced allergic sensitisation related to parental smoking. Arch Dis Child 1992; 67:496–500.

85. Ronchetti R, Macri F, Ciofetta G, Indinnimeo L, Cutrera R, Bonci E, Antognoni G, Martinez FD. Increased serum IgE and increased prevalence of eosinophilia in 9-year-old children of smoking parents. J Allergy Clin Immunol 1990; 86:400–407.

86. Henderson FW, Henry MM, Ivins SS, Morris R, Neebe EC, Leu S, Stewart PW, The physicians of Raleigh Pediatric Associates. Correlates of recurrent wheezing in school-age children. Am J Respir Crit Care Med 1995; 151:1786–1793.

87. Kuehr J, Frischer T, Karmaus W, Meinert R, Barth R, Herrman-Kunz E, Forster J, Urbanek R. Early childhood risk factors for sensitization at school age. J Allergy Clin Immunol 1992; 90:358–363.

88. Arshad SH, Stevens M, Hide DW. The effect of genetic and environmental factors on the prevalence of allergic disorders at the age of two years. Clin Exp Allergy 1993; 23:504–511.

89. Ey JL, Holberg CJ, Aldous MB, Wright AL, Martinez FD, Taussig LM, the GHM Associates. Passive smoke exposure and otitis media in the first year of life. Pediatrics 1995; 95:670–677.

90. Minor TE, Baker JW, Dick EC, DeMeo AN, Ouellette JJ, Cohen M, Reed CE. Greater frequency of viral respiratory infections in asthmatic children as compared with their nonasthmatic siblings. J Pediatr 1974; 85:472–477.

91. Bardin PG, Johnston SL, Pattemore PK. Viruses as precipitants of asthma symptoms. II. Physiology and mechanisms. Clin Exp Allergy 1992; 22:809–822.

92. Rowlands DJ. Rhinoviruses and cells: Molecular aspects. Am J Respir Crit Care Med 1995; 152:S31–S35.

93. Vignola A, Campbell A, Chanez P, Bousquet J, Paul-Lacoste P, Michel FB, Godard P. HLA-DR and ICAM-1 expression on bronchial epithelial cells in asthma and chronic bronchitis. Am Rev Respir Dis 1993; 148:689–694.

94. Salome CM, Peat JK, Britton WJ, Woolcock AJ. Bronchial hyperresponsiveness in two populations of Australian schoolchildren. I. Relation to respiratory symptoms and diagnosed asthma. Clin Allergy 1987; 17:271–281.

95. Pattemore PK, Asher MI, Harrison AC, Mitchell EA, Rea HH, Stewart AW. The interrelationship among bronchial hyperresponsiveness, the diagnosis of asthma, and asthma symptoms. Am Rev Respir Dis 1990; 142:549–554.

96. Nicolai T, von Mutius E, Reitmeir P, Wjst M. Reactivity to cold air hyperventilation in normal and asthmatic children in a survey of 5697 school children in southern Bavaria. Am Rev Respir Dis 1992; 147:565–572.

97. Cockcroft DW, Hargreave FE. Airway hyperresponsiveness. Relevance of random population data to clinical usefulness. Am Rev Respir Dis 1990; 142:497–500.

98. Orehek J. Asthma without airway hyperreactivity: fact or artifact? Eur J Respir Dis 1982; 63:1–4.

99. Park ES, Golding J, Carswell F, Stewart-Brown S. Preschool wheezing and prognosis at 10. Arch Dis Child 1986; 61:642–646.

100. Boulet LP, Cartier A, Thomson NC, Roberts RS, Dolovich J, Hargreave FE. Asthma and increases in nonallergic bronchial responsiveness from seasonal pollen exposure. J Allergy Clin Immunol 1983; 71:399–406.

101. Davé NK, Hopp RJ, Biven RE, Degan J, Bewtra AK, Townley RG. Persistence of increased nonspecific bronchial reactivity in allergic children and adolescents. J Allergy Clin Immunol 1990; 86:147–153.

102. Cockcroft DW, Ruffin RE, Dolovich J, Hargreave FE. Allergen-induced increase in non-allergic bronchial reactivity. Clin Allergy 1977; 7:503–513.

103. Sedgwich JB, Calhoun WJ, Gleich GJ, Kita H, Abrams JS, Schwartz LB, Volovitz B, Ben-Yaakov M, Busse WW. Immediate and late airway response of allergic rhinitis patients to segmental antigen challenge. Characterization of eosinophil and mast cell mediators. Am Rev Respir Dis 1991; 144:1274–1281.

104. Burrows B, Martinez FD, Halonen M, Barbee RA, Cline MG. Association of asthma with serum IgE levels and skin-test reactivity to allergens. N Engl J Med 1989; 320:271–277.

105. Sears MR, Burrows B, Flannery EM, Herbison GP, Hewitt CJ, Holdaway MD. Relation between airway responsiveness and serum IgE in children with asthma and in apparently normal children. N Engl J Med 1991; 325:1067–1071.

106. Clough JB, Williams JD, Holgate ST. Effect of atopy on the natural history of symptoms, peak expiratory flow, and bronchial responsiveness in 7- and 8-year-old children with cough and wheeze. Am Rev Respir Dis 1991; 143:755–760.

107. Kelly WJ. Hudson I. Phelan PD. Pain MC. Olinsky A. Atopy in subjects with asthma followed to the age of 28 years. J Allergy Clin Immunol 1990; 85:548–557.

108. Van Asperen PP, Kemp AS, Mukhi A. Atopy in infancy predicts the severity of bronchial hyperresponsiveness in later childhood. J Allergy Clin Immunol 1990; 85:790–795.

109. Zimmerman B, Feanny S, Reisman J, Hak H, Rashed N, McLaughlin FJ, Levison H. Allergy in asthma. J Allergy Clin Immunol 1988; 81:63–70.

110. Peat JK, Salome CM, Woolcock AJ. Longitudinal changes in atopy during a 4-year period: relation to bronchial hyperresponsiveness and respiratory symptoms in a population sample of Australian schoolchildren. J Allergy Clin Immunol 1990; 85:65–74.

111. Anderson HR, The epidemiological and allergic features of asthma in the New Guinea highlands. Clin Allergy 1974; 4:171–183.

112. Flynn MGL. Respiratory symptoms, bronchial responsiveness, and atopy in Fijan and Indian children. Am J Respir Crit Care Med 1994; 150:415–420.

113. Flynn MGL. Respiratory symptoms of rural Fijian and Indian children in Fiji. Thorax 1994; 49:1201–1204.

114. Braback L, Breborwicz A, Julge K, Knutsson A, Riikjarv MA, Vasar M, Bjorksten B. Risk factors for respiratory symptoms and atopic sensitisation in the Baltic area Arch Dis Child 1995; 72:487–493.

115. von Mutius E, Martinez FD, Fritzsch C, Nicolai T, Roell G, Thiemann HH. Prevalence of asthma and atopy in two areas of West and East Germany. Am J Respir Crit Care Med 1994; 149:358–364.

116. Shaheen SO, Aaby P, Hall AJ, Barker DJP, Heyes CB, Shiell AW, Goudiaby A. Measles and atopy in Guinea-Bissau. Lancet 1996; 347:1792–1796.

117. Matricardi PM, Rosmini F, Ferrigno L, Nisini R, Rapicetta M, Chionne P, Stroffol-

ini T, Pasquini P, D'Amelio R. Cross sectional retrospective study of prevalence of atopy among Italian military students with antibodies against hepatitis A virus. Br Med J 1997; 314:999–1003.

118. Martinez FD, Stern DA, Wright AL, Taussig LM, Halonen M, GHM Associates. Association of non-wheezing lower respiratory tract illnesses in early life with persistently diminished serum IgE levels. Thorax 1995; 50:1067–1072.

119. Romagnani S. Human TH1 and TH2 subsets: Regulation of differentiation and role in protection and immunopathology. Intern Arch Allergy Immunol 1992; 98:279–285.

120. Parronchi P, De Carli M, Manetti R, Simonelli C, Sampognaro S, Piccinni MP et al. IL-4 and IFNs exert opposite regulatory effects on the development of cytolytic potential by TH1 or TH2 human T cell clones. J Immunol 1992; 149:2977–2983.

121. Maggi E-Parronchi P, Manetti R, Simonelli C, Piccinni F, Rugiu FS et al. Reciprocal regulatory effects of IFN-gamma and IL-4 on the in vitro development of human TH1 and TH2 clones. J Immunol 1992; 148:2142–147.

122. Haskins R, Kotch J. Day care and illness: evidence, costs, and public policy. Pediatrics 1986; 77:951–952.

123. Tos M, Poulsen G, Borch J. Tympanometry in 2-year-old children. ORL 1978; 40:77–85.

124. Fiellau-Nikolajsen M. Tympanometry in 3-year-old children: type of care as an epidemiological factor in secretory otitis media and tubal dysfunction in unselected populations of 3-year-old children. ORL 1979; 41:193–205.

125. Rasmussen F, Sundelin C. Use of medical care and antibiotics among preschool children in different day care settings. Acta Paediatr Scand 1990; 79:838–846.

126. Wald ER, Dashefsky B, Byers C, Guerra N, Taylor F. Frequency and severity of infections in day care. J Pediatr 1988; 112:540–546.

127. Anderson LJ, Parker RA, Strikas RA, Farrar JA, Gangarosa EJ, Keyserling HL, Sikes RK. Day-care center attendance and hospitalization for lower respiratory tract illness. Pediatrics 1988; 82:300–308.

128. Pisacane A, Graziano L, Zona G, Granata G, Dolezalova H, Cafiero M, Coppola A, Scarpellino B, Ummarino M, Mazzarella G. Breast feeding and acute lower respiratory infection. Acta Paediatr 1994; 83:714–718.

129. Leventhal JM, Shapiro ED, Aten CB, Berg AT, Egerter SA. Does breast-feeding protect against infections in infants less than 3 months of age? Pediatrics 1986; 78:896–903.

130. Beaudry M, Dufour R, Marcoux S. Relation between infant feeding and infections during the first six months of life. J Pediatr 1995; 126:191–197.

131. Howie PW, Forsyth JS, Ogston SA, Clark A, du Florey CV. Protective effect of breast feeding against infection. Br Med J 1990; 300:11–16.

132. Nafstad P, Jaakkola JJK, Hagen JA, Botten G, Kongerud J. Breastfeeding, maternal smoking and lower respiratory tract infections. Eur Respir J 1996; 9:2623–2629.

133. Braun-Fahrländer C, Ackermann-Liebrich U, Schwartz J, Gnehm HP, Rutishauser M, Wanner HU. Air pollution and respiratory symptoms in preschool children. Am Rev Respir Dis 1992; 145:42–47.

134. Schwartz J, Spix C, Wichmann HE, Malin E. Air pollution and acute respiratory illness in five German communities. Environ Res 1991; 56:1–14.

135. Jaakkola JJ, Paunio M, Virtanen M, Heinonen OP. Low-level air pollution and upper respiratory infections in children. Am J Public Health 1991; 81:1060–1063.

136. von-Mutius E, Sherrill DL, Fritzsch C, Martinez FD, Lebowitz MD. Air pollution and upper respiratory symptoms in children from East Germany. Eur Respir J 1995; 8:723–728.

137. Wjst M, Reitmeir P, Dold S, Wulff A, Nicolai T, von Loeffelholz-Colberg E, von Mutius E. Road traffic and adverse effects on respiratory health in children. Br Med J 1993; 307:596–600.

# 5

## Mechanisms of Virus-Induced Asthma

**RICHARD G. HEGELE and JAMES C. HOGG**

University of British Columbia
Vancouver, British Columbia, Canada

## I. Introduction

Acute viral respiratory tract infections result in increases in airway responsiveness in both normal subjects (1) and asthmatic patients (2,3) and have been implicated in triggering the initial onset of asthma in a subpopulation of predisposed children (4). Persistent (i.e., low-level viral replication) and latent (expression of viral genes without replication of a complete virus) infections have also been postulated to contribute to the pathogenesis of chronic airway inflammation and tissue remodeling in the repair phase of this response that causes the observed structural changes in the airways of asthmatics (5). This chapter will review the respiratory viruses that are commonly implicated in asthma (Table 1) and discuss the various mechanisms by which viral infections are postulated to contribute to the pathogenesis of asthma.

## II. Overview of Viral Infections

Viruses are obligate intracellular parasites, and the steps required to establish an infection in a susceptible host are outlined in Figure 1. The pathology that they

**Table 1**  Viruses Commonly
Implicated in Asthma

Single-stranded RNA viruses:
  Rhinoviruses
  Coronaviruses
  Influenza viruses
  Parainfluenza viruses
  Respiratory syncytial virus (RSV)
Double-stranded DNA viruses:
  Adenovirus
  Cytomegalovirus

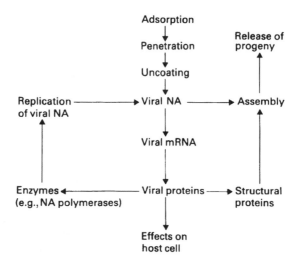

**Figure 1**  Overview of steps involved in the life cycle of viruses. After the initial interaction of a virion with the host cell membrane, the virus is translocated into the cytosol and/or nucleus, where free nucleic acid is used as a template for mRNA transcription. Depending on the interactions between virus and host cell, possible outcomes include assembly of new, complete particles or production of individual viral proteins without assembly of new virions. These viral proteins can have profound effects on the host cell, without the necessity for either viral shedding or cell lysis. (From Ref. 44.)

cause results from both the direct effects of the replicating virus on the cell and the response of the host to this infection. This response has both an innate component, which is fully functional before the viral organisms enter the cell, and an adaptive component, which has memory, specificity, and diversity. The virus first interacts with a cell by binding to specific receptors located on the cell membrane. Unfortunately, the receptors for many of the common respiratory viruses are either unknown or poorly characterized. Exceptions to this include the major group rhinoviruses, which bind to intercellular adhesion molecule-1 (ICAM-1) (6) and the influenza virus, which binds to residues rich in sialic acid. After binding to specific cell surface receptors, viruses penetrate the cell membrane and become uncoated, such that free viral nucleic acid enters the cytoplasm (for most RNA viruses) or nucleus (for most DNA viruses) and undergo transcription into mRNA by viral polymerase enzymes and translation into viral proteins. For many single-stranded RNA viruses, the kinetics of viral replication involve production of complementary mRNA of opposite polarity of the entire viral genome, which can then be used as a template to make new full-length, viral genomic RNA (7). Transcription of individual mRNA species allows for translation into new viral proteins, and the newly synthesized viral genome and proteins assemble into complete particles called virions. The virions can then be released by budding from the cell surface or lysis of the cell to propagate the infection. For RSV, the control over whether the viral polymerase transcribes the entire genome or individual mRNAs for protein synthesis is tightly regulated by the cytoplasmic concentration of the viral nucleocapsid protein, such that a comparatively high concentration of this protein favors the transcription of full-length mRNA, and vice versa. For adenoviruses, a double-stranded DNA virus, the kinetics of viral replication involve the expression of ''early''genes, which use host cell mechanisms to synthesize viral mRNA and proteins that are important to the subsequent replication of viral DNA. The ''late'' genes are responsible for producing structural proteins, which are transported from the cytoplasm to the nucleus for assembly of virions and the complete virus returns to the cytoplasm to be shed or released by cell lysis.

Acute respiratory tract infections such as the common cold, croup, acute bronchiolitis, and pneumonia are primarily produced by this cycle of viral replication (8). The outcome of acute infections ranges from complete resolution to fulminant infections causing death. After the acute infection has passed, the virus is capable of persisting either by low-level replication in the case of RNA viruses (9) or by persistence of circular DNA with or without integration of viral DNA into the host genome (10). In this latter case, viral proteins may be expressed, but a complete virion need not be produced. There is growing evidence that these latent and persistent infections contribute to the production of the chronic inflammation in the airways that may be responsible for diseases such as asthma and COPD. Later in this chapter, we will review evidence that persistent infections can also occur in the lung and will discuss the potential role of these infections in the pathogenesis of asthma.

## III. The Effects of Acute Viral Infections on the Airways

Epidemiological studies have established that acute viral respiratory tract infections can precipitate exacerbations of asthma in both children and adults (for review, see Ref. 11). The mechanisms by which these infections contribute to enhanced airway narrowing must be considered in terms of an inflammatory response of a mucosal surface (12) to an invading virus. Table 2 shows key aspects of the inflammatory response, which we will consider with reference to their potential physical and biochemical effects on the airways.

Plasma- and cell-derived inflammatory mediators released by interaction between the virus and epithelial cell directly affect the airway caliber by increasing smooth muscle shortening. Because the peripheral airways are normally lined by surfactant (13), accumulation of edema fluid on the surface of the airway lumen will substantially increase surface tension and create forces through the Laplace relationship that result in airway narrowing.

These two changes are rapid and act in concert with other inflammatory events in the airway wall. The bronchovasculature consists of two capillary net-

**Table 2**  General Overview of the
Mucosal Inflammatory Response

---

Innate inflammatory response
  Plasma-derived mediators
    Kinins
    Complement
    Coagulation products
    Fibrinolytic system
  Membrane-derived mediators
    Prostaglandins
    Leukotrienes
  Exposure of submucosal nerves
    Neuropeptides
  Systemic response
    Leukocytosis
    Acute phase reactions
Adaptive immune response
  Humoral immunity
  Cell-mediated immunity

---

works (Fig. 2): one located beneath the epithelium internal to the airway smooth (submucosal plexus) and a second located external to the smooth muscle (adventitial plexus)(14). The swelling of the submucosal and adventitial extracellular spaces as a result of fluid exudation from the capillaries has only a small effect on the caliber of the airway lumen. However, when the smooth muscle contracts, it acts in series with the swollen mucosa to markedly reduce airway caliber (15). For example, a 50% increase in submucosal volume due to accumulation of edema fluid acting with a modest degree of smooth muscle contraction (30%) can be shown to result in a 10-fold increase in airway resistance, compared to a normal submucosa with a similar amount of smooth muscle shortening. The expansion of the adventitial interstitial space by edema has an additional negative effect because it uncouples the airway smooth muscle from the afterload exerted by the surrounding lung parenchyma (16). This reduction in afterload allows greater smooth muscle shortening and profoundly affects the reduction in airway caliber.

Airway epithelial cells and type II pneumocytes are major targets for acute viral lower respiratory tract infections (Figs. 3 and 4). Necrosis and sloughing of infected epithelial cells into the lumen change the viscosity of the exudate in the lumen and interfere with the clearance of airway secretions. This combination

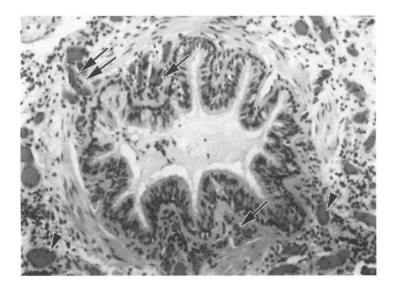

**Figure 2**  Photomicrograph of a bronchiole from an asthmatic patient showing congestion of blood vessels within the submucosal plexus (arrows) and the adventitial plexus external to the airway smooth muscle (arrowheads). (From Ref. 45.)

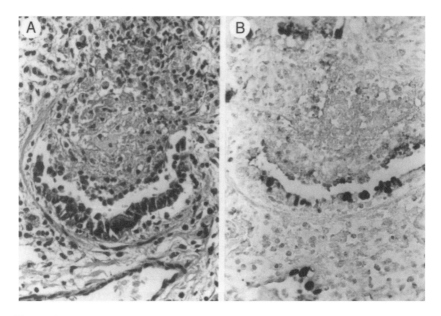

**Figure 3**  Photomicrographs of an airway from a child who died of acute adenoviral bronchiolitis. Note the extensive epithelial cell necrosis and sloughing of inflammatory exudate into the lumen at center (A). In situ hybridization of a serial section with a nonisotopic probe (B) reveals large amounts of adenoviral genome (dark dots) within the nuclei of infected epithelial cells. (From Ref. 46.)

of biochemical and biomechanical events involving cell membranes stimulate the production of membrane-derived mediators, including the prostaglandins and leukotrienes. Many of these mediators modulate smooth muscle activity and influence airways caliber by the mechanisms described above. A further consequence of viral-induced epithelial cell injury is decreased production of neutral endopeptidase (17), an enzyme important for the metabolism of a wide variety of bronchoconstricting neuropeptides, which increase mucus secretion from both the goblet cells and submucosal glands. Moreover, the loss of an intact epithelial barrier from acute viral infection results in exposure of submucosal afferent nerve endings to physical, chemical, biological, and environmental agents that stimulate neurogenic inflammation mediated by peptides such as neurokinin A and substance P.

Alveolar macrophages are also a cellular target for acute viral infections (18,19). In contrast to epithelial cells, viruses infecting alveolar macrophages rarely cause cell lysis. Alveolar macrophages restrict viral replication and act as an effective host-defense mechanism. However, these infected cells secrete

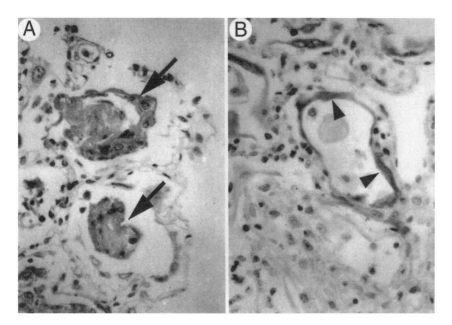

**Figure 4** Photomicrographs of peripheral lung from a child who died of acute RSV bronchiolitis, stained with anti-RSV antibody. Note the positive cytoplasmic immunostaining of sloughed cells within the alveolar lumen (A, arrows) and intact alveolar epithethial lining cells (B, arrowheads). (Courtesy of Dr. James Dimmick, British Columbia's Children's Hospital of British Columbia, Vancouver, British Columbia, Canada.)

inflammatory mediators such as tumor necrosis factor (TNF), various interleukins, colony-stimulating factors, oxygen free radicals, interferons, prostaglandins, and platelet-activating factor. These potent molecules influence airway caliber by acting directly on smooth muscle and by modulating the exudative and cellular components of the inflammatory process. Further information about the effects of respiratory viruses on alveolar macrophage function is available in a recent review article by Lantz et al. (20).

The local generation of plasma- and cell-derived inflammatory mediators results in recruitment and activation of inflammatory cells. For example, interleukin (IL)-4 causes B lymphocytes to express IgE; IL-5 is an important regulator of eosinophils, and IL-8 regulates the migration of neutrophils. Furthermore, activated cells can release preformed and newly synthesized mediators that can stimulate airway narrowing, such as histamine from mast cells and IL-11 (21) from virus-infected lung epithelial and stromal cells.

The specific adaptive humoral and cell-mediated immune responses to viral infection and genetically determined differences in this response have been postulated to be important determinants of clinical outcome. For example, RSV and parainfluenza viruses are reported to induce the production of virus-specific IgE antibodies (22,23) in a subpopulation of children who have recurrent wheezing. In these children, reinfections by these viruses might result in the generation of an allergic response that could modulate airway narrowing via binding of the Fc fragment of IgE to receptors on mast cells, with resultant mediator release and airway smooth muscle contraction. Cell-mediated immunity has also been implicated in the production of "fibrogenic" cytokines, such as transforming growth factor-β (TGF-β), platelet-derived growth factor, and IL-11, which are involved in the repair phase of the inflammatory process responsible for the structural changes observed in the airways in chronic asthma.

Although the general pattern of inflammatory response is becoming much better understood, the details of how any individual virus produces the changes in airway structure responsible for reversible airway narrowing and hyperresponsiveness remain to be worked out. For example, epidemiological studies have implicated pathogens that characteristically cause self-limited upper respiratory tract infections (e.g., rhinoviruses and coronaviruses) as being frequent triggers of acute exacerbations of asthma. To account for these observations, investigators have postulated mechanisms whereby these local infections act from a distance to stimulate the intrapulmonary airways via nerves and trafficking of viral proteins and host effector cells through lymphatic vessels. These mechanisms will probably remain hypothetical until better experimental methods become available to rigorously test them. Gern et al. have recently reported that rhinoviral genome can be identified by the polymerase chain reaction (PCR) testing of bronchoalveolar lavage fluid specimens of experimentally inoculated subjects (24). Should these observations be confirmed, the assumption that rhinoviruses and coronaviruses remain confined to the upper respiratory tract during asthma exacerbations will have to be reconsidered. The detection of viruses in specimens obtained from the lower respiratory tract by using PCR-based methods is a rapidly advancing area in which valuable new information is emerging quickly.

## IV.　Latent Viral Infections

The ability of a virus to remain latent for the lifetime of its human host is best illustrated by the herpes simplex virus (HSV). During an acute infection, this virus enters sensory nerves enervating cells of mucosal membranes and acquires the characteristics of linear or circular DNA. In a fraction of the neurons harboring latent HSV, the virus is periodically reactivated and carried back to the mucosal surface by active transport. The resulting lesions vary considerably in severity depending on the host immune response and can be manifested as barely visible vesicles through severe debilitating lesions in immunosuppressed individuals. The adenovirus provides the best example of latent infection involving respiratory viruses (25,26). This double-stranded DNA virus can infect and replicate at various sites in the respiratory tract as well as the gastrointestinal tract, urinary, bladder, liver, and eye. The adenovirus can produce severe bronchopneumonia and is responsible for approximately 5% of the acute respiratory disease in children under the age of 5. Although there are 49 serotypes, the common ones producing respiratory disease are types 1, 2, 3, 5, and 6. Sporadic cases are usually indistinguishable from other viral infections produced by influenza, parainfluenza, and RSV. A study by Macek and colleagues (27) raised concern that cases of persistent childhood asthma might follow acute adenoviral infection. They described a group of 34 children referred for persistent asthma preceded by an acute illness. This acute illness was attributed to adenoviral bronchiolitis, primarily on clinical grounds, but supported by laboratory evidence of infection in a proportion of the cases. They tested the hypothesis that the asthmatic syndrome that followed this illness was due to adenoviral infection by performing immunohistochemical examination of cytospin preparations of BAL fluid. They demonstrated the adenoviral capsid protein in these preparations in 94% of these children. They concluded that these findings implicated the adenovirus in the pathogenesis of the childhood asthma.

The human adenovirus has a highly ordered structure with an icosohedral shape and its 20 triangular-shaped sides arranged to provide 12 apices (25,26). The surface of each of the 20 sides is covered with a well-organized capsid protein shell made up of hexon macromolecules. The penton molecule is located at each of the 12 apices, and a fiber extending from the penton serves as an attachment to the host cell. Contact is followed by transport into the host by a receptor-mediated endocytosis involving receptors on both the penton molecule and the hexon base. The virus disrupts the endocytic vesicle membrane to gain entry into the cytosol and sheds its external coat to release the DNA. The DNA is transported to the nucleus, where it begins a direct takeover of the transcription and translation capability of the host cells to replicate itself. The host provides the molecular machinery required for transcription, mRNA processing, and translation, but the viral genome produces early proteins that control the rate at which this takes place. One of these early proteins (E1A) can increase host cell replication by allowing the cell to enter its replicative cycle. Another in the E3 region subverts the destruction of the infected cell by cytotoxic T cells by preventing MHC class I molecule expression. When the complete viral genome is replicated and the structural proteins produced, new viruses are assembled in the nucleus and either shed from the cell surface or released in large numbers by cell lysis. Clearance of the virus by the host is not complete, and residual viral DNA can be expressed in this latent infection without replication of the complete virus.

There are several possible mechanisms for the pathogenesis of childhood asthma following an adenoviral infection. One is that the continued stimulation of the immune system by viral proteins results in a chronic inflammatory disease of the airways. The second is that the adenoviral proteins might amplify and prolong the inflammatory response induced by the original infection. Portions of the E1A region of the adenoviral DNA have been commonly demonstrated in human lungs by PCR (28). Immunohistochemistry has revealed that the adenoviral protein is also frequently present (29). An experimental model of latent adenoviral infection in the guinea pig has shown that the persistence of the adenoviral DNA in protein is associated with a choronic bronchiolitis, but the mechanism responsible for this bronchiolitis is incompletely understood (30).

The presence of E1A in cultured epithelial cells increases their susceptibility to lysis by cytokines such as TNF, and proteins included in the E3 region are capable of reversing this effect (31). This means that the virus has the ability to render cells susceptible to cell lysis early in the infection to assist spread and to terminate this lytic process when a more stable symbiotic arrangement between the host and virus occurs. Recent studies with A549 cells transformed by E1A have shown that it upregulates the expression of IL-8 and ICAM-1 (33) following challenge and that this upregulation involves the transcription factor NF-κB (34). These findings suggest several mechanisms whereby latent adenoviral infections might upregulate an inflammatory process and produce the chronic airway changes associated with asthma, but much work remains to be done to fully establish this hypothesis.

## V. Persistent Viral Infections

Persistent viral infections, where there is continuous replication of the virus at a lower level than during an acute infection, are well-described tissue culture phenomena in studies of RNA viruses such as RSV (35). Human (36) and animal studies (37) have also documented persistent viral shedding from the respiratory tract following acute infections. Studies from our laboratory (38) and others (39), where normal juvenile guinea pigs were inoculated with human RSV to follow the natural history of this experimental infection, have shown that RSV continues to replicate in the guinea pig lung for at least 2 months and that the viral genome is present without definite evidence of replication at 4 months after inoculation. Interestingly, persistence of RSV in the guinea pig lung is associated with mild bronchiolitis and long-term increases in airway responsiveness.

Other investigators have developed a rat model of parainfluenza virus infection (40), in which virus-infected, neonatal animals develop sequelae of chronic airway hyperresponsiveness, mast cell hyperplasia of the airway wall, and increased airway wall thickness (41). In contrast to RSV-inoculated guinea pigs, these investigators have not documented persistent parainfluenza virus replication in the lungs, which suggests that the virus could be acting as a "hit-and-run" driver. The subpopulation of children who develop recurrent wheezing and asthma as sequelae of viral respiratory infection in infancy frequently show allergy to one or more environmental antigens (4). Taken together, these observations suggest that asthma may result from complex interactions between the virus, the host, and other antigens in the environment. For example, viral respiratory tract infections during early postnatal life may trigger allergic sensitization to common environmental antigens in a susceptible population (42,43). Much remains to be learned about the role of persistent viral lung infections and/or the interplay between viruses and environmental antigens in the onset of recurrent wheezing and asthma, particularly in children who have a genetic predisposition to developing allergy.

## VI. Summary

In summary, we have provided an overview of the potential mechanisms by which viral respiratory tract infections might contribute to the pathogenesis of increased airway responsiveness in asthma. The distinction between acute, latent, and persistent infection provides an approach for investigators to examine virus-host interactions. An improved understanding of these interactions may lead to innovative strategies for the treatment and prevention of viral-induced airway hyperresponsiveness.

## References

1. Laitinen LA, Elkin RB, Empey DW, Jacobs L, Mills J, Nadel JA. Bronchial hyperresponsiveness in normal subjects during attenuated influenza virus infection. Am J Respir Crit Care Med 1991; 143:358–361.
2. Nicholson KG, Kent J, Ireland DC. Respiratory viruses and exacerbations of asthma in adults. Br Med J 1993; 307:982–986.
3. Johnston SL, Pattemore PK, Sanderson G, Smith S, Lampe F, Josephs L, Symington P, O'Toole S, Myint SH, Tyrrell DAJ, Holgate ST. Community study of role of viral infections in exacerbations of asthma in 9–11 year old children. Br Med J 1995; 310:1225–1229.
4. Frick OL, German DF, Mills J. Development of allergy in children. I. Association with virus infections. J Allergy Clin Immunol 1979; 63:228–241.
5. Hogg JC. The pathology of asthma. In: Holgate ST, Austin KF, Lichtenstein LM, Kay AB, eds. Asthma Physiology, Immunopharmacology and Treatment. Fourth International Symposium. San Diego: Academic Press Ltd., 1993:17–25.
6. Greve JM, Davis G, Meyer AM, Forte CP, Yost SC, Marlor CW, Kamarch ME, McClelland A. The major human rhinovirus receptor is ICAM-1. Cell 1989; 56: 839–847.

7.   Huang YT, Wertz GW. The genome of respiratory syncytial virus is a negative stranded RNA that codes for at least seven mRNA species. J Virol 1982; 43:150–157.

8.   Miller RR. Viral infections of the respiratory tract. In: Thurlbeck WM, Churg AM, eds. Pathology of the Lung. 2d ed. New York: Thieme Medical Publishers, Inc., 1995:195–222.

9.   Oldstone MBA. Viral persistence. Cell 1989; 56:517–520.

10.  Garcia-Blanco M, Cullen BR. Molecular basis of latency in pathogenic human viruses. Science 1991; 254:815–820.

11.  Pattemore PK, Johnston SL, Bardin PG. Viruses as precipitants of asthma symptoms. I. Epidemiology. Clin Exp Allergy 1992; 22:325–336.

12.  Cotran RS, Kumar V, Robbins SL. Inflammation and repair. In: Cotran RS, Kumar V, Robbins SL, eds. Robbins Pathologic Basis of Disease. 5th ed. Philadelphia: WB Saunders Company, 1994:51–92.

13.  Macklem PT, Proctor DF, Hogg JC. The stability of peripheral airways. Respir Physiol 1970; 8:191–203.

14.  Deffeback ME, Widdicombe J. The bronchial circulation. In: Crystal RG, West JB, Barnes RT, Cherniack NS, Weibel ER, eds. The Lung: Scientific Foundations. New York: Raven Press, 1991:741–757.

15.  Moreno RH, Hogg JC, Pare PD. Mechanics of airway narrowing. Am J Respir Crit Care Med 1986; 133:1171–1180.

16.  Macklem PT. Bronchial hyperresponsiveness. Chest 1985; 158S–159S.

17.  Borson DB, Brokaw J, Sekizaw K, McDonald D, Nadel JA. Viral infections increases permeability response to substance P (SP) by decreasing tracheal neutral endopeptidase. FASEB J 1988; 2:A1382.

18.  Mills J. Effects of Sendai virus infection on function of cultured mouse alveolar macrophages. Am J Respir Crit Care Med 1979; 120:1239–1244.

19.  Panuska JR, Cirino NM, Midulla F, Despot JE, McFadden ER Jr., Huang YT. Productive infection of isolated human alveolar macrophages by respiratory syncytial virus. J Clin Invest 1990; 86:113–119.

20.  Lantz RC, Witten ML, Lemen RJ. Pulmonary macrophage and respiratory virus interactions. In: Lipscomb MF, Russell SW, eds. Lung Macrophages and Dendritic Cells in Health and Disease. New York: Marcel Dekker, Inc., 1997:551–570.

21.  Einarsson O, Geba GP, Panuska JR, Zhu Z, Landry M, Elias JA. Asthma-associated viruses specifically induce lung stromal cells to produce interleukin-II, a mediator of airways hyperreactivity. Chest 1995; 107:132S–133S.

22.  Welliver RC, Wong DT, Middleton E Jr., Sun M, McCarthy N, Ogra PL. Role of parainfluenza virus-specific IgE in pathogenesis of croup and wheezing subsequent to infection. J Pediatr 1982; 101:889–896.

23.  Welliver RC, Sun M, Rinaldo D, Ogra PL. Predictive value of respiratory syncytial virus-specific IgE responses for recurrent wheezing following bronchiolitis. J Pediatr 1986; 109:776–780.

24.  Gern JE, Galagan DM, Jarjour NN, Dick EC, Busse WW. Detection of rhinovirus RNA in lower airway cells during experimentally induced infection. Am J Respir Crit Care Med 1997; 155:1159–1161.

25. Shank T. Adenoviridae: the viruses and their replication. Fields BN, Knipe DM, Howley PM, eds. Virology. 3d ed. Philadelphia: Lippincott-Raven Publishers, 1996: 2118–2148.

26. Horowitz. Adenoviruses. In: Fields BN, Knipe DM, Howley PM, eds. Virology. 3d ed. Philadelphia: Lippincott-Raven Publishers, 1996:2149–2171.

27. Macek V, Sorli J, Kopriva S, Marin J. Persistent adenoviral infection and chronic airway obstruction in children. Am J Respir Crit Care Med 1994; 150:7–10.

28. Matsuse T, Hayashi S, Kuwano K, Keunecke H, Jefferies WA, Hogg JC. Latent adenoviral infection in the pathogenesis of chronic airways obstruction. Am J Respir Crit Care Med 1992; 146:177–184.

29. Elliott WM, Hayashi S, Hogg JC. Immunodetection of adenoviral E1A proteins in human lung tissue. Am J Respir Cell Mol Biol 1995; 12:642–648.

30. Vitalis TZ, Keicho N, Itabashi S, Hayashi S, Hogg JC. A model of latent adenovirus 5 infection in the guinea pig (*Cavia procellus*). Am J Respir Cell Mol Biol 1996; 14:225–231.

31. Gooding LR, Wold WSM. Molecular mechanisms by which adenoviruses counteract antiviral immune defences. Crit Rev Immunol 1990; 10:53–71.

32. Keicho N, Elliott WM, Hogg JC, Hayashi S. Adenovirus E1A upregulates interleukin 8 expression induced by endotoxin in pulmonary epithelial cells. Am J Physiol (Lung Cell Mol Physiol) 1997, 16:L1046–L1052.

33. Keicho N, Elliott WM, Hogg JC, Hayashi S. Adenovirus E1A gene dysregulates ICAM-1 expression in transformed pulmonary epithelial cells. Am J Respir Cell Mol Biol 1997; 16:23–30.

34. Keicho N, Higashimoto Y, Bondy GP, Elliott WM, Hogg JC, Hayashi S. Endotoxin-specific NF-kB activation in pulmonary epithelial cells harbouring adenovirus E1A. Am J Respir Crit Care Med 1997; 155:A698.

35. Baldridge P, Senterfit LB. Persistent infection of cells in culture by respiratory syncytial virus. Proc Soc Exp Biol Med 1976; 151:684–688.

36. Hall CB. The shedding and spreading of respiratory syncytial virus. Pediatr Res 1977; 11:236–239.

37. Johnson RA, Prince GA, Suffin SC, Horswood RL, Chanock RM. Respiratory syncytial virus infection in cyclophosphamide-treated cotton rats. Infect Immun 1982; 37: 369–373.

38. Dakhama A, Vitalis TZ, Hegele RG. Persistence of respiratory syncytial virus (RSV) and development of RSV-specific IgG$_1$ antibodies in a guinea pig model of acute bronchiolitis. Eur Respir J 1997; 10:20–26.

39. Riedel F, Obersieck B, Streckert H-J, Philippou S, Krusat T, Marek W. Persistence of airway hyperresponsiveness and viral antigen following respiratory syncytial virus bronchiolitis in young guinea pigs. Eur Respir J 1997; 10:639–645.

40. Castleman WL. Respiratory tract lesions in weanling outbred rats infected with Sendai virus. Am J Vet Res 1983; 44:1024–1031.

41. Uhl EW, Castleman WL, Sorkness RL, Busse WW, Lemanske RF Jr., McAllister PK. Parainfluenza virus-induced persistence of airway inflammation, fibrosis, and dysfunction associated with TGF-β expression in Brown Norway rats. Am J Respir Crit Care Med 1996; 154:1834–1842.

42. Riedel F, Krause A, Slenczka W, Rieger CHL. Parainfluenza-3-virus infection enhances allergic sensitization in the guinea pig. Clin Exp Allergy 1996; 26:603–609.

43. Schwarz J, Hamelmann E, Bradley KL, Takeda K, Gelfand EW. Respiratory syncytial virus infection results in airway hyperresponsiveness and enhanced airway sensitization to allergen. J Clin Invest 1997; 100:226–233.

44. Taussig MJ. Viral infections. In: Processes in Pathology and Microbiology. 2d ed. Oxford: Blackwell Scientific, 1987:215–375.

45. Hogg JC. Pathology of asthma. In: Weiss EB, Stein M, eds. Bronchial Asthma. Boston: Little Brown, 1993:352–355.

46. Hogg JC, Irving WL, Porter H, et al. In situ hybridization studies of adenoviral infections of the lungs and their relationship to follicular bronchiectasis. Am J Respir Crit Care Med 1989; 139:1531–1535.

# 6

## The Use of Experimentally Infected Volunteers in Research on the Common Cold

**JACK M. GWALTNEY, Jr.**

University of Virginia Health Sciences Center
Charlottesville, Virginia

## I. Introduction

The common cold is one of relatively few human illnesses that can be artificially induced in volunteers for research purposes. A human model for studying human disease has the obvious advantage of creating disease in the species of interest, the human. Thus, scientific observations made with the human model require no extrapolations across species with their attendant dangers from differences in anatomy, physiology, and molecular biology. Using the human model, a considerable body of important information about colds has been obtained in this century. Much of the work has focused on rhinovirus, the most important common cold virus. Rhinovirus challenge in humans was initially used to confirm the pathogenicity of the virus and subsequently has been employed to investigate routes of transmission, mechanisms of pathogenesis, and responses to traditional and experimental treatments.

## II. History

Walter Kruse is credited with first using experimental challenge to investigate the common cold (Fig. 1). As his challenge inoculum, he used nasal discharge

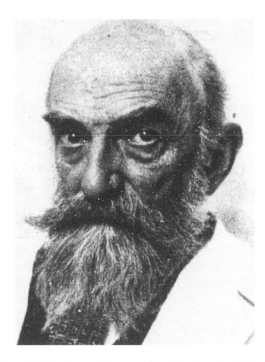

**Figure 1**  Professor Walter Kruse, Director of the Hygienic Institute, Leipzig, who reported the first common cold challenge studies in 1914.

from persons with colds. The material was diluted in saline and filtered to remove bacteria before instillation in the nose. In two experiments reported in 1914, 19 of 48 staff and students of the Hygienic Institute in Leipzig developed colds after experimental challenge (1) (Fig. 2). This provided the first direct evidence of the infectious nature of colds. This challenge method was adopted by A. R. Dochez and associates in New York and used for a series of experiments in chimpanzees and humans in the 1920s (2). In addition to inocula prepared from nasal discharge, these investigators used material passed in chick embryo, which was thought to contain an infectious agent, and also control broths. Consistent rates of illness were not produced in their volunteers.

Common cold challenge studies in volunteers came into prominence when Christopher Andrewes established the Common Cold Research Unit in Salisbury, England, in 1946 (3) (Fig. 3). Dr. Andrewes was later knighted for his work on the common cold, most of it done with experimental challenge in volunteers. He conducted a number of innovative studies during the 1940s and 1950s on the

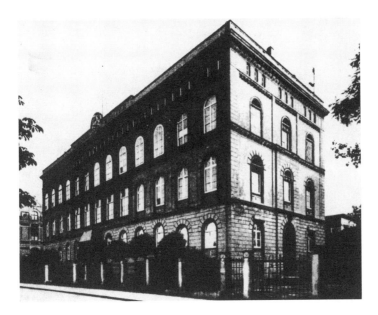

**Figure 2** Hygienic Institute, Leipzig, which was the site of the first common cold experiments using artificial virus challenge.

etiology, transmission, and pathogenesis of common colds. During this period, none of the common cold viruses had been discovered, and he still had to work with challenge inocula of unknown potency and with subjects with unknown immune status to the challenge material. In an admirable admission of his frustration, he states that the results of work from 1946 to 1960 were "difficult to interpret" because of these problems. Some of Andrewes's inocula were later shown to contain strains of rhinovirus, which was first isolated in cell culture by Pelon and Mogabgab at the Great Lakes Naval Research Station (4) and Price at Johns Hopkins (5) in 1956. In 1958, Andrewes was joined at the Common Cold Research Unit by David Tyrrell, who later became director of the unit and continued the research until 1990, when the unit was closed (6). The availability of inoculum pools prepared with known respiratory viruses greatly facilitated progress in the field.

In the United States, challenge studies using volunteers have been conducted during the past 50 years by George Jackson at the University of Illinois; Vernon Knight, Robert Couch, Gordon Douglas, and their colleagues at the National Institute of Allergy and Infectious Diseases and later at Baylor University; Jack Gwaltney, Owen Hendley, Frederick Hayden, and Birgit Winther at the

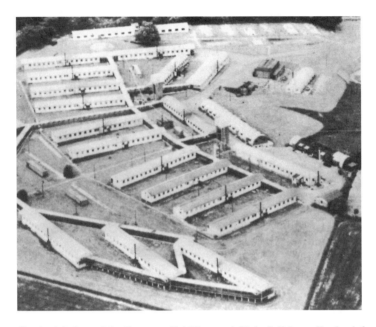

**Figure 3** Aerial view of the Common Cold Research Unit, Salisbury, England, founded by Sir Christopher Andrewes in 1946.

University of Virginia; Elliot Dick and his colleagues at the University of Wisconsin; and Ronald Turner at the University of Charleston. These investigators have used experimental challenge with rhinovirus and other respiratory viruses to investigate transmission, pathogenesis, treatment, and prevention of colds and related illnesses.

## III. Methodology

### A. Inoculum Preparation

The first challenge inocula were prepared from collections of nasal discharge, which were unmodified except for dilution in saline and passage through filters to exclude bacteria and other large microorganisms (1–3). After discovery of the rhinovirus and other respiratory viruses in the late 1950s, it was possible to harvest cold viruses from cell culture, providing a more certain and specific infectious source for making challenge inocula.

Using methods of cultivation developed at the Common Cold Research Unit (7), rhinovirus has been grown in human embryonic lung cells (8) and other cell cultures of diploid karyotype to prepare challenge inocula. Virus is harvested at low passage to avoid possible attenuation of the pathogenicity of the virus. The number of serial passages required to attenuate a rhinovirus is not well established. In one instance, only a single passage appeared to result in attenuation of pathogenicity (9), while with other strains 10–25 cell culture passages did not lead to significant attenuation (R.B. Conch and J.M. Gwaltney, Jr., personal communication). Rhinovirus challenge inocula retain virulence after storage at $-70°C$ for months or years, although infectivity titers may decline by a log or more after prolonged storage.

In 1964, Knight et al. published a suggested methodology to ensure that extraneous agents were not present in viral challenge pools to be used for common cold studies (10). Safety testing procedures were updated in 1992 by Gwaltney et al. to deal with new infectious agents that had been discovered (11). Rhinovirus challenge pools have been given safely to thousands of subjects in England and the United States over the past five decades without reports of serious complications. While a small percentage of subjects may develop clinically recognized sinusitis and otitis media, more serious respiratory illness such as pneumonia has not occurred, nor has illness been recognized from possible extraneous infectious agents in the challenge inocula.

## B. Challenge Procedures

The standard method of inoculation is to give a small amount of coarse drops containing the virus into the nose. In a standard technique, 0.25 ml of inoculum is given per nostril, sometimes repeated once, using a 1-ml pipette with the subject in the supine position (12). A variant on this method has been to give 50 µl of the inoculum per nostril, using a calibrated pipette (13).

In studying sites of initiation of infection, rhinovirus has been given by drops into the eye (14,15) or mouth (14) and into the upper airway by artificially generated small particle aerosols (16,17). In other novel transmission experiments, rhinovirus has been deposited into the nose or onto the conjunctival membrane from the finger (18,19) and into the mouth by prolonged kissing (20). Also, transmission has been reported by means of exposure to natural aerosols presumably created by the coughs of experimentally infected subjects (21).

It was originally believed that the illness produced after artificial aerosol inoculation was different from that after intranasal inoculation, with aerosol leading to more coughing and a tracheobronchitis (16). Further work with strains of other rhinovirus types did not produce tracheobronchitis after small particle aerosol exposure, but illness was confined predominately to the upper respiratory tract (17).

## C.  Measurement of Infection

The traditional criteria used for the diagnosis of experimental rhinovirus infection are viral recovery from respiratory secretions in cell culture and a $\geq$fourfold rise in serum-neutralizing antibody titer to the challenge virus. Virus recovery is a very sensitive indicator of experimental rhinovirus infection, with $\geq$90% of challenged subjects shedding virus on one or more of the first 5 days after intranasal inoculation (22).

The seroconversion rate is a less sensitive measure of infection and varies among the different rhinovirus serotypes. For example, with type 39, the rate averaged 50% in 56 antibody-free subjects who shed virus (23) compared to 82% in 50 antibody-free subjects who shed Hank's strain, a rhinovirus not identified by antisera to the known types (24). The reasons for the differences in seroconversion rates among the different rhinovirus serotypes is unknown. Most challenged subjects are diagnosed by viral shedding with or without antibody response, but a small percentage from whom virus is not recovered have a diagnostic antibody rise.

Methods for detecting viral nucleic acid are now also available for diagnosing infection. A PCR assay was found to be of equal or greater sensitivity than viral isolation in cell culture for detecting rhinovirus in nasal washings of experimentally infected volunteers (25). Also, in situ hybridization has been used to identify rhinovirus replication in cells from the upper respiratory tract of subjects with experimental colds (26).

## D.  Measurement of Illness

*Subjective Measurements*

The illness associated with common cold viruses is largely subjective in nature. A method developed by Jackson et al. (27) has been used frequently to measure the presence of cold symptoms and to provide criteria to make the diagnosis of a cold. In this method, a series of respiratory and general symptoms are recorded daily by an investigator after the virus challenge has been administered. The symptoms are sneezing, rhinorrhea, nasal obstruction, sore throat, cough, malaise, and chilliness. The original criteria for diagnosing the occurrence of a cold were a total symptom score of 14 or greater summed over 6 days and the subject's impression of having had a cold, and/or rhinorrhea reported for $\geq$3 days. The original work was done with inocula prepared from nasal discharge specimens, which may have contained a variety of agents. For rhinovirus work, the criteria have been modified to require a total symptom score of $\geq$five or $\geq$six summed over 5 or 6 days with the other criteria staying the same (12,28). Other refinements of the Jackson symptom-recording method by more frequent recording of symptoms or by use of visual analogs have been tried and have not substantially improved on the Jackson method. Such refinements tend to attempt more precision than the nature of the data sets warrant.

### Objective Measurement

#### Measurement of Nasal Discharge Weights

Recording of nasal discharge weight has been a useful objective measure of the severity of experimental cold illness (29,30). In this method, used nasal tissues are collected in airtight containers over 24-hour periods. The weight of nasal discharge is determined by subtracting the weight of an equal number of unused tissues from the weight of those used by the subject. Nasal discharge weights have correlated with rhinorrhea severity scores in the rhinovirus challenge model (31). Other objective measurements of nasal function used with the model have been nasal air-flow resistance and mucus transport times (30).

#### Imaging of the Paranasal Sinuses

Rhinovirus infection has recently been shown to routinely involve the paranasal sinuses as well as the nasal cavity. This was first demonstrated by sinus MRI in volunteers with experimental rhinovirus colds (32). Thus, sinus imaging provides another objective measurement of rhinovirus disease, which can be used with the challenge model. The sinus abnormalities most frequently observed are occlusion of the infundibulum and opacities in the sinus cavities (33). The abnormality in the sinus cavity is thought to represent thick secretions adherent to the sinus wall because of the irregular distribution along the wall and because the material sometimes contains bubbles that would not be present if due to mucosal swelling.

#### Eustachian Tube Function and Middle Ear Pressure

Rhinovirus infection is also frequently associated with abnormalities in eustachian tube function and middle ear pressure (34). In one study of volunteers with experimental rhinovirus colds, tubal function was present in only 50% of ears (35). Middle ear underpressures of less than $-50$ mmH$_2$O occurred in 50% of infected volunteers. More recently, middle ear effusions were observed to develop in volunteers who presented with negative pressures before virus challenge and had worsening underpressures after infection (36). Measurements of middle ear dysfunction have been used to evaluate the effectiveness of antiviral treatment in subjects with experimental rhinovirus colds (37).

#### Pulmonary Function and Lower Airway Responsiveness

Pulmonary function and lower airway response to inhaled histamine and immediate and late reactions to inhaled allergen are other objective measures that have been used with the rhinovirus challenge model (38–41). An increase in airway responsiveness to histamine has been noted during the time of the acute infection in patients with allergic rhinitis (42). Also, rhinovirus infection increased the immediate response to inhaled allergen and the probability of late asthmatic reactions. The amounts of reduction in the allergen concentrations required to drop the $FEV_1$ by 20% for immediate response and by 15% for the late reaction were the standards used.

Airway response to inhaled allergen was also measured by a method called segmental bronchoprovocation (40). With this technique, specific segments of the lung are lavaged after allergen challenge. Longitudinal sampling by this method has provided specimens for measuring mast cell mediator release products and cellular influxes.

## IV. Applications of the Rhinovirus Challenge Model

### A. Studies of Etiology and Pathogenesis

*Infection, Incubation Period, and Immunity*

In 1958, Tyrrell and Byone reported giving a cell culture harvest of JH rhinovirus to volunteers but only observed colds in 6 of 58 challenged subjects (43). The following year, Jackson et al. presented data showing development of colds in 48 (30%) of 159 rhinovirus challenged volunteers versus 17 (18%) of 96 volunteers challenged with a control inoculum ($p \leq 0.05$) (44). These findings, which completed Koch's criteria, confirmed rhinovirus as a human pathogen that causes colds. In these studies, the immune status of the volunteers to the challenge virus was not determined before inoculation.

In following years, British investigators continued to use volunteers with undetermined antibody status before challenge, later stratifying the subjects into groups based on antibody levels determined retrospectively on serum specimens collected prior to virus challenge. American investigators have tended to pre-screen volunteers for antibody and work only with those having known prechallenge antibody levels of $\leq 1:2$ or $\leq 1:4$ to the challenge virus.

Experimental challenge has subsequently been used to determine the human infectious $dose_{50}$ for rhinovirus. This was found to be as low as 0.1 $TCID_{50}$ for one serotype (45) and for others ranged from 0.4 to 5.7 $TCID_{50}$ (12). In the latter study, artificial challenge was used to determine the levels of serum-neutralizing antibody that are protective for varying challenge doses of rhinovirus. With a low virus challenge (0.05–50 $TCID_{50}$), an antibody titer of $\geq 1:64$ was associated with resistance to infection. In another similar study, large viral challenges (10,000 $TCID_{50}$) resulted in infection of volunteers with prechallenged antibody levels of up to 1:512 (46). Under natural conditions, serum antibody levels of 1:8 are usually protective, suggesting that natural rhinovirus infection results from exposure to relatively low amounts of virus (0.5–80 $TCID_{50}$) (12).

The original challenge studies showed that the usual incubation period for rhinovirus colds was quite brief, less than 24 hours (44). Subsequent monitoring of the time to onset of viral shedding and symptoms has revealed that the cycle of viral replication in nasal cells is similar in duration to that in cell culture and that symptoms appear shortly after virus is recovered in nasal secretions. Following intranasal challenge with rhinovirus type 39, the median period to first virus recovery was 10 hours, and mean total symptom scores for virus-challenged subjects became significantly higher than those for sham-challenged controls at 16 hours (47). Nasal obstruction and rhinorrhea appeared within 2 hours of virus challenge, suggesting nonspecific nasal irritation from the prechallenge nasal wash and viral inoculum. Sore or scratchy throat developed between 10 and 12 hours after virus challenge.

Awareness of perhaps the most basic feature of rhinovirus pathogenesis—the inability of the normal nose in the nonimmune individual to withstand rhinovirus challenge—became apparent as a result of experience with the challenge model. In contrast to intranasal challenge with pathogenic respiratory bacteria, which are routinely cleared by the defense mechanisms in the upper airway, challenge of susceptible volunteers with rhinovirus almost always leads to infection. In 14 studies done over a 10-year period in different seasons of the year and with different rhinovirus serotypes, 321 of 343 (94%) nonimmune subjects became infected after intranasal challenge (22). Of 277 of these volunteers for whom clinical information was available, 205 (74%) met the modified Jackson criteria (12,27,28) for having a cold.

### Portal of Entry, Sites of Infection, and Histopathology

Volunteer studies were used to determine that the nose and eye, but not the mouth, were efficient portals of entry for rhinovirus infection (14,15,18). Another volunteer study suggested that rhinovirus infection usually begins in the nasopharynx and spreads anteriorly, resulting in a patchy distribution of infection in the nasal passages (15). Rhinovirus antigen and ribonucleic acid were shown to be present in a small proportion of the ciliated cells present in the nasal secretions of experimentally infected volunteers (26,48,49). The sparse distribution of virus probably explains why cytopathic changes of the nasal epithelium are not identifiable in nasal mucosal biopsies from volunteers with rhinovirus colds (15). A more recent study with specimens from experimentally infected volunteers using in situ hybridization confirmed the presence of virus in nasal ciliated epithelial cells and also in nonciliated cells from the nasopharynx (26). Also with this technique, only a very small proportion of cells was seen to be infected.

### Role of Inflammatory Mediators

Because of the finding that rhinovirus did not produce discernible damage to the nasal epithelium, it was proposed that rhinovirus illness may largely result from the release of inflammatory mediators and activation of neurological reflexes

(49,50). This idea has been investigated by measuring mediator concentrations in the nasal secretions of volunteers with experimental colds and by using drugs with known mechanisms of action as pharmacological probes to block cold symptoms in subjects with experimental infection.

Nasal secretions have been shown to contain bradykinin (51), histamine (52), interleukin-1 (53), and interleukin-6 (54). Treatment with first-generation antihistamines (28,30) has reduced sneezing and rhinorrhea in experimentally infected volunteers, implicating parasympathetic reflexes and possibly histamine in rhinovirus pathogenesis. Similar reductions in nasal secretions volumes have occurred during treatment with anticholinergic compounds like atropine methonitrate (55) and ipratropium bromide (56). Naproxen treatment of volunteers with experimental rhinovirus colds has also reduced symptoms, suggesting a pathogenic role for prostaglandins (57).

### Relationship to Stress and Other Psychosocial Factors

The rhinovirus challenge model has also been used to examine the possible effects of stress and other psychosocial factors on susceptibility to infection and illness (58–60). Because of the uniformly high infection rate (~95%) after experimental challenge of antibody-free volunteers (22), stress appears to exert an effect primarily on development of illness rather than initiation of infection.

### B. Transmission

Experimentally infected volunteers have been used to investigate routes of respiratory virus transmission since Andrewes's early work at the Common Cold Research Unit. Early attempts to transmit colds by exposing potential recipients to artificially infected donors by aerosol or close contact were not successful (61–63). Reliable transmission of experimental rhinovirus infection was first achieved between married couples by D'Alessio et al. (64), by Holmes et al. in an antarctic hut environment (65), and by Gwaltney et al. using a hand-contamination self-inoculation method (18,19) (Fig. 4). Dick also developed an aerosol transmission model, which used experimentally infected subjects with severe cough as the viral donors (66).

The challenge models, while extremely useful in investigating transmission under highly controlled conditions, do not provide the ultimate answer to the question of how colds are transmitted under natural conditions (63). The latter question must be answered by intervention studies in the natural setting involving persons with natural colds.

### C. Clinical Trials of Cold Treatments

### Traditional Treatments

The rhinovirus challenge model has been used to test traditional cold remedies including decongestants (13,67), antihistamines (28,30), anticholinergics (55,56),

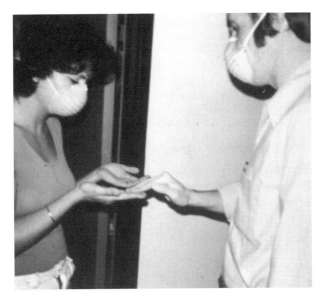

**Figure 4**   Volunteers transferring rhinovirus by hand contact in an experiment conducted in 1975 by Drs. Jack Gwaltney and Owen Hendley in Charlottesville, Virginia.

and nonsteroidal anti-inflammatory drugs (NSAIDs) (57). These studies have either confirmed earlier natural cold studies or established for the first time the usefulness of these drugs for treating certain cold symptoms. Pseudoephedrine was shown to improve nasal patency and relieve the symptom of nasal obstruction. First-generation antihistamines reduced nasal mucus weights and the severity of rhinorrhea and sneezing (28). Anticholinergics also were effective in reducing nasal mucus weights and rhinorrhea (56). Naproxen reduced headache, malaise, and myalgia severity scores and appeared to also reduce coughing (57).

*Experimental Treatments*

A variety of intranasally and orally administered experimental treatments have been tested using the challenge model. The list includes compounds having classical antiviral activity, interferons, capsid binders, and antibody to rhinovirus receptor (ICAM-1) (68–70). Also tested have been home remedies and unconventional treatments and preventatives such as vitamin C (71,72), zinc lozenges (73), inhalation of warm air (74), and nasal tissues treated with virucidal chemicals (75). More recently, a clinical trial was conducted with a combination treatment, which contained interferon and two anti-inflammatory compounds (76).

Of the items tested, topical interferon (77) and some of the capsid binders (70) reduced viral concentrations in nasal secretions but did not substantially reduce illness severity scores. Antireceptor antibody showed promise in reducing symptom scores (69) as did the combined antiviral–anti-inflammatory treatment, which also reduced viral shedding (76). Large doses of vitamin C had a modest therapeutic effect, presumably due to a weak anticholinergic action (71,72). The other treatments tested in the model were not effective.

## V. Performance of the Rhinovirus Challenge Model

### A. Standardization and Consistency

Large clinical data sets have become available for evaluating the performance of the model. The mean ($\pm$SD) total symptom score, using modified Jackson criteria of scoring (12,27,28), was 16.4 ($\pm$12.7) in 151 subjects in 14 experiments conducted over a 5-year period (31). The mean ($\pm$SD) total nasal discharge weight of a 4-day collection was 23 ($\pm$22) grams for the group. In these studies, rhinovirus type 39 or Hank's strain, a previously characterized but unnumbered rhinovirus, were used.

Two other large data sets are composed of results with Hank's strain and type 16 rhinoviruses (J. M. Gwaltney Jr., unpublished data). The mean ($\pm$SE) total symptom score was 16.4 ($\pm$1.5) for Hank's strain and 19.3 ($\pm$1.1) for type 16. The mean ($\pm$SE) total nasal discharge weight of a four-day collection was 18.1 ($\pm$2.8) grams and 23.7 ($\pm$2.3) grams for Hank's strain and type 16, respectively. The mean total symptom score of type 16 colds was significantly greater than that for Hank's strain colds on day 3 (Fig. 5). This was due to higher severity scores for sore throat, cough, headache, and malaise with the type 16 colds. The scores for sneezing, rhinorrhea, and nasal obstruction were remarkably similar for the two viruses. In these experiments, the viral inoculum given was less (10–30 $TCID_{50}$) for Hank's strain virus than for type 16 (300–10,000 $TCID_{50}$). Therefore, it is not possible to know if the greater virulence of type 16 virus is an inherent characteristic of the virus or due to the larger inoculum.

### B. Variance

Although the mean symptom scores and mucus weights obtained with the rhinovirus challenge model are very consistent, the interindividual variation in these parameters is considerable. The total symptom severity scores of 58 volunteers with experimental rhinovirus infection calculated by the modified Jackson method (12,27,28) ranged from 1 to 44 (78). The mode that was 7 represented only 12% of the group. Nasal discharge weights showed similar wide individual variations.

The interaction of variance and effect size and their influence on statistical significance has been examined with a data set from the challenge model (78) (Fig. 6). When an effect size of 40% was held constant, the variance could be

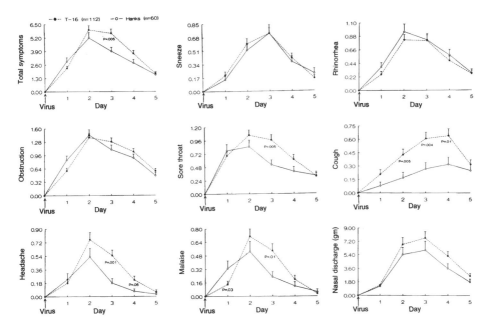

**Figure 5** Daily symptom severity scores and nasal discharge weights in volunteers with colds due to type 16 or Hank's strain rhinovirus.

increased by approximately 250% and still yield a probability of $p < 0.05$. In contrast, reducing the magnitude of the effect size by 50% (to 20%) while holding the variance constant resulted in a probability of $p = 0.1$. Thus, simultaneous increases in variance and decreases in effect size attenuate the significance levels of statistical tests in a nonlinear fashion. This indicates that reducing factors that adversely influence effect size such as noncompliance in dosing and inaccurate reporting of symptoms is more important than attempting to restrict variance by restricting enrollment to subjects with a predetermined level of severity of illness. Also, as discussed below, both natural and experimental colds most often are perceived as a mild illness. Restricting enrollment to only those illnesses perceived as moderate or severe markedly restricts sample size and compromises the external validity of study results. Also, it is often not possible to determine a cold's ultimate severity in its early stages, thus delaying start of treatment and missing the crucial period when evaluation should be performed.

## C. Similarity of Experimental and Natural Rhinovirus Colds

A frequently raised question is whether experimental rhinovirus colds are similar to natural rhinovirus colds. The concern has been raised that experimental colds

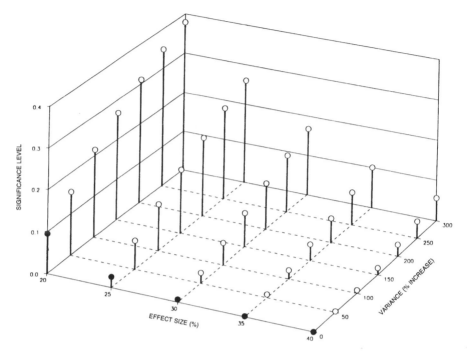

**Figure 6** Interaction of variance and effect size and their influence on statistical significance in a data set from volunteers with experimental rhinovirus infection.

may be milder than their natural counterpart. That the latter question is raised is not surprising, since most experimental colds are diagnosed by the modified Jackson method (12,27,28), which employs predetermined criteria set to detect illness of very mild severity. The usual self-diagnosed natural cold experienced by the naive observer is more severe than the average cold diagnosed by the Jackson method. Thus, an unconscious selection bias occurs in the naive observer, who judges the severity of colds by his or her own personal experience with self-diagnosed natural colds in themselves and others.

The fact is that natural rhinovirus colds can be quite mild. Epidemiological studies have shown that 25% of natural rhinovirus infections are not associated with any reported illness and others are very mild (79). Mild natural colds may not be recognized as such and, thus, escape attention, although they would be counted by the modified Jackson criteria. So far, there have been no comparisons of the severity of natural and experimental rhinovirus colds in similar populations using the same method of symptom recording and identical criteria for diagnosis. However, when similar diagnostic criteria were applied to one data set from patients with natural rhinovirus colds and to another from volunteers with experimental rhinovirus colds, the frequency of occurrence by day of the individual symptoms was similar (80) (Fig. 7). Where differences were observed, the experimental colds most often had a greater prevalence of symptoms, especially nasal obstruction, presumably due to nasal manipulation in the experimental setting. The severity of symptoms was not reported in the natural cold data set, and, therefore, severity could not be directly compared in this evaluation although severity would be expected to have a relationship with frequency of occurrence. The comparison suggested that when similar diagnostic criteria are used, natural and experimental rhinovirus colds are more similar than different.

Data sets from subjects with experimental rhinovirus colds and from patients with self-diagnosed natural colds of undetermined etiology show that in both instances most persons perceive cold symptoms as mild, although the criteria used to diagnose a cold were different (S. Johnson, unpublished data). For example, on the day on which sneezing was most prevalent and severe, only 4% of

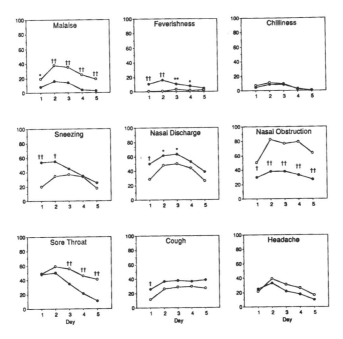

**Figure 7** Comparison of symptom prevalence in volunteers with experimental rhinovirus colds (O—O) and patients with natural rhinovirus colds (●—●). Colds were diagnosed by the same criteria in both groups. $*p < 0.05$; $**p < 0.01$; $\dagger p < 0.005$; $\ddagger p < 0.001$. (From Ref. 80.)

patients with experimental colds and 9% of patients with natural colds judged sneezing as either "severe" or "very severe" (Fig. 8). On the same day, only 16% of patients with experimental colds and 27% of patients with natural colds judged rhinorrhea as "severe" or "very severe." The "very severe" category was rarely reported. The difference in the proportion of symptoms judged as severe in the two groups was probably due to the different methods of diagnosis used and also to the probability that the natural cold data set included cases of influenza and adenovirus illness, which are more severe on average than a rhinovirus cold.

In these data sets, 39% of patients with experimental colds reported no rhinorrhea compared to only 10% of patients with natural colds. This indicates that when self-diagnosing, persons usually do not consider a natural illness to be a cold unless it includes the symptoms of rhinorrhea. In reality, both natural and experimental "colds" of proven rhinovirus etiology may not include the symptom of rhinorrhea. In the two large data sets described above, only 61% of persons with experimental rhinovirus infection and 44% of those with natural rhinovirus colds reported the symptom of rhinorrhea on the day on which this symptom was most prevalent (Fig. 7) (80). In both data sets, the diagnosis of a "cold" was based on predetermined criteria, which were designed to capture mild illness, and not on self-diagnosis by the patients. Thus, some illnesses had primarily

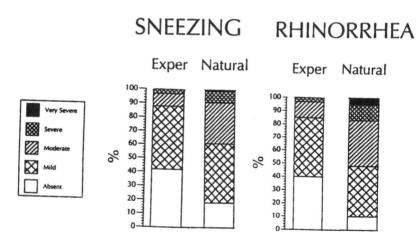

**Figure 8** Symptom severity in persons with experimental rhinovirus colds and with natural colds of undetermined etiology. Comparisons were made on the day on which maximum prevalence and severity of symptoms were reported. The experimental colds were diagnosed by modified Jackson criteria (12,27,28), and the natural colds were self-diagnosed. (Data kindly supplied by Dr. Susan Johnson.)

sore or scratchy throat and others had sneezing and/or nasal obstruction without rhinorrhea or with rhinorrhea of brief duration. The importance of recognizing that the method of diagnosis determines the characteristics of the illness recorded cannot be overemphasized, especially when making comparisons between different data sets.

### D. Correlation of Results from Clinical Trials in Patients with Experimental and Natural Colds

Several opportunities are available for comparing the results of clinical trials using the rhinovirus challenge model and studies employing the natural cold method. In seven instances involving antihistamines (28,30,81,82), interferons (83–88), a decongestant (13,89), an anticholinergic (50,90), and a capsid binder (91,92), there was concordance in the results. This indicates that the model is a good predictor of what will happen on testing under natural conditions (Table 1). These findings suggest that if an experimental treatment or prophylactic does not give positive results with the challenge model, it may not be worth the time and expense to subsequently test it in patients with natural colds. However, special circumstances may sometimes alter this principle.

Since experimental colds diagnosed by modified Jackson criteria (12,27,28) are on average milder than self-diagnosed natural colds, the question has been raised whether the therapeutic effects observed in volunteers with mild colds will also be seen in those with colds of greater severity. Results of testing an antihistamine in the rhinovirus challenge model showed equal or greater therapeutic effect sizes in a subset of volunteers with moderate or severe illness compared to those with illness of lesser severity (28).

**Table 1**  Correlation of Clinical Trials Results Using the Rhinovirus Challenge Model and the Natural Cold Method

|  | Positive effect observed | |
| --- | --- | --- |
| Agent tested | RV model (Ref.) | Natural cold (Ref.) |
| Chlorpheniramine therapy | Yes (30) | Yes (81) |
| Clemastine therapy | Yes (28) | Yes (82) |
| Pseudoephedrine therapy | Yes (13) | Yes (89) |
| Ipratropium therapy | Yes (56) | Yes (90) |
| IFN-α prophylaxis | Yes (84,84) | Yes (85,86) |
| IFN-α therapy | No[a] (87) | No (88) |
| Pirodavir therapy | No (91) | No (92) |

[a] May have had modest effect on some nasal symptoms.

## VI.  Advantage and Disadvantage of Experimental Colds in Research

Experimental colds have several advantages over natural colds in their usefulness in research. Foremost is that experimental challenge provides a known cause of infection and a known time of exposure to the infectious agent. Knowing the specific viral etiology of the infection allows information to be collected on clinical expression, pathophysiological responses, therapeutic effects, and other experimental parameters for a specific infectious agent of interest. While the etiology of a substantial proportion of natural colds can be determined, this requires considerable effort in the laboratory. Also, the etiology of up to a third of natural colds cannot be diagnosed (93). Recruiting natural cold patients is an inefficient way of acquiring virus-specific cases for study. It is only practical with rhinovirus because of the low prevalence of the other cold viruses and/or the lack of readily available methods for their identification. Also, diagnosis of natural colds is possible only in retrospect after cell culture is positive or serology completed. Nucleic acid probe techniques may help with this problem in the future, but these methods still require considerable time and effort.

Knowing the precise time at which infection occurs is extremely important in clinical trials of cold treatments where early treatment is essential to achieve meaningful results. Rhinovirus cold symptoms peak in intensity on average on the first through the third day after virus challenge (Fig. 5). It is during this period that maximum therapeutic benefit can be expected to be observed when an effective treatment is being tested. If treatment is started too late in the illness, potentially beneficial treatment effects may be missed or underestimated. Therapeutic trials done in patients with natural colds have the problem of subjects entering the study late in the course of illness (80). Recruiting subjects early in their illness is not easy for logistical reasons. Falling symptom scores in placebo groups in published natural cold treatment trials indicate that patients were often enrolled in the advanced stages of the illness and were, thus, not optimal for study (78,81,94–97). Even when free-living volunteers were asked to keep a prospective record of cold symptoms, up to a third delayed in reporting the onset of illness and thus did not enter the study in the first or second day of illness as requested (78).

Challenge studies have other advantages since subjects are often (but not always) cloistered during the experiment. These advantages include supervised compliance with medication and complete and accurate recording of clinical data and collection of specimens.

A major disadvantage of the challenge model is that it does not reflect the diverse viral etiology of natural colds. Extrapolations of observations to viruses other than the ones studied may not be valid. Also, while it is possible to study the efficacy of cold treatments under optimum conditions in the challenge model, the effectiveness of the test treatment in the clinic setting cannot be predicted with certainty due to the variables associated with patient behavior.

## VII. Conclusion

Experimentally infected volunteers have been used to study the common cold for over 80 years. The early challenge studies provided the first valid scientific evidence of the infectious nature of colds. Subsequent studies have provided invaluable information on incubation periods, routes of transmission, clinical manifestations, pathogenesis, and methods of treatment. As new scientific discoveries led to the development of new technologies such as viral growth in cell culture, antibody assessment, antiviral development, CT and MRI examinations, cytokine measurements, and nucleic acid probes, the challenge model has provided a means for their fruitful application, and the discovery of important new knowledge has been the result. With medicine now entering the era of molecular biology, the common cold challenge model offers an unusual opportunity to study an important human pathogen in its natural host, the human. For this purpose, the model, when used with large sample sizes, produces consistent parameters of illness and allows sampling of tissues and secretions from the sites of disease. With available technology, it should now be possible to relate individual cold symptoms to specific mediators and to improve prospects for better cold treatments.

## References

1. Kruse W. Die Erregung von Husten und Schnupfen (the etiology of cough and nasal catarrh). Munch Med Wochenschr 1914; 61:1574.
2. Dochez AR, Shibley GS, Mills KC. Studies in the common cold. IV. Experimental transmission of the common cold to anthropoid apes and human beings by means of a filtrable agent. J Exp Med 1930; 52:701–716.
3. Andrewes C. The Common Cold. New York: WW Norton, 1965.
4. Pelon W, Mogabgab WJ, Phillips WJ, Pierce WE. A cytopathogenic agent isolated from naval recruits with mild respiratory illness. Proc Soc Exp Biol Med 1957; 94: 262–267.
5. Price WH. The isolation of a new virus associated with respiratory clinical disease in humans. Proc Natl Acad Sci USA 1956; 42:892–896.
6. Tyrrell DAJ. Common Colds and Related Diseases. Baltimore: The Williams & Wilkins Co., 1965.
7. Tyrrell DAJ, Parsons R. Some virus isolations from common colds. III. Cytopathic effects in tissue cultures. Lancet 1960; i:239–242.
8. Hayflick L, Moorehead PS. The serial cultivation of human diploid cell strains. Exp Cell Res 1961; 25:585–621.

9. Douglas RG Jr, Couch RB. Attenuation of rhinovirus type 15 for humans. Nature 1969; 223(202):213–214.

10. Knight V. The use of volunteers in medical virology. In: Melnick JL, ed. Progress in Medical Virology. Vol. 6. Basel: Karger, 1964:1–26.

11. Gwaltney JM Jr, Hendley O, Hayden FG, McIntosh K, Hollinger FB, Melnick JL, Turner RB. Updated recommendations for safety-testing of viral inocula used in volunteer experiments on rhinovirus colds. In: Melnick JL, ed. Progress in Medical Virology. Vol. 39. Basel: Karger, 1992:256–263.

12. Hendley JO, Edmondson WP Jr, Gwaltney JM Jr. Relations between naturally acquired immunity and infectivity of two rhinoviruses in volunteers. J Infect Dis 1972; 125:243–248.

13. Sperber SJ, Sorrentino JV, Riker DK, Hayden FG. Evaluation of an alpha agonist alone and in combination with a nonsteroidal anti-inflammatory agent in the treatment of experimental rhinovirus colds. Bull NY Acad Med 1989; 65:145–160.

14. Bynoe ML, Hobson D, Horner J, Kipps A, Schild GC, Tyrrell DA. Inoculation of human volunteers with a strain of virus from a common cold. Lancet 1961; 1:1194–1196.

15. Winther B, Gwaltney JM Jr, Mygind N, Turner RB, Hendley JO. Sites of rhinovirus recovery after point inoculation of the upper airway. JAMA 1986; 256:1763–1767.

16. Cate TR, Couch RB, Fleet WF, Griffith WR, Gerone PJ, Knight V. Production of tracheobronchitis in volunteers with rhinovirus in a small-particle aerosol. Am J Epidemiol 1965; 81:95–105.

17. Couch RB, Cate TR, Douglas RG Jr, Gerone PJ, Knight V. Effect of route of inoculation on experimental respiratory viral disease in volunteers and evidence for airborne transmission. Bacteriol Rev 1966; 80:517–529.

18. Hendley JO, Wenzel RP, Gwaltney JM Jr. Transmission of rhinovirus colds by self-inoculation. N Engl J Med 1973; 288:1361–1364.

19. Gwaltney JM Jr, Moskalski PB, Hendley JO. Hand-to-hand transmission of rhinovirus colds. Ann Intern Med 1978; 88:463–467.

20. D'Alessio DJ, Meschievitz CK, Peterson JA, Dick CR, Dick EC. Short-duration exposure and the transmission of rhinoviral colds. J Infect Dis 1984; 150:189–194.

21. Dick EC, Jennings LC, Mink KA, Wartgow CD, Inhorn SL. Aerosol transmission of rhinovirus colds. J Infect Dis 1987; 156:442–448.

22. Gwaltney JM Jr, Hayden FG. Letter. Response to psychological stress and susceptibility to the common cold. NEJM 1992; 326:644–645.

23. Alper CM, Doyle WJ, Skoner DP, Buchman CA, Seroky JT, Gwaltney JM, Cohen SA. Prechallenge antibodies: Moderators of infection rate, signs, and symptoms in adults experimentally challenged with rhinovirus type 39. Laryngoscope 1996; 106:1298–1305.

24. Alper CM, Doyle WJ, Skoner DP, Buchman CA, Cohen S, Gwaltney JM Jr. Prechallenge antibodies moderate disease expression in adults experimentally exposed to Hank's strain rhinovirus. Laryngoscope 1996; 106:1298–1305.

25. Arruda E, Hayden FG. Detection of human rhinovirus RNA in nasal washings by PCR. Mol Cell Probes 1993; 7:373–379.

26. Arruda E, Boyle TR, Winther B, Pevear DC, Gwaltney JM Jr, Hayden FG. Localiza-

tion of human rhinovirus replication in the upper respiratory tract by in situ hybridization. J Infect Dis 1995; 171:1329–1333.

27. Jackson GG, Dowling HF, Spiesman IG, Boand AV. Transmission of the common cold to volunteers under controlled conditions. I. The common cold as a clinical entity. Arch Intern Med 1958; 101:267–278.

28. Gwaltney JM Jr, Park J, Paul RA, Edelman DA, O'Connor RR, Turner RB. Randomized controlled trial of clemastine fumarate for treatment of experimental rhinovirus colds. Clin Infect Dis 1996; 22:656–662.

29. Samo TC, Greenberg SB, Couch RB Jr, Quarles J, Johnson PE, Hook S, Harmon MW. Efficacy and tolerance of intranasally applied recombinant leukocyte A interferon in normal volunteers. J Infect Dis 1983; 148:535–542.

30. Doyle WJ, McBride TP, Skoner DP, Maddren BR, Gwaltney JM Jr, Uhrin M. A double-blind, placebo-controlled clinical trial of the effect of chlorpheniramine on the response of the nasal airway, middle ear and eustachian tube to provocative rhinovirus challenge. Pediatr Infect Dis J 1988; 7:229–238.

31. Parekh HH, Cragun KT, Hayden FG, Hendley JO, Gwaltney JM Jr. Nasal mucus weights in experimental rhinovirus infection. Am J Rhinol 1992; 6, 3:107–110.

32. Turner BW, Cail WS, Hendley JO, Hayden FG, Doyle WJ, Sorrentino JV, Gwaltney JM Jr. Physiologic abnormalities in the paranasal sinuses during experimental rhinovirus colds. J Allergy Clin Immunol 1992; 90:474–478.

33. Gwaltney JM Jr., Phillips CD, Miller RD, Riker DK. Computed tomographic study of the common cold. N Engl J Med 1994; 330:25–30.

34. Doyle WJ, McBride TP, Hayden FG, Gwaltney JM Jr. The response of the nasal airway, middle ear and eustachian tube to experimental rhinovirus infection. Am J Rhinol 1988; 2:149–154.

35. McBride TP, Doyle WJ, Hayden FG, Gwaltney JM Jr. Alterations of eustachian tube, middle ear, and nose in rhinovirus infections. Arch Otolaryngol Head Neck Surg 1989; 115:1054–1059.

36. Buchman CA, Doyle WJ, Skoner D, Fireman P, Gwaltney JM. Otologic manifestations of experimental rhinovirus infection. Laryngoscope 1994; 104:1295–1299.

37. Sperber SJ, Doyle WJ, McBride TP, Sorrentino JV, Riker DK, Hayden FG. Otologic effects of interferon beta serine in experimental rhinovirus colds. Arch Otolaryngol Head Neck Surg 1992; 118:933–936.

38. Blair HT, Greenberg SB, Stevens PM, Bilunos PA, Couch, RB. Effects of rhinovirus infection on pulmonary function of healthy human volunteers. Am Rev Respir Dis 1976; 114:95–102.

39. Halperin SA, Eggleston PA, Hendley JO, Suratt PM, Gröschel DHM, Gwaltney JM, Jr. Pathogenesis of lower respiratory tract symptoms in experimental rhinovirus infection. Am Rev Respir Dis 1983; 128:806–810.

40. Calhoun WJ, Dick EC, Schwartz LB, Busse WW. A common cold virus, rhinovirus 16, potentiates airway inflammation after segmental antigen bronchoprovocation in allergic subjects. J Clin Invest 1994; 94:2200–2208.

41. Fraenkel DJ, Bardin PG, Sanderson G, Lampe F, Johnston SL, Holgate ST. Lower airway inflammation during rhinovirus colds in normal and in asthmatic subjects. Am J Respir Crit Care Med 1995; 151:879–886.

42. Lemanske RF Jr, Dick EC, Swanson CA, Vrtis RF, Busse WW. Rhinovirus upper

respiratory infection increases airway hyperactivity and late asthmatic reactions. J Clin Invest 1989; 83:1–10.

43. Tyrrell DAJ, Bynoe ML. Inoculation of volunteers with JH strain of new respiratory virus. Lancet 1958; 2:931–933.

44. Jackson GG, Dowling HF, Mogabgab WJ. Infectivity and interrelationships of 2060 and JH viruses in volunteers. J Lab Clin Med 1960; 55:331–341.

45. Douglas RG Jr. Pathogenesis of rhinovirus common colds in human volunteers. Ann Otol Rhinol Laryngol 1970; 79:563–571.

46. Mufson MA, Ludwig WM, James HD, Gauld LW, Rourke JA, Hopler JC, Chanock RM. Effect of neutralizing antibody on experimental rhinovirus infection. JAMA 1963; 186:578–584.

47. Harris JM II, Gwaltney JM Jr. The incubation periods of experimental rhinovirus infection and illness. Clin Infect Dis 1996; 23:1286–1290.

48. Bardin PG, Johnston SL, Sanderson G, Robinson BS, Pickett MA, Fraenkel DJ, Holgate ST. Detection of rhinovirus infection of the nasal mucosa by oligonucleotide in situ hybridization. Am J Respir Cell Mol Biol 1994; 10:207–213.

49. Turner RB, Hendley JO, Gwaltney JM Jr. Shedding of infected ciliated epithelial cells in rhinovirus colds. J Infect Dis 1982; 145:849–853.

50. Gwaltney JM Jr, Hendley JO, Mygind N. Symposium on Rhinovirus Pathogenesis: summary. Acta Oto-Laryngol (Stockh) 1984; 413(suppl):43–45.

51. Naclerio RM, Proud D, Kagey-Sobotka A, Lichtenstein LM, Hendley JO, Gwaltney JM Jr. Kinins are generated during experimental rhinovirus colds. J Infect Dis 1988; 157:133–142.

52. Igarashi Y, Skoner DP, Doyle WJ, White MV, Fireman P, Kaliner MA. Analysis of nasal secretions during experimental rhinovirus upper respiratory infections. J Allergy Clin Immunol 1993; 92:722–731.

53. Proud D, Gwaltney JM Jr, Hendley JO, Dinarello CA, Gillis S, Schleimer RP. Increased levels of interleukin-1 are detected in nasal secretions of volunteers during experimental rhinovirus colds. J Infect Dis 1994; 169:1007–1013.

54. Zhu Z, Tang W, Ray A, Wu Y, Einarsson O, Landry M, Gwaltney J Jr, Elias JA. Rhinovirus stimulation of interleukin-6 in vivo and in vitro: evidence for NF-κB-dependent transcriptional activation. J Clin Invest 1966; 97:421–430.

55. Gaffey MJ, Gwaltney JM Jr, Dressler WE, Sorrentino JV, Hayden FG. Intranasally administered atropine methonitrate treatment of experimental rhinovirus colds. Am Rev Respir Dis 1987; 135:241–244.

56. Gaffey MJ, Hayden FG, Boyd JC, Gwaltney JM Jr. Ipratropium bromide treatment of experimental rhinovirus infection. Antimicrob Agents Chemother 1988; 32:1644–1647.

57. Sperber SJ, Hendley JO, Hayden FG, Riker DK, Sorrentino JV, Gwaltney JM Jr. Effects of naproxen on experimental rhinovirus colds. A randomized, double-blind, controlled trial. Ann Intern Med 1992; 117:37–41.

58. Cohen S, Tyrrell DAJ, Smith AP. Psychological stress and susceptibility to the common cold. N Engl J Med 1991; 325:606–612.

59. Stone AA, Bovbjerg DH, Neale JM, Napoli A, Valdimarsdottir H, Cox D, Hayden FG, Gwaltney JM Jr. Development of common cold symptoms following experimen-

tal rhinovirus infection is related to prior stressful life events. Behav Med 1992; 18: 115–120.

60. Cohen S, Gwaltney JM Jr, Doyle WJ, Skoner DP, Fireman P, Newsom JT. State and trait negative affect as predictors of objective and subjective symptoms of a common cold. J Personality Soc Psychol 1995; 68:159–169.

61. Gwaltney JM Jr. Epidemiology of the common colds. Ann NY Acad Sci 1980; 353: 54–60.

62. D'Alessio DJ, Meschievitz CK, Peterson JA, Dick CR, Dick EC. Short-duration exposure and the transmission of rhinoviral colds. J Infect Dis 1984; 150:189–194.

63. Hendley JO, Gwaltney JM Jr. Mechanisms of transmission of rhinovirus infections. Epidemiol Rev 1988; 10:242–258.

64. D'Alessio DJ, Peterson JA, Dick CR, Dick EC. Transmission of experimental rhinovirus colds in volunteer married couples. J Infect Dis 1976; 133:26–36.

65. Holmes MJ, Reed SE, Stott EJ, Tyrrell DAJ. Studies of experimental rhinovirus type 2 infections in polar isolation and in England. J Hyg (Camb) 1976; 76:379–393.

66. Dick EC, Jennings LC, Mink KA, Wartgow CD, Inhorn SL. Aerosol transmission of rhinovirus colds. J Infect Dis 1987; 156:442–448.

67. Doyle WJ, Riker DK, McBride TP, Hayden FG, Hendley JO, Swarts JD, Gwaltney JM. Therapeutic effects of an anticholinergic-sympathomimetic combination in induced rhinovirus colds. Annl Otol Rhinol Laryngol 1993; 102:521–527.

68. Sperber SJ, Hayden FG. Chemotherapy of rhinovirus colds. Antimicrob Agents Chemother 1988; 32:409–419.

69. Hayden FG, Gwaltney JM Jr, Colonno RJ. Modification of experimental rhinovirus colds by receptor blockade. Antiviral Res 1988; 9:233–247.

70. Arruda E, Hayden FG. Clinical studies of antiviral agents for picornaviral infections. In: Jeffries DJ, De Clercq E, eds. Antiviral Chemotherapy. New York: John Wiley & Sons Ltd, 1995:321–355.

71. Walker GH, Bynoe ML, Tyrrell DAJ. Trial of ascorbic acid in prevention of colds. Br Med J 1967; 1:603–606.

72. Schwartz AR, Togo Y, Hornick RB, Tominaga S, Gleckman RA. Evaluation of the efficacy of ascorbic acid in prophylaxis of induced rhinovirus 44 infection in man. J Infect Dis 1973; 128:500–505.

73. Farr BM, Conner EM, Betts FR, Oleske J, Minnefor A, Gwaltney JM Jr. Two randomized controlled trials of zinc gluconate lozenge therapy of experimentally induced rhinovirus colds. Antimicrob Agents Chemother 1987; 31:1183–1187.

74. Hendley JO, Abbott RD, Beasley PB, Gwaltney JM Jr. Effect of inhaltion of hot humidified air on experimental rhinovirus (RV) infections. JAMA 1994; 271:1112–1113.

75. Hayden GF, Hendley JO, Gwaltney JM Jr. The effect of placebo and virucidal paper handkerchiefs on viral contamination of the hand and transmission of experimental rhinoviral infection. J Infect Dis 1985; 152:403–407.

76. Gwaltney JM Jr. Combined antiviral and antimediator treatment of rhinovirus colds. J Infect Dis 1992; 166:776–782.

77. Hayden FG. Use of interferons for prevention and treatment of respiratory viral

infections. In: Mills J, Corey L, eds. Antiviral Chemotherapy: New Directions for Clinical Application and Research. New York: Elsevier 1986:28–40.

78. Gwaltney JM Jr, Buier RM, Rogers JL. The influence of signal variation, bias, noise, and effect size on statistical significance in treatment studies of the common cold. Antiviral Res 1996; 29:287–295.

79. Gwaltney JM Jr. Rhinoviruses. In: Evans AS, Kaslow RA, eds. Viral Infection of Humans: Epidemiology and Control. 4th ed. New York: Plenum Press, 1997:815–838.

80. Rao SR, Hendley JO, Hayden FG, Gwaltney JM Jr. Symptom expression in natural and experimental rhinovirus colds. Am J Rhinol 1995; 9:49–52.

81. Howard JC Jr, Kantner TR, Lilienfield LS, Princiotto JV, Krum RE, Crutcher JE, Belman MA, Danzig MR. Effectiveness of antihistamines in the symptomatic management of the common cold. JAMA 1979; 242:2414–2417.

82. Turner RB, Sperber SJ, Sorrentino JV, O'Connor RR, Rogers J, Batouli AM, Gwaltney JM Jr. Effectiveness of clemastine fumarate for treatment of rhinorrhea and sneezing associated with the common cold. Clin Inf Dis 1997; 25:574–583.

83. Scott GM, Phillpotts RJ, Wallace J, Gauci CL, Greiner J, Tyrrell DAJ. Prevention of rhinovirus colds by human interferon alpha-2 from *Escherichia coli*. Lancet 1982; 2:186–188.

84. Hayden FG, Gwaltney JM Jr. Intranasal interferon-a$_2$ for prevention of rhinovirus infection and illness. J Infect Dis 1983; 148:543–550.

85. Hayden FG, Albrecht JK, Kaiser DL, Gwaltney JM Jr. Prevention of natural colds by contact prophylaxis with intranasal alpha$_2$-interferon. N Engl J Med 1986; 314:71–75.

86. Douglas RM, Moore BW, Miles HB, Davies LM, Graham NMH, Ryan P, Worswick DA, Albrecht JK. Prophylactic efficacy of intranasal alpha$_2$-interferon against rhinovirus infections in the family setting. N Engl J Med 1986; 814:65–70.

87. Hayden FG, Gwaltney JM Jr. Intranasal interferon-$\alpha_2$ treatment of experimental rhinoviral colds. J Infect Dis 1984; 150:174–180.

88. Hayden FG, Kaiser DL, Albrecht JK. Intranasal recombinant alfa-2b interferon treatment of naturally occurring common colds. Antimicrob Agents Chemother 1988; 32:224–230.

89. Bye CE, Cooper J, Empey DW, Fowle ASE, Hughes DTD, Letley E, O'Grady J. Effects of pseudoephedrine and triprolidine, alone and in combination, on symptoms of the common cold. Br Med J 1980; 281:189–190.

90. Hayden FG, Diamond L, Wood, PB, Korts DC, Wecker MT. Effectiveness and safety of intranasal ipratropium bromide in common colds. Ann Intern Med 1996; 125:89–97.

91. Hayden FG, Andries K, Janssen PAJ. Safety and efficacy of intranasal pirodavir (R77975) in experimental rhinovirus infection. Antimicrob Agents Chemother 1992; 36:727–732.

92. Hayden FG, Hipskind GJ, Woerner DH, Eisen GF, Janssens M, Janssen PAJ, Andries K. Intranasal pirodavir (R77;975) treatment of rhinovirus colds. Antimicrob Agents Chemother 1995; 39:290–294.

93. Gwaltney JM Jr. The Common Cold. In: Mandell GL, Bennett JE, Dolin R, eds. Principles and Practice of Infectious Diseases. 4th ed. New York: Churchill Livingstone, 1995:581–566.

94. Crutcher JE, Kantner TR. The effectiveness of antihistamines in the common cold. J Clin Pharmacol 1981; 21:9–15.

95. Virtanen A. Slow release combined preparation (dexchlorpheniramine + pseudo-ephedrine) for symptomatic treatment of the common cold. J Laryngol Otol 1983; 97:159–163.

96. Gaffey MJ, Kaiser DL, Hayden FG. Ineffectiveness of oral terfenadine in natural colds: evidence against histamine as a mediator of common cold symptoms. Pediatr Infect Dis J 1988; 7:223–228.

97. Berkowitz RB, Connell JT, Dietz AJ, Greenstein SM, Tinkelman DG. The effectiveness of the nonsedating antihistamine loratadine plus pseudoephedrine in the symptomatic management of the common cold. Ann Allergy 1989; 63:336–339.

# 7

# Overview of Experimental Animal Respiratory Viral Provocation Models

**GERT FOLKERTS, HENK J. VAN DER LINDE, and FRANS P. NIJKAMP**

Utrecht University
Utrecht, The Netherlands

## I. Introduction

The major clinical symptoms of asthma are paroxysms of dyspnea, wheezing, and cough. These symptoms vary from mild to severe and may even be unremitting (status asthmaticus). A characteristic feature of most asthmatic patients is that their airways have an increased tendency to narrow on exposure to a variety of chemical, pharmacological, or physical stimuli, a phenomenon called "airway hyperresponsiveness." Although its etiology is still unclear, it is well known that viral respiratory infections can induce or aggravate airway hyperresponsiveness. A number of excellent reviews have been written on virus-induced airway hyperresponsiveness from a clinical point of view (1–6). However, most of the basic research concerning this issue has been performed in animals. Airway dysfunction after a viral infection has been measured in a variety of animal species, including the mouse (7), rat (8,9), guinea pig (10–17), ferret (18), feline (19), dog (20,21), lamb (22,23), and calf (24). In most of the studies human-relevant viruses were used, like parainfluenza (PI) virus (8,10–15,17,25), influenza virus (7,21,26), adenoviruses (27), and respiratory syncytial virus (RSV) (9,22–24,28). The onset of airway dysfunction is observed as soon as 2–3 days after infection in the mouse, feline, and dog (19,25,29), and airway hyperresponsiveness was detected up to 13–16 weeks after virus inoculation in rats (30). The pathogenesis of virus-induced airway hyperresponsiveness can be investigated more thoroughly in animals, since a number of experimental setups can easily be performed in animals and are either impossible or not ethical to perform in humans. The goal of this chapter is to bring together the fundamental observations in animal models with respiratory tract infections to unravel the pathogenesis of virus-induced airway hyperresponsiveness in humans. This may finally lead to an improvement in the management of airway diseases like asthma.

## II. Airway Hyperresponsiveness to Histamine and Histamine Release

Isolated trachea, bronchi, and lung parenchyme strips from virus-infected guinea pigs responded with an increased contraction in response to histamine (17,31–33). Hyperresponsiveness to histamine was also observed in vivo in guinea pigs (15,17,34–39), dogs (25,27,40), lambs (23), and calves (24). Nakazawa et al. (15) suggested that this hyperresponsiveness could simply be explained by a virus-induced diminished activity of histamine *N*-methyltransferase, an enzyme that breaks down histamine (Fig. 1). In virus-treated guinea pigs histamine *N*-methyltransferase activity was decreased by more than 50% in isolated trachea, bronchi, and lungs. Although this might offer an explanation for an increased histamine *sensitivity*, it is not likely to be the cause of an increased *maximal response* after a histamine dose-response curve, since an excess of histamine is likely under these experimental conditions. Instead, histamine itself might be indirectly responsible for the airway hyperresponsiveness, since antihistamines can prevent virus-induced inflammatory reactions (37). In addition, clinical studies indicated that the concentration of histamine in bronchoalveolar lavage fluid is related to the level of methacholine responsiveness (41), and airway obstruction (42).

Histamine can be released from basophils and mast cells, and there is now abundant evidence that these cells are activated during a viral infection. Ida et al. (43) found that isolated human basophils released more histamine after IgE stimulation when these cells were incubated with respiratory viruses and suggested a role for interferon. Furthermore, interferon, a cytokine produced in the lungs after viral infections (44–47), augments the in vitro chemotactic response of basophils to complement factor C5 (48). Complement is activated in vitro (49) and in vivo (50) by viruses. In T-lymphocyte–depleted fractions of leukocyte suspensions, virus incubation did not enhance histamine release (51). This suggests that T lymphocytes and their cytokine products play an integral role in the process by which viruses enhance basophil histamine release. Since interferon did not alter the calcium ionophore A23187–induced histamine release from leukocyte suspension (52), other mechanisms probably also play a significant role

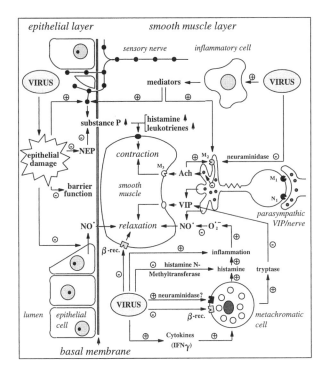

**Figure 1**  Schematic overview of possible targets of viruses to modulate airway responsiveness.

in virus-induced hypersensitivity reactions (52,53). Moreover, inactivated respiratory viruses could augment in vitro IgE-mediated histamine release in both the presence and the absence of interferon (53).

Clementsen et al. (54) found that neuraminidase, an enzyme expressed on the surface of influenza A, was responsible for the potentiating effect on basophil histamine release. Monoclonal antibodies directed against the viral neuraminidase, carbohydrates, or hemagglutinin prevented the potentiating effect of viruses on basophil histamine release (55–57). Therefore, sugar groups and binding of virus to the basophil cell surface by hemagglutinin seems to be necessary for neuraminidase to cause its effect (Fig. 1). It is likely that similar mechanisms also occur in vivo, since peripheral blood basophils isolated from guinea pigs infected with PI-3 virus showed an increased histamine release upon immunological stimulation (58).

Moreover, data pointing to mast cell activation have been obtained. Basal and stimulated histamine release from mast cells isolated from airways of calves

7 days after inoculation with PI-3 virus were significantly increased (59). Besides the enhanced activation of metachromatic cells, their numbers are increased as well. Sorden and Castleman (60) demonstrated in different rat strains that mast cell numbers increased after viral infection, and this effect was associated with both local mast cell proliferation and increases in blood mast cell precursors (61). Increases in bronchiolar mast cell numbers at times from 30 to 90 days after virus inoculation of neonatal rats were associated with airway hyperresponsiveness to methacholine and airway inflammation (30,62). In virally infected guinea pigs, airway hyperresponsiveness also coincided with mast cell activation as demonstrated by more surface microvilli, relatively more high electron-dense granules, and increased histamine concentrations in bronchoalveolar lavage fluid (38). In humans a positive correlation exists between airway responsiveness and the relative numbers of mast cells recovered by bronchoalveolar lavage (63). An increased spontaneous histamine release by bronchoalveolar lavage mast cells is seen only in those subjects with enhanced bronchial responsiveness (63). Gaddy and Busse (64) have demonstrated that the amount of histamine release from basophils is directly associated with the degree of airway responsiveness in individuals with asthma. Infants with acute bronchiolitis have higher tryptase and IgE concentration (65). Plasma histamine levels were increased and correlated with the disease severity (66). In infants with an RSV infection, histamine in nasopharyngeal secretions was detected significantly more often and in higher concentrations in patients with wheezing. Peak titers of RSV-IgE and concentrations of histamine correlated significantly with the degree of hypoxia (67,68).

Antihistamines were commonly administered for upper respiratory tract infections, but their efficacy could not be easily demonstrated (69). Three placebo-controlled, double-blind studies identified either a slight or no beneficial effect after oral and nasal antihistamines on mild and moderately ill patients with upper respiratory tract infections (70–72). However, in these studies antihistamines were administered *after* the infection. At this time, histamine has already exerted its effect. Histamine receptor antagonists might be effective when administered prophylactically. Indeed, guinea pigs pretreated with the antiallergic drug nedocromil or with the $H_1$-receptor antagonists oxatomide or levocabastine one day before viral inoculation not only inhibited the development of airway hyperresponsiveness but also airway inflammation (37). This might be of importance, since inflammatory cells can release a range of mediators that may interfere with airway responsiveness.

### III. Parasympathetic Nerves

Efferent parasympathetic nerves arise in the brain stem and pass down the vagus nerves to synapse in the ganglia situated in the airway wall. Short postganglionic cholinergic nerves supply bronchial or vascular muscle, mucus glands, and probably mast cells. Nerves staining positive for acetylcholinesterase are abundant in the submucosa and the smooth muscle of the trachea, bronchi, and bronchioles. Acetylcholine release from preganglionic fibers in airway parasympathetic ganglia activates nicotinic ($N_1$) cholinergic receptors on ganglion cells (73). Acetylcholine subsequently activates muscarinic ($M_3$) receptors on airway smooth muscle, which results in contraction (Fig. 1). Drugs that block cholinergic receptors were effective in a group of asthmatic patients. Therefore, cholinoceptors may play a role in airway hyperresponsiveness (74). A number of receptors ($M_2$, $H_3$, $\beta_2$) located presynaptically inhibit acetylcholine release (75–78) (Fig. 1). Evidence has been found that presynaptic $M_2$ receptors in asthmatics are deficient, since selective $M_2$ receptor agonists could inhibit reflex bronchoconstriction in healthy persons but were ineffective in asthmatics (79).

Airway hyperresponsiveness after a viral respiratory tract infection is observed after cholinoceptor stimulation. Guinea pig tracheal contractions were enhanced in vitro (33,80,81), and an increased airway responsiveness in vivo was observed in rats (8,62), guinea pigs (14,34,36,39), and dogs (21). Similar results were obtained when the vagal nerve was stimulated of rats (8) and guinea pigs (34,82) in vivo and of the isolated trachea of cats in vitro (19). Reflex bronchoconstriction was also enhanced in guinea pigs (39) and lambs (22).

A role for the parasympathetic nerve in virus-induced airway hyperresponsiveness was published in 1985 by Buckner et al. (34). They infected guinea pigs with parainfluenza 3 virus and stimulated the vagus nerve. The airway obstruction due to vagal nerve stimulation was significantly enhanced in virus-treated animals and could be prevented by the muscarinic receptor antagonist atropine and the ganglion blocker hexamethonium. Moreover, airway hyperresponsiveness was observed after stimulation with nicotine (a drug that can stimulate parasympathetic ganglia). Isolated lung parenchymal strips from infected animals did not respond with an enhanced contraction after nicotine- or electrical field stimulation, which points to a defect in the central airways. A simple explanation for this cholinergic hyperresponsiveness is a diminished activity of cholinesterase. However, there are no data that support this suggestion. Another hypothesis was put forward in 1990, when Killingsworth et al. (19) found that respiratory viral infections in cats resulted in an enhanced tracheal contraction after stimulation of the vagus nerve. In contrast, exogenously applied acetylcholine did not enhance tracheal reactivity, and therefore it was concluded that the defect was probably presynaptically located. In parainfluenza virus–infected guinea pigs a selective dysfunction of inhibitory muscarinic receptors on pulmonary parasympathetic nerves was found (82). These receptors (muscarinic $M_2$ subtype) normally provide a negative feedback whereby acetylcholine released from the vagus nerve turns off further release of acetylcholine (83). Similar results were obtained by Sorkness et al. (8); the parasympathetic hyperresponsiveness after a viral infection in rats was sustained up to 8 weeks after the inoculation and was associated both with $M_2$ autoreceptor malfunction and with muscarinic $M_2$-independent mechanisms. Among others, two mechanisms may contribute to the muscarinic $M_2$-receptor dysfunction. First, the enzyme neuraminidase, expressed in large quantities on the viral coat of both influenza and parainfluenza viruses, may directly act on the muscarinic $M_2$-receptor (Fig. 1). Using [$^3$H]QNB-binding studies (which binds to all muscarinic receptors), it was demonstrated that parainfluenza virus and neuraminidase reduces the affinity of carbachol for muscarinic receptors in guinea pig lung and heart (84). A neuraminidase inhibitor completely blocked virus-induced changes in carbachol affinity in these tissues. In an elegant set of experiments, Haddad and Gies (85) showed that neuraminidase reduced the number of super-high-affinity [$^3$H]oxotremorine muscarinic $M_2$-receptor binding sites in guinea pig lungs. The dysfunction of inhibitory muscarinic $M_2$ receptors may be an effect of viral neuraminidase, which cleaves sialic acid residues from the muscarinic $M_2$ receptors, thereby decreasing agonist affinity for the receptors. Alternatively, inflammatory cells and their products may be important participants in loss of muscarinic $M_2$-receptor function. In ozone-exposed or antigen-challenged guinea pigs, depletion of inflammatory cells with cyclophosphamide protects the function of the neural $M_2$ muscarinic receptors (86,87). Furthermore, administration of heparin to the antigen-challenged guinea pigs acutely restores neuronal muscarinic $M_2$-receptor function, probably by binding to and neutralizing positively charged inflammatory cell proteins such as eosinophil major basic protein (86). Since eosinophils and eosinophil-product could be involved in the virus-induced airway hyperresponsiveness (see epithelial damage and dysfunction), it was investigated whether inflammatory cells are essential to virus-induced loss of neuronal $M_2$ muscarinic receptors. Fryer et al. (12) tested the effect of leukocyte depletion on $M_2$ muscarinic-receptor function in parainfluenza virus–infected guinea pigs. They concluded that heparin did not reverse virus-induced loss of muscarinic $M_2$-receptor function, even in those guinea pigs with a lower viral titer. Leukocyte depletion protected $M_2$ receptor function only in animals with mild viral infection. It appears that viruses have both an indirect, leukocyte-dependent effect on muscarinic $M_2$ receptors and in animals with a more severe infections a leukocyte-independent effect on muscarinic $M_2$ receptors. The failure of heparin to restore muscarinic $M_2$-receptor function in the airways indicates that the leukocyte-dependent loss of muscarinic $M_2$-receptor function is not mediated by positively charged inflammatory proteins (Fig. 1). Although the virus-induced dysfunction of the $M_2$ receptor is obvious, an enhanced release of acetylcholine after nicotine or electrical field stimulation has not yet been demonstrated in airways of infected animals.

The parasympathetic nerve may also be involved in reflex bronchoconstriction. Empey et al. (88) showed during a viral respiratory infection in healthy young subjects that bronchial hyperresponsiveness to histamine could be inhibited by prior administration of an atropine aerosol, implying a vagus reflex–mediated effect. Further, the airway hyperresponsiveness after histamine in virus-infected and artificially ventilated guinea pigs was inhibited by vagotomy (cutting the nevus vagus), by hexamethonium, and by 5 mg/kg atropine, but not by 1 mg/kg atropine (34). In spontaneously breathing anesthetized guinea pigs, atropine could only block the virus-induced airway hyperresponsiveness at low doses of histamine, but not at high doses of this agent (89). These results suggest that the airway hyperresponsiveness to histamine after a viral infection is partly mediated by the parasympathetic nerves.

## IV. Nonadrenergic Noncholinergic Nerves

Inhibitory nonadrenergic noncholinergic (iNANC) nerves relax airway smooth muscle. These nerves have been demonstrated in vitro by electrical field stimulation after adrenergic and cholinergic receptor blockade (90). In human airways smooth muscle, the NANC inhibitory system is the only neural bronchodilator pathway, since there is no sympathetic innervation. Current evidence suggests that nitric oxide (NO) and/or the neuropeptide vasoactive intestinal peptide (VIP) may mediate iNANC effects (Fig. 1). VIP immunoreactivity is localized to nerves and ganglia in airways and pulmonary vessels (91,92). VIP immunoreactivity is present in ganglion cells in the posterior trachea and around intrapulmonary bronchi, diminishing in frequency as the airways become smaller. The pattern of distribution largely follows that of cholinergic nerves. A striking depletion of VIP-immunoreactivity nerves has been reported in patients with severe asthma (93). VIP receptors are located in high density in pulmonary vascular smooth muscle and in airway smooth muscle of large, but not small, airways. VIP receptors are also present in high density in airway epithelium and submucosal glands (94). Binding of VIP to its receptor activates adenylyl cyclase, and VIP stimulates cyclic AMP formation in lung fragments (95). VIP is more potent than isoproterenol in relaxing human bronchi, making it one of the most potent endogenous bronchodilators (96). Interestingly, mast cell tryptase is particularly active in degrading VIP (97,98), and tryptase concentrations were elevated in asthmatic airways and in infants with an acute bronchiolitis (42,65,99) (Fig. 1). Indeed, inhibitory NANC responses were dramatically decreased in rats infected with human RSV (9). Beside the inactivation of VIP by tryptase, NO may be inactivated by oxidants, such as the superoxide anion released from activated inflammatory cells (Fig. 1). Inflammatory cell numbers are increased in the airways after a viral infection (33,36), and viruses are potent stimulators to release reactive oxygen species from inflammatory cells (37) and isolated granulocytes (100). It was demonstrated in an isolated tracheal tube preparation of guinea pigs that the hyperresponsiveness after a viral infection was associated with decreased NO production

(16,17). Interestingly, incubation of naive tracheas in vitro with bronchoalveolar cells obtained from guinea pigs 4 days after a viral infection caused an increased reactivity to histamine. It cannot be excluded that the release of reactive oxygen species, and consequently the inactivation of NO, are responsible for the decreased NO concentration and, hence, airway hyperresponsiveness (101).

Besides efferent nerves there also exists an afferent mechanism in the airways that responds to inhaled irritants, chemical particles, and stretch. C-fiber endings are nonmyelinated and localized between and beneath the airway epithelial cells (102). When C-fiber endings are stimulated, peptides are released via axon reflexes. These mediators, such as substance P, neurokinin A and B, and calcitonin gene–related peptide have the potential to constrict airway smooth muscle, dilate bronchial arteries, cause leakiness of postcapillary venules, increase mucus secretion, release mediators from mast cells, and may recruit inflammatory cells into the airway mucosa. Therefore, neuropeptides may contribute to the deterioration of airway function (90). Substance P is localized to sensory nerves in the airways of several species, including humans (90,103,104). Substance P is predominantly synthesized in the nodose ganglion of the vagus nerve and then transported down the vagus nerve to peripheral branches in the airways. Treatment of animals with capsaicin (present in red peppers), bradykinin, histamine, nicotine receptor agonist, and electric nerve stimulation causes acute release of substance P, neurokinin (NK) A/B, and calcitonin gene–related peptide from sensory nerves in the airways (105,106). These tachykinins mediate their effects via specific receptors, and each tachykinin appears to selectively activate a distinct receptor: $NK_1$ receptors are activated preferentially by substance P, $NK_2$ receptors by NKA, and $NK_3$ receptors by NKB (107). Substance P receptors are present in high density in airway smooth muscle from trachea down to small bronchioles and vascular endothelium. Submucosal glands in human airways are also labeled. Tachykinins are subject to degradation by at least two enzymes: angiotensin-converting enzyme (ACE, EC 3.4.15.1, kininase I) and neutral endopeptidase (NEP, EC 3.4.24.11, enkephalinase). NEP has been shown by enzymological methods to be present in the airway epithelium (104). Immunological methods have confirmed the presence of NEP in the epithelial layer (108). Inhibitors of NEP by phosphoramidon or thiorphan markedly potentiate the bronchoconstrictor effect of tachykinins in vitro (104,109) and in vivo after inhalation (109,110). NEP inhibition also potentiates mucus secretion in response to tachykinins (90). NEP inhibition enhances excitory NANC- and capsaicin-induced bronchoconstriction caused by the release of tachykinins from airway sensory nerves. Tachykinins cause contraction of airway smooth muscle by stimulating phosphoinositide hydrolysis and increase the formation of inositol (1,4,5) triphosphate, which releases calcium ions from intracellular stores in airway smooth muscle (111).

Airway hyperresponsiveness to capsaicin and substance P after a viral respiratory infection was described for the first time by Saban et al. (112). Bronchi obtained from virus-infected animals responded with an enhanced contraction to substance P in the presence and absence of indomethacin. The contractile responses to leukotriene $C_4$ or $D_4$ were not changed by the infection. Jacoby et al. (18,26) incubated ferret tracheal segments with human influenza virus and measured tracheal responsiveness 4 days later. Although an increased contraction to substance P was observed in infected tissues, there was no effect of cyclooxygenase and lipoxygenase inhibition. In contrast, evidence was obtained that the hyperresponsiveness to substance P was due to a 50% decrease in the activity of NEP. Similar results were obtained by Dusser et al. (113). A 40% decrease in NEP activity and a greater bronchoconstriction to substance P was observed in infected animals compared to controls. Further, phosphoramidon, a neutral endopeptidase inhibitor, did not further increase pulmonary resistance in infected animals but did increase resistance in uninfected controls. It was reported that guinea pigs infected with Sendai virus showed airway hyperresponsiveness not only when substance P was administered intravenously or by inhalation, but also after stimulation of the vagus nerve in the presence of atropine and propranolol (14). In the above-mentioned studies, the observed effects were associated with epithelial destruction (Fig. 1). Moreover, epithelial damage exposes sensory nerve endings and cause excessive release of sensory neuropeptides (90). Trachea from PI-3– infected animals were characterized by reductions in substance P-like immunoreactivity compared to controls. Substance P release occurred during critical periods of respiratory viral infection and was temporally correlated with airway hyperresponsiveness (13). Guinea pigs pretreated in vivo with the antitussive drug levodropropizine, a drug that interferes with the sensory neuropeptide system, prevented the development of virus-induced airway inflammation and hyperresponsiveness to histamine (Fig. 2A and B) and methacholine in vivo (Fig. 2C and 2D) (80). The role of sensory neuropeptides was further investigated by Ladenius et al. (81) in guinea pigs in which the sensory nerves were depleted by pretreatment with capsaicin. The virus-induced tracheal hyperresponsiveness to both histamine and cholinoreceptor stimulation was completely prevented when the sensory nerves were depleted of their peptides. Interestingly, the increased tracheal contraction in response to substance P was only partly reduced. The hyperresponsiveness to substance P is caused by two phenomena. First, NEP activity is disturbed in virus-treated animals, and this explains one part of the increased tracheal contraction to substance P. Second, the induction of nonspecific airway hyperresponsiveness (also to substance P) might be due to a continuous release of tachykinins by the exposed sensory nerves after virus-induced epithelial damage. There are data supporting this suggestion. Capsaicin aerosols that cause endogenous release of neuropeptides *acutely* increase in vivo guinea pig

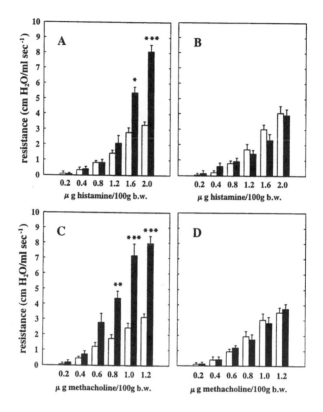

**Figure 2**   Changes in pulmonary lung resistance to intravenously administered histamine (A and B) or methacholine (C and D) in guinea pigs 4 days after inoculation with control solution (open bars) or PI-3 virus (solid bars). Animals were pretreated with (A and C) saline (1 ml/kg) or (B and D) the antitussive drug levodropropizine (10 mg/kg). *$p <$ 0.05; **$p <$ 0.01; ***$p <$ 0.005. (From Ref. 80.)

airway responsiveness to histamine (114), acetylcholine, and neurokinin A (115). The intravenous administration of substance P also resulted in potentiation of histamine responses in the airways (114). Exogenously administered substance P increased acetylcholine-induced bronchospasm in the guinea pig (114,116). Tamura et al. (117) reported that neurokinin A augmented methacholine responses for as long as 4 weeks in Japanese monkeys.

Besides the effect of tachykinins on airway reactivity, viral infections intensify neurogenic plasma extravasation in airway mucosa (118,119) and potentiate the increase in airway blood flow produced by substance P (120).

## V.  β₂-Receptors

Szentivanyi proposed that an imbalance between the parasympathetic and sympathetic system was the fundamental abnormality in asthma (121). The abnormal β-adrenergic function could be a feature of all varieties of asthma: allergic, nonallergic, and during respiratory infections (122). Indeed, blocking of the β-adrenergic receptors increases the responsiveness of the bronchi of humans (123) and animals (124). Motojima et al. (125) reported that there was a correlation between β-adrenergic receptor density and the threshold response to acetylcholine in patients with asthma. This effect was probably due to an enhanced mediator release.

It is nearly impossible to obtain airway tissue from patients with an upper respiratory tract infection. Therefore, investigators used isolated human granulocytes and animal models to study the effect of viral infections on β-receptors.

Granulocytes from patients with asthma responded less well to β-adrenoceptor stimulation than granulocytes from control subjects, and furthermore, β-adrenoceptor response diminished during a flare of asthma with a clinical viral upper respiratory tract infection (126,127). β-Adrenoceptor function on human granulocytes has compromised in a similar fashion after incubation of these cells in vitro with respiratory viruses (100,126). Moreover, a loss of β-receptor agonist–induced inhibition of bronchial contraction to antigen in vitro was found in guinea pigs infected with parainfluenza in vivo (10). A change in β-receptor number or function on basophils and mast cells could be the cause of this finding. A loss of β-adrenoceptor binding sites was obtained in pulmonary parenchyma of guinea pigs infected with Sendai virus (Fig. 1) (11). The change in β-receptor binding sites or function after a viral respiratory infection may be caused by various T-lymphocyte–derived cytokines (128). In contrast, an increase in β-receptor number was demonstrated in the murine trachea at several time points after a respiratory infection with influenza A/PR-8/34 (7). Interestingly, infected mouse tracheal segments were approximately two times less sensitive to β-adrenoceptor stimulation and to the adenylyl cyclase activator forskolin. Similar data were obtained by Scarpace and Bender (129).

These results indicate that besides changes in the β-adrenoceptor numbers, a decreased function of the second messenger system could also contribute to the defect of β-receptor function after a viral respiratory infection.

## VI.  Epithelial Damage and Dysfunction

Guinea pigs infected with PI-3 virus demonstrated depleted goblet cells 4 days after inoculation (38). This seems to be an active process since mucin mRNA is not detectable in pathogen-free rats but is present in rats with acquired Sendai virus (130). Moreover, the mucociliary system is impaired after a viral infection (131). In humans and guinea pigs with a respiratory infection, the cilia on the airways were absent (38,132,133), and this resulted in mucus plugging in the deeper airways (28,33).

From the data discussed above it is likely that viral infections can cause airway epithelial inflammation and damage. The epithelial damage, and thus loss of the barrier function, observed after the viral infection may contribute to the development of airway hyperresponsiveness (Fig. 1). The epithelial damage may be induced by mediators released by inflammatory cells, like oxygen species and cationic proteins. Indeed, bronchoalveolar cells obtained from guinea pigs release oxygen radicals upon stimulation with PI-3 virus (33). It is likely that cellular antioxidant enzymes may protect airway epithelial cells against damage. Indeed, Jacoby and Choi (134), showed in primary cultures of human epithelial cells that influenza virus and IFN-γ increases mRNA for the antioxidant enzymes manganese superoxide dismutase and indoleamine 2,3-dioxygenase. These enzymes are likely to be important protective mechanisms in viral airway infections. Cationic proteins released by eosinophils can also induce epithelial damage and airway hyperresponsiveness (135–137). After experimentally induced infection with rhinovirus in the nose of humans, an airway hyperresponsiveness was associated with an increase in epithelial eosinophils (138). In guinea pigs, the increase in airway responsiveness paralleled the increase in numbers of eosinophils in bronchoalveolar lavage fluid 4, 8, and 16 days after the viral respiratory infection (36). A similar association was found in infected animals pretreated with antiinflammatory agents (37). Interleukin (IL)-5 was first described as a factor that induces differentiation and proliferation of bone marrow eosinophils (139–141). Subsequently, IL-5 has been shown to have several other properties, including the ability to activate or prime eosinophils (142–144) and to prolong their survival in vitro (145). Interestingly, pretreatment of guinea pigs with antibodies to IL-5 partly reduced the number of eosinophils in blood and bronchoalveolar lavage and prevented the development of airway hyperresponsiveness after the viral respiratory tract infection (146). Further, the total number of eosinophils from lung homogenates was increased in rats that had neonatal infections and demonstrated airway hyperresponsiveness. These changes persist at least into young adults (30,61,62). Virus-specific CD8$^+$ cells contributed to the airway eosinophilia (147). Concentrations of eosinophilic cationic protein are significantly increased in infants with bronchiolitis (148). RSV, directly added to eosinophils, activates and primes these cells to release various inflammatory mediators (149). Eosinophil activation was also characterized by piecemeal degranulation and extrusion of granule contents in the environment (150). Guinea pigs with a viral respiratory tract infection have more eosinophils in their lumen. Eosinophils that have migrated into the lumen of the airways showed piecemeal degranulation (146). It is therefore likely that cationic proteins released by eosinophils after a viral infection may contribute to epithelial damage. Last, but not least, the replication of respiratory viruses in the epithelial layer may contribute to the cytopathological effects (151–154).

Beside the loss of neutral endopeptidase(s), an enzyme that degrades tachykinines, after virus-induced epithelial damage, the release of epithelium-derived relaxing factors, like prostaglandin $E_2$ and NO, may be decreased (35, 155). Prostaglandin $E_2$ does not seem to play a critical role, since isolated tracheas obtained from guinea pigs 4 days after a PI-3 virus infection produce similar amounts of this lipid mediator after histamine stimulation as control preparations did (38). Moreover, pretreatment of guinea pigs with a cyclooxygenase inhibitor in vivo does not modulate the virus-induced airway inflammation or airway hyperresponsiveness (37). In contrast, the release of nitric oxide in tracheal tubes of virus-infected animals was diminished by 75% compared to controls (16,17) (Fig. 3). Interestingly, incubation of healthy tracheal tubes with a nitric oxide synthesis inhibitor also enhanced the reactivity for histamine in intact, but not epithelium-denuded preparations, indicating that NO is derived from the epithelial layer (156). Further, potassium and bradykinin added to the inside of tracheal tubes induces an NO- and epithelium-dependent relaxation (16,157), whereas potassium added to the ouside induces a contraction (16). These results further suggest that NO can be produced by the epithelial layer. Inhalation of low doses of L-arginine prevented the virus-induced airway hyperresponsiveness (17). From the results described above, it is likely that after a viral infection a deficiency in endogenous nitric oxide is due to a dysfunction of the constitutive nitric oxide synthase. Among others, four possible mechanisms may account for the NO deficiency in virally infected airways. First, the decreased NO production can be explained by substrate limitation, e.g., a decreased concentration of L-arginine in virus-treated animals. However, intracellular levels of arginine are already high, and the supply of arginine is normally not rate-limiting for the constitutive enzyme (158). On the other hand, we cannot exclude the possibility that the activity of arginase, the enzyme that breaks down arginine, is increased. Arginase is widely distributed in the body including the lungs (159) and is elevated during growth of tissues and tumors (160). Whether arginase activity is increased in the lungs during viral respiratory infections needs to be investigated. Second, a likely explanation for the lack in NO in virus-treated animals is a diminished activity or availability of the constitutive nitric oxide synthase due to epithelial damage. The constitutive nitric oxide synthase is present in rat airway epithelial cells but not in human airway epithelium (161). A cause of this discrepancy might be that the specimens of the human airways were taken from diseased lungs versus the healthy airways of the rat. Indeed, in biopsies of human airways, immunoreactivity to inducible nitric oxide synthase was seen in the epithelium in 22 of 23 asthmatic cases but only in 2 of 14 nonasthmatic controls (162). Although in diseased airways the inducible nitric oxide synthase is present and under basal

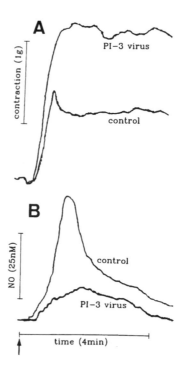

**Figure 3**  Individual tracings of the histamine ($10^{-3}$ M)–induced contraction (A) and nitric oxide release (B) of perfused isolated tracheal tubes obtained from control and virus-infected guinea pigs. In a preparation obtained from a virus-infected animal, the histamine-induced contraction was enhanced and NO production was markedly suppressed compared to the control tissue. Arrow indicates addition of histamine. (From Ref. 17.)

conditions the NO concentration in exhaled air is higher in asthmatic patients and in persons suffering a viral respiratory infection (163,164), it cannot be excluded that the NO released by the activity of the constitutive enzyme is diminished during bronchoconstriction. In healthy humans nitric oxide concentrations in exhaled air are increased after breath-holding or exercise (165). Further, inhalation of nitric oxide diminishes the airways contractions induced by cholinoceptor agonists in guinea pigs, rabbits, and humans (166–168). A third mechanism by which the concentration of NO can be decreased is inactivation of NO by products released from inflammatory cells, i.e., superoxide anions (169,170). Indeed, agents that generate superoxide, induce an enhanced reactivity of tracheal tubes (171). Besides decreasing the NO concentration, the reactive peroxynitrite (ONOO—) is produced by the interaction of superoxide anions with NO, which accordingly may lead to "additional" epithelial damage and airway hyperresponsiveness (172). Moreover, isolated guinea pig epithelial cells themselves can release reactive oxygen species (173). Fourth, during viral infections interferon is produced (174–176). This might stimulate inducible nitric oxide synthase, and the high amount of nitric oxide production could inactivate the constitutive nitric oxide synthase and, hence, the NO production after histamine stimulation (177,178).

In conclusion, it is clear that a number of interesting results have been obtained in animal models with a viral respiratory infection. These results can form a basis for more specific clinical investigations to elucidate the pathophysiology and mechanisms behind virus-induced airway obstruction and hyperresponsiveness in humans. This may finally lead to an improvement in the management of airway diseases like asthma.

### References

1. Folkerts G, Busse WW, Nÿkamp FP, Sorkness R, Gern JE. Virus-induced airway hyperresponsiveness and asthma. Am J Respir Crit Care Med 1998; 157:1708–1720.
2. Busse WW. Respiratory infections: their role in airway responsiveness and the pathogenesis of asthma. J Allergy Clin Immunol 1990; 85:671–683.
3. Bardin PG, Johnston SL, Pattemore PK. Viruses as precipitants of asthma symptoms. II. Physiology and mechanisms. Clin Exp Allergy 1992; 22:809–822.
4. Pattemore PK, Johnston SL, Bardin PG. Viruses as precipitants of asthma symptoms. Clin Exp Allergy 1992; 22:325–336.
5. Sterk PJ. Virus-induced airway hyperresponsiveness in man. Eur Respir J 1993; 6:894–902.
6. Folkerts G, Nijkamp FP. Virus-induced airway hyperresponsiveness: role of inflammatory cells and mediators. Am J Respir Crit Care Med 1995; 151:1666–1674.
7. Henry PJ, Rigby PJ, Mackenzie JS, Goldie RG. Effect of respiratory tract viral infection on murine airway β-adrenoceptor function, distribution and density. Br J Pharmacol 1991; 104:914–921.
8. Sorkness R, Clough JJ, Castleman WL, Lemanske RFJ. Virus-induced airway obstruction and parasympathetic hyperresponsiveness in adult rats. Am J Respir Crit Care Med 1994; 150:28–34.
9. Colasurdo GN, Hemming VG, Prince GA, Loader JE, Graves JP, Larsen GL. Human respiratory syncytial virus affects nonadrenergic noncholinergic inhibition in cotton rat airways. Am J Phys 1995; 12:L1006–L1011.
10. Buckner CK, Clayton DE, Ain-Shoka AA, Busse WW, Dick EC, Shult P. Parainfluenza 3 infection blocks the ability of a β- adrenergic receptor agonist to inhibit antigen-induced contraction of guinea pig isolated airway smooth muscle. J Clin Invest 1981; 67:376–384.
11. Ohashi Y, Motojima S, Yamanouchi K, Makino S. Changes in bronchial response after Sendai virus infection in guinea pigs. Ann Allergy 1988; 61:109.
12. Fryer AD, Yarkony KA, Jacoby DB. The effect of leukocyte depletion on pulmo-

nary $M_2$ muscarinic receptor function in parainfluenza virus-infected guinea-pigs. Br J Pharmacol 1994; 112:588–594.

13. Kudlacz EM, Shatzer SA, Farrell AM, Baugh LE. Parainfluenza virus type 3 induced alterations in tachykinin NK1 receptors, substance P levels and respiratory functions in guinea pig airways. Eur J Pharmacol 1994; 270:291–300.

14. Elwood W, Lotvall JO, Barnes PJ, Chung KF. Airway hyperresponsiveness to acetylcholine and to tachykinins after respiratory virus infection in the guinea pig. Ann Allergy 1993; 70:231–236.

15. Nakazawa H, Sekizawa K, Morikawa M, Yamauchi K, Satoh M, Maeyama K, Watanabe T, Sasaki H. Viral respiratory infection causes airway hyperresponsiveness and decreases histamine N-methyltransferase activity in guinea pigs. Am J Respir Crit Care Med 1994; 149:1180–1185.

16. Folkerts G, Linde van der H, Verheyen AKCP, Nijkamp FP. Endogenous nitric oxide modulation of potassium-induced changes in guinea pig airway tone. Br J Pharmacol 1995; 115:1194–1198.

17. Folkerts, Linde van der HJ, Nijkamp FP. Virus-induced airway hyperresponsiveness in guinea pigs is related to a deficiency in nitric oxide. J Clin Invest 1995; 95:26–30.

18. Murray TC, Jacoby DB. Viral infection increases contractile but not secretory responses to substance P in ferret trachea. J Appl Physiol 1992; 72:608–611.

19. Killingsworth CR, Robinson NE, Adams T, Maes RK, Berney C, Rozanski E. Cholinergic reactivity of tracheal smooth muscle after infection with feline herpesvirus I. J Appl Physiol 1990; 69:1953–1960.

20. Lemen RJ. Clues to the mechanism of virus-induced asthma from animal models. Semin Respir Med 1990; 11:321–329.

21. Inoue H, Horio S, Ichinose M, Ida S, Hida W, Takishima T, Ohwada K, Homma M. Changes in bronchial reactivity to acetylcholine with type C influenza virus in dogs. Am Rev Respir Dis 1986; 133:367–371.

22. Lindgren C, Jing L, Graham B, Grogaard J, Sundell H. Respiratory syncytial virus infection reinforces reflex apnea in young lambs. Pediatr Res 1992; 31:381–385.

23. Wagner MH, Evermann JF, Gaskin J, McNicol K, Small P, Stecenko AA. Subacute effects of respiratory syncytial virus infection on lung function in lambs. Pediatr Pulmonol 1991; 11:56–64.

24. LeBlanc PH, Baker JC, Gray PR, Robinson NE, Derksen FJ. Effects of bovine respiratory syncytial virus on airway function in neonatal calves. Am J Vet Res 1991; 52:1401–1406.

25. Lemen RJ, Quan SF, Witten ML, Sobonya RE, Ray CG, Grad R. Canine parainfluenza type 2 bronchiolitis increases histamine responsiveness in beagle puppies. Am Rev Respir Dis 1990; 141:199–207.

26. Jacoby DB, Tamaoki J, Borson DB, Nadel JA. Influenza infection causes airway hyperresponsiveness by decreasing enkephalinase. J Appl Physiol 1988; 64(6): 2653–2658.

27. Quan SF, Witten ML, Grad R, Sobonya RE, Ray CG, Dambro NN, Lemen RJ. Acute canine adenovirus 2 infection increases histamine airway reactivity in beagle puppies. Am Rev Respir Dis 1990; 141:414–420.

28. Hegele RG, Robinson PJ, Gonzalez S, Hogg JC. Production of acute bronchiolitis

in guinea-pigs by human respiratory syncytial virus. Eur Respir J 1993; 6:1324–1331.

29. Walden SM, Proud D, Lichtenstein LM, Kagey-Sobotka A, Naclerio RM. Antigen-provoked increase in histamine reactivity. Am Rev Respir Dis 1991; 144:642–648.

30. Sorkness R, Lemanske RFJ, Castleman WL. Persistent airway hyperresponsiveness after neonatal viral bronchiolitis in rats. J Appl Physiol 1991; 70:375–383.

31. Folkerts G, Esch B van, Nijkamp FP. Does stimulation of broncho-alveolar cells by viruses lead to respiratory airway hyperreactivity in the guinea pig? Eur J Pharmacol 1990; 183:188–189.

32. Folkerts G, Janssen M, Nijkamp FP. Parainfluenza-3 induced hyperreactivity of the guinea pig trachea coincides with an increased number of bronchoalveolar cells. Br J Clin Pharmacol 1990; 30:159S–161S.

33. Folkerts G, Verheyen A, Nijkamp FP. Viral infection in guinea pigs induces a sustained non-specific airway hyperresponsiveness and morphological changes of the respiratory tract. Eur J Pharmacol 1992; 228:121–130.

34. Buckner CK, Songsiridej V, Dick EC, Busse WW. In vivo and in vitro studies on the use of the guinea pig as a model for virus-provoked airway hyperreactivity. Am Rev Respir Dis 1985; 132:305–310.

35. Folkerts G, Engels F, Nijkamp FP. Endotoxin-induced hyperreactivity of the guinea pig isolated trachea coincides with decreased prostaglandin $E_2$ production by the epithelial layer. Br J Pharmacol 1989; 96:388–394.

36. Folkerts G, Esch B van, Janssen M, Nijkamp FP. Virus-induced airway hyperresponsiveness in guinea pigs in vivo: study of broncho-alveolar cell number and activity. Eur J Pharmacol 1992; 228(4):219–227.

37. Folkerts G, De Clerck F, Reijnart I, Span P, Nijkamp FP. Virus-induced airway hyperresponsiveness in the guinea-pig: possible involvement of histamine and inflammatory cells. Br J Pharmacol 1993; 108:1083–1093.

38. Folkerts G, Verheyen AKCP, Geuens GMA, Folkerts HF, Nijkamp FP. Virus-induced changes in airway responsiveness, morphology, and histamine levels in guinea pigs. Am Rev Respir Dis 1993; 147:1569–1577.

39. Kudlacz EM, Baugh LE, Porter WP, Kenny MT, Farrell AM. A time-course study of airway hyperresponsiveness in conscious parainfluenza virus type 3-infected guinea pigs. Lab Anim Sci 1993; 43:445–453.

40. Quan SF, Witten ML, Grad R, Ray CG, Lemen RJ. Changes in lung mechanics and histamine responsiveness after sequential canine adenovirus 2 and canine parainfluenza 2 virus infection in beagle puppies. Pediatr Pulmonol 1991; 10:236–243.

41. Casale TB, Wood D, Richerson HB, Trapp S, Metzger WJ, Zavala D, Hunninghake GW. Elevated bronchoalveolar lavage fluid histamine levels in allergic asthmatics are associated with methacholine bronchial responsiveness. J Clin Invest 1987; 79:1197–1203.

42. Jarjour NN, Calhoun WJ, Schwartz LB, Busse WW. Elevated bronchoalveolar lavage fluid histamine levels in allergic asthmatics are associated with increased airway obstruction. Am Rev Respir Dis 1991; 144:83–87.

43. Ida S, Hooks JJ, Siraganian RP, Notkins AL. Enhancement of IgE-mediated histamine release from human basophils by viruses: role of interferon. J Exp Med 1977; 145:892–906.

44. Hall CB, Douglas RG, Simons RL, Geiman JM. Interferon production in children with respiratory syncytial, influenza, and parainfluenza virus infections. J Pediatr 1978; 93:28–33.

45. Schwartz LB, Kawahara MS, Hugi TE, Vik DT, Fearon DT, Austen KF. Generation of C3a anaphylatoxin from human C3 by mast cell tryptase. J Immunol 1983; 130: 1891–1895.

46. Söderberg M, Hellström S, Lundgren R, Bergh A. Bronchial epithelium in humans recently recovering from respiratory infectious caused by influenza or mucoplasma. Eur Respir J 1990; 3:1023–1028.

47. Graighead JE. Growth of parainfluenza type 3 virus and interferon production in infant and adult mice. Br J Exp Pathol 1966; 23:235–241.

48. Lett-Brown MA, Aelvoet M, Hooks JJ, Georgiades JA, Thueson DO, Grant JA. Enhancement of basophil chemotaxis in vitro by virus-induced interferon. J Clin Invest 1981; 67:547–552.

49. Smith TF, McIntosh K, Fishaut M, Henson PM. Activation of complement by cells infected with respiratory syncytial virus. Infec Immun 1981; 33:43–48.

50. Bjornson AB, Mellencamp MA, Schiff GM. Complement is activated in the upper respiratory tract during influenza virus infection. Am Rev Respir Dis 1991; 143: 1062–1066.

51. Huftel MA, Swensen CA, Borchering WR, Dick EC, Hong R, Kita H, Gleich GJ, Busse WW. The effect of T-cell depletion on enhanced basophil histamine release after in vitro incubation with live influenza a virus. Am J Respir Cell Mol Biol 1992; 7:434–440.

52. Busse WW, Swenson CA, Borden EC, Treuhaft MW, Dick EC. Effect of influenza A virus on leukocyte histamine release. J Allergy Clin Immunol 1983; 71:382–388.

53. Chonmaitree T, Lett-Brown MA, Tsong Y, Goldman AS, Baron S. Role of interferon in leukocyte histamine release caused by common respiratory viruses. J Infec Dis 1988; 157:127–132.

54. Clementsen P, Jensen CB, Jarlov JO, Hannoun C, Norn S. Virus enhances histamine release from human basophils. Agents Actions 1988; 23:165–167.

55. Norn S, Clementsen P, Kristensen KS, Hannoun C, Jarlov JO. Carbohydrates inhibit the potentiating effect of bacteria, endotoxin and virus on basophil histamine release. Agents Actions 1990; 30:53–63.

56. Clementsen P, Douglas AR, Skehel JJ, Hannoun C, Bach-Mortensen N, Norn S. Influenza A virus enhances IgE-mediated histamine release from human basophil leukocytes. Examination of the effect of viral neuraminidase and haemagglutinin. Agents Actions 1989; 27:58–61.

57. Clementsen P, Norn S, Kristensen KS, Hannoun C. Influenza A virus enhances basophil histamine release and the enhancement is abolished by carbohydrates. Allergy 1990; 45:471–476.

58. Graziano FM, Tilton R, Hirth T, Segaloff D, Mullins D, Dick E, Buckner C, Busse WW. The effects of parainfluenza 3 infection on guinea pig basophil and lung mast cell histamine release. Am Rev Respir Dis 1989; 139:715–720.

59. Ogunbiyi PO, Black WD, Eyre P. Parainfluenza 3 virus-induced enhancement of

histamine release from calf lung mast cell: effect of levamisole. J Vet Pharmacol Ther 1988; 11:338–344.

60. Sorden S, Castleman WL. Brown norway rats are high responders to bronchiolitis, pneumonia, and bronchiolar mastocytosis induced by parainfluenza virus. Exp Lung Res 1991; 17:1025–1045.

61. Sorden SD, Castleman WL. Virus-induced increases in bronchiolar mast cells in brown Norway rats are associated with both local mast cell proliferation and increases in blood mast cell precursors. Lab Invest 1995; 73:197–204.

62. Castleman WL, Sorkness RL, Lemanske RFJ, McAllister PK. Viral bronchiolitis during early life induces increased numbers of bronchiolar mast cells and airway hyperresponsiveness. Am J Pathol 1990; 137(4):821–831.

63. Djukanovic R, Roche WR, Wilson JW, Beasley CRW, Twentyman OP, Howarth PH, Holgate ST. Mucosal inflammation in asthma. Am Rev Respir Dis 1990; 142: 434–457.

64. Gaddy H, Busse WW. Enhanced IgE-dependent basophil histamine release and airway reactivity in asthma. Am Rev Respir Dis 1986; 134:969–974.

65. Everard ML, Fox G, Walls AF, Quint D, Fifield R, Walters C, Swarbrick A, Milner AD. Tryptase and IgE concentrations in the respiratory tract of infants with acute bronchiolitis. Arch Dis Child 1995; 72:64–69.

66. Skoner DP, Fireman P, Caliguiri L, Davis H. Plasma elevations of histamine and a prostaglandin metabolite in acute bronchiolitis. Am Rev Respir Dis 1990; 142: 359–364.

67. Welliver RC, Wong DT, Sun M, Middelton EJ, Vaugan RS, Ogra PL. The development of respiratory syncytial virus-specific IgE and the release of histamine in nasopharyngeal secretions after infection. N Engl J Med 1981; 305(15):841–846.

68. Welliver RC. Role of virus-specific immunoglobulin E antibody responses in obstructive airway disease. Semin Respir Med 1990b; 11:330–335.

69. Welliver RC. The role of antihistamines in upper respiratory tract infections. J Allergy Clin Immunol 1990a; 86:633–637.

70. Crutcher JE, Kantner TR. The effectiveness of antihistamines in the common cold. J Clin Pharmacol 1981; 21:9–15.

71. Gaffey JM, Gwaltney JM, Sastre A, Dressler WE, Sorrentino JV, Hayden FG. Intransally and orally administered antihistamine treatment of experimental rhinovirus colds. Am Rev Respir Dis 1987; 136:556–560.

72. Gaffey MJ, Kaiser DL, Hayden FG. Ineffectiveness of oral terfenadine in natural colds: evidence against histamine as a mediator of common cold symptoms. Pediatr Infect Dis J 1988; 7:223–228.

73. Barnes PJ. Neural control of human airway in health and disease. Am Rev Respir Dis 1986; 134:1289–1314.

74. Holgate ST. Anticholinergics in acute bronchial asthma. Postgrad Med J 1987; 63(suppl 1):35–39.

75. Maclagan J. Presynaptic control of airway smooth muscle. Am Rev Respir Dis 1987; 136:S54–S57.

76. Patel HJ, Barnes PJ, Takahashi T, Tadjkarimi S, Yacoub MH, Belvisi MG. Evi-

dence for prejunctional muscarinic autoreceptors in human and guinea pig trachea. Am J Respir Crit Care Med 1995; 152:872–878.

77. Ichinose M, Barnes PJ. Inhibitory histamine $H_3$-receptors on cholinergic nerves in human airways. Eur J Pharmacol 1989; 163:383–386.

78. Rhoden KJ, Meldrum LA, Barnes PJ. Inhibition of cholinergic neurotransmission in human airways by $\beta_2$-adrenoceptors. J Appl Physiol 1988; 65:700–705.

79. Minette PAH, Lammers J, Dixon CMS, Mccusker MT, Barnes PJ. A muscarinic agonist inhibits reflex bronchoconstriction in normal but not in asthmatic subjects. Am J Physiol 1989; 67:2461–2465.

80. Folkerts G, Linde van der H, Omini C, Nijkamp FP. Virus-induced airway inflammation and hyperresponsiveness in the guinea pig is inhibited by levodropropizine. N-S Arch Pharmacol 1993; 348:213–219.

81. Ladenius ARC, Folkerts G, Linde van der HJ, Nijkamp FP. Potentiation by viral respiratory infection of ovalbumin-induced guinea pig tracheal hyperresponsiveness: role for tachykinins. Br J Pharmacol 1995; 115:1048–1052.

82. Fryer AD, Jacoby DB. Parainfluenza virus infection damages inhibitory $M_2$ muscarinic receptors on pulmonary parasympathetic nerves in the guinea-pig. Br J Pharmacol 1991; 102:267–271.

83. Jacoby DB, Fryer AD. Abnormalities in neural control of smooth muscle in virus-infected airways. TIPS 1990; 11:393–395.

84. Fryer AD, El-Fakahany EE, Jacoby DB. Parainfluenza virus type 1 reduces the affinity of agonists for muscarinic receptors in guinea-pig lung and heart. Eur J Pharmacol 1990; 181:51–58.

85. Haddad EB, Gies JP. Neuraminidase reduces the number of super-high-affinity [$^3$H]oxotremorine-M binding sites in lung. Eur J Pharmacol 1992; 211:273–276.

86. Fryer AD, Jacoby DB. Function of pulmonary $M_2$ muscarinic receptors in antigen challenged guinea-pig is restored by heparin and poly-1-glutamate. J Clin Invest 1992; 90:2292–2298.

87. Gambone LM, Fryer AD. Inflammatory cell depletion preserves neuronal $M_2$ receptor function in guinea pigs exposed to ozon. Am Rev Respir Dis 1992; 145: A614.

88. Empey DW, Laitinen LA, Jacobs L, Gold WM, Nadel JA. Mechanisms of bronchial hyperreactivity in normal subjects after upper respiratory tract infection. Am Rev Respir Dis 1976; 113:131–139.

89. Folkerts G, Nijkamp FP. Bronchial hyperreactivity induced by parainfluenza 3 virus is partly prevented by atropine. Agents Actions 1989; 26:68–70.

90. Barnes PJ, Baraniuk JN, Belvisi MG. Neuropeptides in the respiratory tract. Am Rev Respir Dis 1991; 144:1391–1399.

91. Lundberg JM, Fahrenkrug J, Hokfelt T, Martling CR, Larsson OT K, Anggard A. Coexistence of peptide histidine isoleucine (PHI) and VIP in nerves regulating blood flow and bronchial smooth muscle tone in various mammals including man. Peptides 1984; 5:593–606.

92. Dey RD, Shannon WA, Said SI. Localization of VIP-immunoreactive nerves in airways and pulmonary vessels of dogs, cats and human subjects. Cell Tissue Res 1981; 220:231–238.

93. Ollerenshaw S, Jarvis D, Woolcock A, Sullivan C, Scheibner T. Absence of Immunoreactive vasoactive intestinal polypeptide in tissue from lungs of patients with asthma. N Engl J Med 1989; 320:1244–1248.

94. Baraniuk JN, Okayama M, Lundgren JD. Vasoactive intestinal polypeptide (VIP) in human nasal mucosa. J Clin Invest 1990; 86:825–831.

95. Frandsen EK, Krishina GA, Said SI. Vasoactive intestinal polypeptide promotes cyclic adenosine 3′,5′monophosphate accumulation in guinea trachea. Br J Pharmacol 1978; 62:367–369.

96. Palmer JBD, Cuss FMC, Barnes PJ. VIP and PHM and their role in nonadrenergic inhibitory responses in isolated human airways. J Appl Physiol 1986; 61:1322–1328.

97. Caughey GH, Leidig F, Vizo NF, Nadel JA. Substance P and vasoactive intestinal peptide degradation by mast cell tryptase and chymase. J Pharmacol Exp Ther 1988; 244:133–137.

98. Tam EK, Caughey GH. Degradation of airway neuropeptides by human lung tryptase. Am J Respir Cell Mol Biol 1990; 3:27–32.

99. Pavia D, Bateman JRM, Clarke SW. Deposition and clearance of inhaled particles. Bull Eur Phys Respir 1980; 16:335–366.

100. Busse WW, Vrtis RF, Steiner R, Dick EC. In vitro incubation with influenza virus primes human polymorphonuclear leukocyte generation of superoxide. Am J Respir Cell Mol Biol 1991; 4:347–354.

101. Folkerts G, Verheyen A, Janssen M, Nijkamp PP. Virus-induced airway hyperresponsiveness in the guinea pig can be transferred by bronchoalveolar cells. J Allergy Clin Immunol 1992; 90:364–372.

102. Laitinen A. Ultrastructural organization of intraepithelial nerves in the human airway tract. Thorax 1985; 40:488–492.

103. Lundberg JM, Hokfelt T, Martling CR, Saria A, Cuello C. Substance P immunoreactive sensory nerves in the lower respiratory tract of various mammals including man. Cell Tissue Res 1984; 235:251–261.

104. Borson DB. Roles of neural endopeptidase in airways. Am J Physiol 1991; 260:L212–L225.

105. Lundberg JM, Saria A, Lundblad L. Bioactive peptides in capsaicin-sensitive C-fiber afferents of the airways: functional and pathophysiological implications. In: Kaliner M, Barnes PJ, eds. The Airways: Neural Control in Health and Disease. New York: Marcel Dekker, 1987:417–445.

106. Saria A, Martling CR, Yan Z, Theodorsson-Norheim E, Gamse R, Lundberg JM. Release of multiple tachykinins from capsaicin-sensitive nerves in the lung by bradykinin, histamine, dimethylphenylpiperainium, and vagal nerve stimulation. Am Rev Respir Dis 1988; 137:1330–1335.

107. Rhoden KJ, Barnes PJ. Effect of hydrogen peroxide on guinea pig tracheal smooth muscle in vitro: role of cyclo-oxygenase and airway epithelium. Br J Pharmacol 1989; 98:325–330.

108. Sekizawa K, Tamaoki J, Graf PD, Basbaum CB, Borson DB, Nadel JA. Enkephalinase inhibitor potentiates mammalian tachykinin-induced contraction in ferret trachea. J Pharmacol Exp Ther 1987; 243:1211–1217.

109. Black JL, Johnson PRA, Armour CL. Potentiation of the contractile effects of neu-

ropeptides in human bronchus by an enkephalinase inhibitor. Pulm Pharmacol 1988; 1:21–23.

110. Lötvall JO, Skoogh B-E, Barnes PJ, Chung KF. Effects of aerosolised substance P on lung resistance in guinea-pigs: a comparison between inhibition of neutral endopeptidase and angiotensin-converting enzyme. Br J Pharmacol 1990; 100:69–72.

111. Grandordy BM, Frossard N, Rhoden KJ, Barnes PJ. Tachykinin-induced phospho-inositide breakdown in airway smooth muscle and epithelium: relationship to contraction. Mol Pharmacol 1988; 33:515–519.

112. Saban R, Dick EC, Fishleder RI, Buckner CK. Enhancement by parainfluenza 3 infection of the contractile response to substance P and capsaicin in airway smooth muscle of the guinea pig. Am Rev Respir Dis 1987; 136:586–591.

113. Dusser DJ, Jacoby DB, Djorkic TD, Rubinstein I, Borson DB, Nadel JA. Virus induces airway hyperresponsiveness to tachykinins: role of neutral endopeptidase. J Appl Physiol 1989; 67:1504–1511.

114. Umeno E, Hirose T, Sishima S. Pretreatment with aerosolized capsaicin potentiates histamine-induced bronchoconstriction in guinea pigs. Am Rev Respir Dis 1992; 146:159–162.

115. Hsiue TR, Garland A, Ray DW, Hershenson MB, Leff AR, Solway J. Endogenous sensory neuropetide release enhances nonspecific airway responsiveness in guinea pigs. Am Rev Respir Dis 1992; 146:148–153.

116. Omini C, Brunelli G, Hernandez A, Daffonichia L. Bradykinin and substance P potentiate acetylcholine-induced bronchospasm in guinea pig. Eur J Pharmacol 1989; 163:195–197.

117. Tamura G, Sakai K, Taniguchi Y, Iijima H, Honma M, Katsumata U, Maruyama N, Aizawa T, Takishima T. Neurokinin A-induced bronchial hyperresponsiveness to metacholine in Japanese monkeys. Tohoku J Exp Med 1989; 159:69–73.

118. McDonald DM. Respiratory tract infections increase susceptibility to neurogenic inflammation in the rat trachea. Am Rev Respir Dis 1988; 137:1432–1440.

119. McDonald DM. Infections intensify neurogenic plasma extravasation in the airway mucosa. Am Rev Respir Dis 1992; 146:S40–S44.

120. Yamawaki I, Geppetti P, Bertrand C, Chan B, Massion P, Piedimonte G, Nadel JA. Viral infection potentiates the increase in airway blood flow produced by substance P. J Appl Physiol 1995; 79:398–404.

121. Szentivanyi A. The β-adrenergic theory of the atopic abnormality in bronchial asthma. J Allergy 1968; 42:203–232.

122. Nijkamp FP, Engels F, Henricks PAJ, Van Oosterhout AJM. Mechanisms of β-adrenergic receptor regulation in lungs and its implications for physiological responses. Phys Rev 1992; 72:323–367.

123. Reed CE, Cohen M, Enta T. Reduced effect of epinephrine on circulating eosinophils in asthma and after β-adrenergic blockade or bordetella pertussis vaccine. J Allergy 1970; 46:90.

124. Ishihara T, Mue S, Ohmi T. Bronchial responses to inhaled histamine and methacholine after influenza virus vaccination in monkeys. Tohoku J Exp Med 1983; 140:335.

125. Motojima S, Fukuda T, Makino S. Measurement of β-adrenergic receptors on lym-

phocytes in normal subjects and asthmatics in relation to β-adrenergic hyperglycemia response and bronchial responsiveness. Allergy 1983; 38:331.

126. Busse WW. Decreased granulocyte response to isoproterenol in asthma during upper respiratory infections. Am Rev Respir Dis 1977; 115:783–791.

127. Bush RK, Busse WW, Flaherty D. Effects of experimental rhinovirus 16 infection on airways and leukocyte function in normal subjects. J Allergy Clin Immunol 1978; 61:80–87.

128. Van Oosterhout AJM, Stam WB, Vanderscheuren RGJRA, Nijkamp FP. Effects of cytokines on β-adrenoceptor function of human peripheral blood mononuclear cells and guinea pig trachea. J Allergy Clin Immunol 1992; 90:340–348.

129. Scarpace PJ, Bender BS. Viral pneumonia attenuates adenylate cyclase but not β-adrenergic receptors in murine lung. Am Rev Respir Dis 1989; 140:1602–1606.

130. Jany B, Gallup M, Tsuda T, Basbaum C. Mucin gene expression in rat airways following infection and irritation. Biochem Biophys Res Commun 1991; 181: 1–8.

131. Lindberg S. Morphological and functional studies of the mucociliary system during infections in the upper airways. Acta Otolaryngol Suppl Stockh 1994; 515:22–24.

132. Hers JFPH. Disturbances of the ciliated epithelium due to influenza virus. Am Rev Respir Dis 1966; 93:162–171.

133. Walsh JJ, Dietlein LF, Low FN, Burch GE, Mogabgab WJ. Bronchotracheal response in human influenza. Arch Intern Med 1961; 108:376–382.

134. Jacoby DB, Choi AM. Influenza virus induces expression of antioxidant genes in human epithelial cells. Free Rad Biol Med 1994; 16:821–824.

135. Hamann KJ, Strek ME, Baranowski SL, Munoz NM, Williams FC, White SR, Vita A, Leff AR. Effects of activated eosinophils cultured from human umbilical cord blood on guinea pig trachealis. Am J Physiol 1993; 265:L301–L307.

136. White SR, Ohno S, Monoz NM, Gleich GJ, Abrahams C, Solway J, Leff AR. Epithelium-dependent contraction of airway smooth muscle caused by eosiniphil MBP. Am J Physiol 1990; 259:L294–L303.

137. Kimpen JLL, Garofalo R, Welliver RC, Ogra PL. Activation of human eosinophils in vitro by respiratory syncytial virus. Pediatr Res 1992; 32:160–164.

138. Fraenkel DJ, Bardin PG, Sanderson G, Lampe F, Johnston SL, Holgate ST. Lower airways inflammation during rhinovirus colds in normal and in asthmatic subjects. Am J Respir Crit Care Med 1995; 151:879–886.

139. Sanderson CJ, Warren DG, Strath M. Identification of a lymphokine that stimulates eosinophil differentiation in vitro. Its relationship to interleukin 3, and functional properties of eosinophils produced in cultures. J Exp Med 1985; 162:60–74.

140. Clutterbuck EJ, Sanderson CJ. Human eosinophil hematopoiesis studied in vitro by means of murine eosinophil differentiation factor (IL-5): production of functionally active eosinophils from normal human bone marrow. Blood 1988; 71:646–651.

141. Yamaguchi T, Suda T, Suda J, Eguchi M, Miura Y, Harada N, Tominaga A, Takatsu K. Purified interleukin 5 supports the terminal differentiation and proliferation of murine eosinophilic precursors. J Exp Med 1988; 167:43–56.

142. Sehmi R, Wardlaw AJ, Cromwell O, Kurihara K, Waltmann P, Kay AB. Interleukin-5 selectively enhances the chemotactic response of eosinophils obtained from normal but not eosinophilic subjects. Blood 1992; 79:2952–2959.

143. Warringa RAJ, Mengelers HJJ, Kuijper PHM, Raaijmakers JAM, Bruijnzeel PLB, Koenderman L. In vivo priming of platelet-activating factor-induced eosinophil chemotaxis in allergic asthmatic individuals. Blood 1992; 79:1836–1841.

144. Coeffier E, Joseph D, Vargaftig BB. Activation of guinea pig eosinophils by human recombinant IL-5. Selective priming to platelet-activating factor and interference of its antagonists. J Immunol 1991; 147:2595–2602.

145. Tai PC, Sun L, Spry CJF. Effects of IL-5, granulocyte/macrophage colony-stimulating factor (GM-CSF) and IL-3 on the survival of human blood eosinophils in vitro. Clin Exp Immunol 1991; 85:312–316.

146. Oosterhout AJM, Ark van I, Folkerts G, Linde van der HJ, Savelkoul HFJ, Verheyen AKCP, Nijkamp FP. Antibody to interleukin-5 inhibits virus-induced airway hyperresponsiveness to histamine in guinea pigs. Am J Respir Crit Care Med 1995; 151:177–183.

147. Coyle AJ, Erard F, Bertrand C, Walti S, Pircher H, Le Gros G. Virus-specific CD8+ cells can switch to interleukin 5 production and induce airway eosinophilia. J Exp Med 1995; 181:1229–1233.

148. Garofalo R, Kimpen JL, Welliver RC, Ogra PL. Eosinophil degranulation in the respiratory tract during naturally acquired respiratory syncytial virus infection. J Pediatr 1992; 120:28–32.

149. Chand N, Harrison JE, Rooney S, Pillar J, Jakubicki R, Nolan K, Diamantis W, Sofia RD. Anti-IL-5 monoclonal antibody inhibits allergic late phase bronchial eosinophilia in guinea pigs: a therapeutic approach. Eur J Pharmacol 1992; 211:121–123.

150. Kimpen JLL. Respiratory syncytial virus: immunology and immunopathogenesis. Ph.D. Dissertation, University of Groningen, Groningen, The Netherlands, 1993.

151. Winther B, Gwaltney JM, Hendley JO. Respiratory virus infection of monolayer cultures of human nasal epithelial cells. Am Rev Respir Dis 1990; 141:839–845.

152. Becker S, Soukup J, Yankaskas JR. Respiratory syncytial virus infection of human primary nasal and bronchial epithelial cell cultures and bronchoalveolar macrophages. Am J Respir Cell Mol Biol 1992; 6:369–374.

153. Massion PP, Funari CCP, Ueki I, Ikeda S, McDonald DM, Nadel JA. Parainfluenza (Sendai) virus infects ciliated cells and secretory cells but not basal cells of rat tracheal epithelium. Am J Respir Cell Mol Biol 1993; 9:361–370.

154. Subauste MC, Jacoby DB, Richards SM, Proud D. Infection of a human respiratory epithelial cell line with rhinovirus—induction of cytokine release and modulation of susceptibility to infection by cytokine exposure. J Clin Invest 1995; 96:549–557.

155. Folkerts G, Nijkamp FP. Airway epithelium: more than just a barrier! TIPS 1998; 19:334–341.

156. Nijkamp FP, Van der Linde HJ, Folkerts G. Nitric oxide synthesis inhibitors induce airway hyperresponsiveness in the guinea pig in vivo and in vitro. Am Rev Respir Dis 1993; 148:727–734.

157. Figini M, Ricciardolo FLM, Javdan P, Nijkamp FP, Emanueli C, Pradelles P, Folkerts G, Geppetti P. Evidence that epithelium-derived relaxing factor released by bradykinin in the guinea pig trachea is nitric oxide. Am J Respir Crit Care Med 1996; 153:918–923.

158. McCall T, Vallance P. Nitric oxide takes centre-stage with newly defined roles. TIPS 1992; 13:1–6.

159. Aminlari M, Vaseghi T. Arginase distribution in tissues of domestic animals. Comp Biochem Physiol 1992; 103B:385–389.

160. Taylor AA, Stewart GR. Tissue and subcellular localization of enzymes of arginine metabolism in pisum sativum. Biochem Biophys Res Commun 1981; 101:1281–1289.

161. Kobzik L, Bredt DS, Lowenstein CJ, Drazen J, Gaston B, Sugarbaker D, Stamler JS. Nitric oxide synthase in human and rat lung: Immunocytochemical and histochemical localization. Am J Respir Cell Mol Biol 1993; 9:371–377.

162. Springall DR, Hamid OA, Buttery LKD, Chanez P, Howarth P, Bousquet J, Holgate ST, Polak JM. Nitric oxide synthase induction in airways of asthmatic subjects. Am Rev Respir Dis 1993; 147:A515.

163. Kharitonov SA, Yates D, Robbins RA, Logan-Sinclair R, Shinebourne EA, Barnes PJ. Increased nitric oxide in exhaled air of asthmatic patients. Lancet 1994; 343:133–135.

164. Kharitonov SA, Yates D, Barnes PJ. Increased nitric oxide in exhaled air of normal human subjects with upper respiratory tract infections. Eur Respir J 1995; 8:295–297.

165. Persson MG, Wiklund NP, Gustafsson LE. Endogenous nitric oxide in single exhalations and the change during exercise. Am Rev Respir Dis 1993; 148:1210–1214.

166. Dupuy PM, Shore SA, Drazen JM, Frostell C, Hill WA, Zapol WM. Bronchodilator action of inhaled nitric oxide in guinea pigs. J Clin Invest 1992; 90:421–428.

167. Högman M, Frostell C, Arnberg H, Hedenstierna G. Inhalation of nitric oxide modulates methacholine-induced bronchoconstriction in the rabbit. Eur Respir J 1993; 6:177–180.

168. Högman M, Frostell CG, Hedenström H, Hedenstierna G. Inhalation of nitric oxide modulates adult human bronchial tone. Am Rev Respir Dis 1993; 148:1474–1478.

169. Barnes PJ, Belvisi MG. Nitric oxide and lung disease. Thorax 1993; 48:1034–1043.

170. Nijkamp FP, Folkerts G. Nitric oxide and bronchial reactivity. Clin Exp Allergy 1994; 24:905–914.

171. Sadeghi-Hashjin G, Folkerts G, Henricks PAJ, Van de Loo PGF, Van der Linde HJ, Dik IEM. Induction of guinea pig airway hyperresponsiveness by inactivation of guanylate cyclase. Eur J Pharmacol 1996; 302:109–115.

172. Sadeghi-Hashjin G, Folkerts G, Henricks PAJ, Verheyen AKCP, Linde HJ van der, Ark I van, Coene A, Nijkamp FP. Peroxynitrite induces airway hyperresponsiveness in guinea pigs in vitro and in vivo. Am J Respir Crit Care Med 1996; 153:1860–1864.

173. Kinnula VL, Adler KB, Ackley NJ, Crapo JD. Release of reactive oxygen species by guinea pig tracheal epithelial cells in vitro. Am J Physiol 1992; 262:L708–L712.

174. McIntosh K. Interferon in nasal secretions from infants with viral respiratory tract infections. J Pediatr 1978; 93:33–36.

175. Harmon AT, Harmon MW, Glezen WP. Evidence of interferon production in the hamster lung after primary or secondary exposure to parainfluenza virus type 3. Am Rev Respir Dis 1982; 125:706–711.

176. Fitzpatrick FA, Stringfellow DA. Virus and interferon effects on cellular prostaglandin biosynthesis. J Immunol 1980; 125:431–437.
177. Rengasamy A, Johns RA. Regulation of nitric oxide synthase by nitric oxide. Mol Pharmacol 1993; 44:124–128.
178. De Kimpe SJ, Van Heuven-Nolsen D, Van Amsterdam JGC, Radomski MW, Nijkamp FP. Induction of nitric oxide release by interferon-γ inhibits vasodilation and cyclic GMP increase in bovine isolated mesenteric arteries. J Pharmacol Exp Ther 1994; 268:910–915.

# 8

# Role of Allergy and Airway Hyperresponsiveness in Virus-Induced Asthma

**JAMES E. GERN, ROBERT F. LEMANSKE, Jr., and WILLIAM W. BUSSE**

University of Wisconsin Medical School
Madison, Wisconsin

## I. Epidemiology of Viral Infections and Asthma

### A. Infants

Viral respiratory infections can profoundly influence airway function and asthma through two distinct pathways (Fig. 1). First, in infancy, infections with respiratory viruses, particularly respiratory syncytial virus (RSV), can provoke episodes of wheezing, which can be recurrent (Fig. 1A). Infants with reduced lung function are at greatest risk for developing wheezing with RSV infection (1), yet only a subset of wheezing infants will go on to develop persistent asthma. Risk factors for the development of persistent asthma after wheezing in infancy include an elevated serum IgE level at the age of 9 months and the development of allergen-specific IgE (2), suggesting that atopy may influence pulmonary physiology after wheezing induced by viral infection.

There are also data to suggest that RSV infections that cause wheezing may increase the risk of allergen sensitization. For example, Sigurs and colleagues prospectively identified infants with wheezing RSV infections requiring hospitalization and a control group of normal infants (3). Upon reevaluation at the age of 3 years, infants who had wheezing illnesses due to RSV were more likely to have allergen-specific IgE (32% vs. 9%) and asthma (23% vs. 1%), defined as

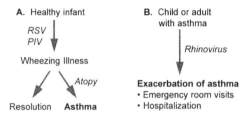

**Figure 1**   The relationship between viral infections and asthma (see text).

three or more episodes of wheezing, even though the groups had similar family histories of atopy and asthma. Although not all studies have found that RSV increases the risk of allergy (4,5), these findings, if confirmed, suggest that severe RSV infections in infancy can modify the immune response induced by subsequent exposure to allergens. Given the close relationship between allergen sensitization and the development of asthma, early exposure to respiratory viruses could also be an important factor in determining whether asthma develops.

### B.   Children and Adults

In children or adults with existing asthma (Fig. 1B), respiratory viruses frequently cause exacerbations of asthma (6–9). Initial studies designed to establish this relationship identified respiratory pathogens in association with wheezing episodes by serology or culture (7,10). However, many of the respiratory viruses, particularly rhinovirus (RV), are difficult to culture. The use of reverse transcription–polymerase chain reaction (RT-PCR) assays, which are much more sensitive for detecting RV than standard cell culture techniques (11,12), has underscored the importance of RV in causing exacerbations of asthma. For example, Johnston and colleagues determined that 80–85% of school-aged children with wheezing episodes tested positive for a virus, and the virus most commonly detected was rhinovirus (8). In adults with asthma, Nicholson and colleagues used similar techniques to demonstrate that 44% of severe and 54% of less severe episodes of wheezing were associated with RV infection (9). Moreover, virus-induced asthma may be severe: seasonal patterns of upper respiratory virus prevalence correlate closely with hospital admissions for asthma, especially in children (13). Furthermore, RV and other respiratory viruses are frequently detected in children hospitalized for asthma (12). Together, these studies indicate that RV infections are the most common cause of asthma exacerbations in children and also contribute substantially to the morbidity of asthma in adults.

In addition to epidemiological studies linking respiratory viral infections to exacerbations of asthma, there is clinical evidence that implicates that respiratory allergies are a risk factor for developing lower airway effects during infections with common cold viruses. For example, Duff and colleagues evaluated risk factors for wheezing in infants and children that presented to a hospital emergency department (14). Wheezing children older than 2 years of age were more likely to have respiratory allergies (odds ratio [OR] = 4.5) or have a confirmed viral infection (OR = 3.7) compared to children without wheezing. Children with the greatest risk (OR = 10.8) for wheezing were those who had both respiratory allergies and a viral infection. These findings indicated that viral infections and respiratory allergies may have synergistic inflammatory effects on lower airway physiology that greatly increase the likelihood of wheezing.

Together, these studies indicate that respiratory viral infections frequently trigger bronchospasm in patients with asthma and suggest that there may be specific interactions between respiratory allergy and viral infections to either initiate or propagate this process. Since bronchospasm in asthma is a result of airway inflammation and hyperresponsiveness, the effects of viral infections on these conditions are of special interest. In this chapter, we will explore potential mechanisms by which respiratory viruses, and particularly RV, enhance airway responsiveness and/or inflammation in the context of asthma.

## II. Interactions Between Viruses and Allergy

### A. Studies of the Upper Airway

Allergic inflammation in the upper airway shares many features with bronchial inflammation in asthma and provides a convenient model to study interactions between respiratory viruses and allergy. Two groups of investigators have experimentally infected adult volunteers with RV to test the hypothesis that individuals with respiratory allergies develop more severe symptoms during viral upper respiratory infection (URI). Bardin and colleagues inoculated 22 subjects (11 nonatopic, 5 atopic, and 6 both atopic and asthmatic) with type 16 RV (RV16), and 17 individuals developed clinical colds (15). There were no differences between atopic and nonatopic subjects in terms of viral shedding or symptom scores, and IgE levels did not correlate with the severity of the cold. One difference between the groups was their susceptibility to RV infection. Although the study was intended to include only subjects who lacked RV16-neutralizing antibody, 10 subjects unexpectedly developed virus-specific antibody between the screening visit and time of viral inoculation. In contrast to the normal control subjects, those with atopy developed severe colds despite the presence of neutralizing antibody. These data suggest that atopic individuals may be more susceptible to RV infection.

Doyle and colleagues experimentally infected atopic and nonatopic volunteers with a different RV serotype, RV39 (16). In 38 subjects studied outside of the pollen season, all were successfully infected as indicated by viral shedding after inoculation, and all but 6 developed typical cold symptoms. Although allergic individuals developed cold symptoms slightly earlier, there were no differences in the severity of symptoms between the two groups. The effect of RV infection on nasal responsiveness was studied in these same subjects by performing paired histamine provocation tests 2 months before and then again 8–13 days after RV inoculation. RV infection increased sneezing, weight of secretions, and rhinorrhea after nasal histamine challenge in both allergic and nonallergic subjects, and there were no differences between the two groups (17). Although the clinical symptoms were similar, there were some allergy-related differences in the systemic immune response to RV infection. For example, total IgE levels rose significantly in atopic subjects, but not in controls (18). In addition, peripheral blood mononuclear cells from allergic subjects had a lower baseline proliferative response to RV39, but both groups had vigorous responses 3 weeks after viral inoculation (19).

The upper airway provides a readily accessible model that can be used to study interactions between atopy and viral infections, and together these studies of experimentally infected volunteers have provided clues regarding lower airway pathology in virus-induced exacerbations of asthma. In the absence of allergen exposure, RV39 infection produced similar intensity of cold symptoms in allergic and nonallergic individuals. Several features of RV infection, however, were distinct in allergic individuals. First, allergy may increase susceptibility to RV infection and is possibly related to increased expression of ICAM-1, the cellular receptor for 90% of RV serotypes, by nasal epithelial cells in allergic rhinitis. Second, acute RV infection in allergic subjects increased serum levels of total IgE, and there is convincing evidence to link total IgE to both asthma prevalence and severity (20,21). A key question yet to be addressed by studies of the upper airway is whether RV infection alters the airway response to allergen exposure. If RV infection does amplify allergen-induced responses, this interaction could contribute to increased airway inflammation and respiratory symptoms.

### B.  Studies of the Lower Airway

To study the effect of RV infection on lower airway physiology, we conducted a study involving 10 patients with allergic rhinitis (22). None of the subjects had detectable levels of neutralizing antibody specific for RV16, which was the virus used for inoculation. Baseline measures of pulmonary function were measured along with assessments of airway responses to inhaled histamine and the immediate and late reactions to inhaled allergen. Four weeks after initial evaluations, the subjects were inoculated with RV16. Airway physiology was retested 48 hours later, near the peak of the subjects' cold symptoms.

In subjects inoculated with RV16, there was an increase in airway responsiveness to histamine at the time of the acute viral respiratory infection. An increase in lower airway responsiveness during viral respiratory infections has also been noted with other viruses (23–25) and in some (26–28) but not all (29,30) other studies with RV. In addition, RV infection increased the immediate response to allergen, as indicated by the decrease in the concentration of allergen required to drop the $FEV_1$ by 20%. In addition to enhancing the early response to allergen, RV infection increased the probability of late asthmatic reaction (LAR). Before virus inoculation, only one subject had a LAR to inhaled antigen as indicated by a drop in $FEV_1$ of greater than 15% approximately 4–6 hours post–allergen challenge. However, at the time of the viral respiratory infection, 8 of the 10 subjects developed a LAR after allergen challenge. Furthermore, when 7 of these individuals were evaluated 4 weeks later, 5 continued to manifest the LAR.

To determine the effects of RV infection on mast cell and basophil mediator release, we performed a second study of similar design involving eight additional subjects (31). Airway responsiveness to histamine, methacholine, and allergen were again increased during RV infection, and this effect was most pronounced in the subset of patients that developed a LAR after allergen inhalation. Furthermore, those patients that developed a LAR to allergen after RV infection also had an enhanced increase in plasma histamine levels after the inhaled allergen challenge.

Thus, our observations showed that RV infection not only increased airway responsiveness, but also changed the pattern of the allergic airway response. During RV infection, patients exhibited an increase in airway reactivity and had a greater likelihood of developing a late asthmatic reaction after exposure to allergen. These findings raise the possibility that RV infections increase the intensity of those factors provoked by allergen inhalation that determine and regulate the lower airway responsiveness and inflammation.

Cheung and colleagues have extended these results by inoculating 14 subjects with mild asthma with either RV16 or placebo and then measuring effects on pulmonary function and methacholine responsiveness (32). Airway hyperresponsiveness (AHR) increased during the acute infection in the seven subjects who were given RV16, and returned to baseline levels by one week after the inoculation. The maximal response to inhaled methacholine was significantly greater during the acute RV16 infection but, in contrast to AHR, remained elevated 7 and 15 days after inoculation (Fig. 2). These results indicate that RV infections can enhance both the sensitivity of the lower airway and the magnitude of bronchoconstriction in response to inhaled irritants in asthma and that these effects can persist for weeks after the acute infection.

### C. The Use of Animal Models to Determine the Mechanisms of Virus-Induced Airway Hyperresponsiveness

To study the effects of virus infection on airway physiology, a number of mammalian species have been studied including the guinea pig (33–37), ferret (38),

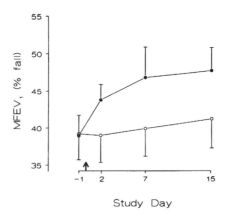

Study Day

**Figure 2** The maximal response to inhaled methacholine (MFEV$_1$, mean $\pm$ SEM) in subjects inoculated with RV16 (closed circles) or placebo (open circles). The arrow indicates placebo or virus inoculation. In the virus-treated group, there was a significant increase in MFEV$_1$ on days 2, 7, and 15 after inoculation as compared with the values at entry ($p = 0.009$). (From Ref. 32.)

dog (39), mouse (40–44) and rat (45–52). Although the precise mechanism by which viruses can enhance airway hyperresponsiveness is unknown, a number of factors have been observed that may be relevant to these changes. First, airway tone could be enhanced due to effects on sympathetic (40), parasympathetic (47,53), or noncholinergic/nonadrenergic (NANC) (35,38) pathways. The parasympathetic pathway could be upregulated through inhibitory effects of the virus on M$_2$ receptor feedback inhibition of acetylcholine release from postganglionic neurons (37). The NANC system could contribute through the downregulation of neutral endopeptidase activity, which would leave neurokinin (substance P) procontractile activity of bronchial smooth muscle unopposed (35,37).

Second, tissue inflammation may also play a role. Virus-induced airway hyperresponsiveness can be passively transferred in vitro using bronchial alveolar lavage cells from infected guinea pigs (36). Depletion of leukocytes with cyclophosphamide partially reverses viral effects on blockade of M$_2$ muscarinic receptors, suggesting that both the virus and the inflammatory response to the virus contribute to parasympathetic dysfunction (53). In addition, treatment of guinea pigs with anti-IL-5 monoclonal antibody before inoculation with parainfluenza virus prevents the development of hyperresponsiveness. These effects may be related to the production of cytokines, such as IL-5, IL-11, and TGF-$\beta$, which may influence airway tone, responsiveness, or remodeling (48,54,55). Nitric oxide (NO) may be an important mediator in virus-induced hyperresponsiveness, as administering the NO precursor L-arginine to parainfluenza virus–infected guinea pigs prevented AHR (56). Alternately, it has been suggested that viral infection could increase histamine-induced airway responsiveness by reducing the activity of histamine methyltransferase, an enzyme in respiratory epithelial cells that modulates contractile responses to histamine (57). Finally, respiratory infections may enhance neurogenic inflammation, which may secondarily affect airway responses by alterations in airway geometry (51,52). Together, these animal models of viral infections suggest a number of mechanisms that could lead to increased AHR. Additional studies are needed to determine which of these potential mechanisms contribute to AHR and/or exacerbations of asthma in humans.

### D. The Use of Bronchoscopy to Study Airway Responses to Allergen

Determining the biology of the airway response to inhaled allergen is very difficult without the direct sampling of airway secretions and tissues. Based on previous observations, we hypothesized that RV infections promote the development of the allergic reaction by increasing those factors involved in producing both the immediate and late-phase reactions to allergen. To evaluate this possibility, both normal and allergic rhinitis patients without serological evidence of RV16 infection were identified, and lower airway responses to allergen were measured one month before, during, and one month after an experimental RV infection (27). Bronchoscopy was performed on two occasions separated by 48 hours during each phase of the study (Fig. 3). At the first occasion, segmental allergen challenge was performed and lavage fluid analyzed for mast cell mediator release products. Forty-eight hours later, the same segments were lavaged and their contents analyzed for mediators and cellular components. Four to six weeks later, the subjects were experimentally infected with RV16, and the bronchoscopic procedures were repeated. The duration of RV-induced changes was determined by performing one last set of studies 4–6 weeks after the RV infection.

Infection with RV16 enhanced both the early and late response to segmental antigen challenge. During the acute RV infection, subjects with allergic rhinitis had an increased release of histamine after allergen challenge (Fig. 4). Interestingly, this increased secretion of histamine was still noted 4–6 weeks after the RV infection. In addition, RV infection produced changes in the recruitment of inflammatory cells into the airway 48 hours after allergen challenge. In allergic individuals infected with RV, there was an increase in airway leukocytes, and these cells were predominantly eosinophils (Fig. 5). Furthermore, in preliminary evaluations, we also detected increased lower airway levels of tumor necrosis factor-$\alpha$ (TNF-$\alpha$) in association with the RV infection. Thus, these data show that RV infection may intensify both the immediate and late responses to allergen

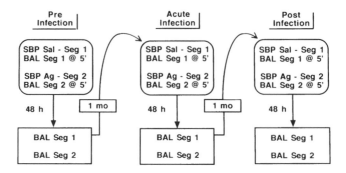

**Figure 3**  Experimental design: the pulmonary response to antigen challenge was examined during three study periods—1 month before (preinfection), during (acute infection), and 1 month after (postinfection) experimental infection with RV16. On the first 2 days in each period, a bronchoscopy was performed and segmental challenge with saline was accomplished, followed by bronchoalveolar lavage (BAL) 5 minutes later. Segmental challenge with antigen and subsequent BAL were then performed similarly in a separate bronchopulmonary segment. Forty-eight hours later, the two segments were lavaged again. (From Ref. 27.)

challenge, and this is accompanied by increasing mast cell or basophil mediator release and the recruitment of eosinophils to the lower airway.

### E.  Does RV Infection Cause Increased Lower Airway Responses in Allergic Individuals?

Since AHR is a key feature of asthma, several studies have addressed the possibility that RV infections may enhance AHR to a greater degree in the presence of allergy or asthma. The effect of naturally occurring colds on AHR in atopic versus nonatopic subjects was evaluated by Trigg and associates, who evaluated 15 volunteers with allergic rhinitis and 15 matched controls over a 9-month period of time (58). Twenty clinical ''colds'' were reported, but viruses were detected on only eight occasions, and only three of these episodes were associated with RV infection, precluding subgroup analysis.

Experimental infection provides an opportunity to perform detailed measurements of airway physiology under controlled conditions and evaluate separate effects of allergy and viral infection. We experimentally infected (RV16) 18 volunteers with allergic rhinitis and 13 normal controls and measured effects on the lower airway response to histamine (59). All subjects were successfully infected, as indicated by increased upper respiratory symptoms and culture of RV16 from nasal secretions. The change in histamine $PD_{20}$ ($\Delta PD_{20}$) caused by RV infection was significantly different in allergic subjects compared to nonallergic controls

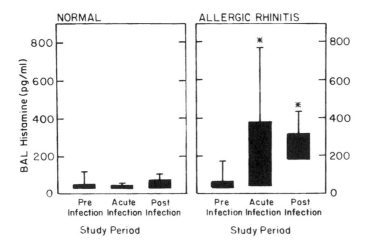

**Figure 4** BAL histamine concentrations 48 hours after segmental antigen challenge in subjects experimentally infected with RV16. Data for normal subjects ($n = 5$) and those with allergic rhinitis ($n = 7$) are shown separately, and whisker bars represent the 5th and 95th percentiles. For subjects with allergic rhinitis, there was a significant potentiating effect of RV16 infection (*$p < 0.001$, ANOVA), with higher histamine concentrations observed during the acute infection and postinfection periods compared with preinfection. (From Ref. 27.)

($\Delta PD_{20} = -0.40$ vs. $-0.03$ log units; $p = 0.04$) (Fig. 6). This relationship was strengthened after adjusting for initial $PD_{20}$ and $FEV_1$ (mean $\Delta PD_{20} = -0.43$ vs. $0.01$ log units; $p < 0.01$). The virus-induced $\Delta PD_{20}$ was also influenced by baseline lung function: there was a positive correlation between initial $FEV_1$ and $\Delta PD_{20}$, indicating that RV16 tended to increase the sensitivity to methacholine in subjects with lower baseline $FEV_1$.

Fraenkel and colleagues experimentally infected 17 volunteers, including 6 with atopic asthma and 11 normal controls, with RV16, and then measured effects on bronchial responses to histamine 5 days after inoculation (28). Although RV infection increased histamine responsiveness in the group as a whole, subgroup analyses suggested that the response of the allergic/asthmatic and normal control subgroups may have been different. When analyzed separately, subjects with allergic asthma had a significant increase in histamine responsiveness, but this was not the case with the normal controls. In a second study by the same group, experimental infection with RV16 increased AHR in a group of 25 subjects (60). Subgroup analysis, however, revealed that AHR was selectively enhanced in the 17 atopic subjects, and not in the 8 nonatopic subjects. Together, these studies suggest that host factors such as allergy and baseline $FEV_1$ influence

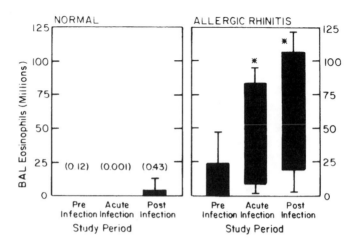

**Figure 5**  BAL eosinophils 48 hours after segmental antigen challenge in subjects experimentally infected with RV16. Data for normal subjects ($n = 5$) and those with allergic rhinitis ($n = 7$) are shown separately, and whisker bars represent the 5th and 95th percentiles. Eosinophil recruitment was low in normal subjects during all periods, and median values are shown in parentheses. For the subjects with allergic rhinitis, eosinophil recruitment was potentiated by RV16 during the acute infection and postinfection periods when compared with preinfection (*$p < 0.005$, ANOVA). (From Ref. 27.)

the changes in lower airway physiology caused by RV infection and raise the possibility that these factors contribute to the increased lower airway effects of RV infection in subjects with asthma.

Not all studies utilizing experimental RV infection have found consistent effects on AHR. For example, Halperin et al. infected 19 asthmatic volunteers with one of two RV serotypes (RV39 and Hanks serotype) and found changes in airway responsiveness to histamine in only four of these subjects (61). Interestingly, the four subjects who developed increased bronchial responsiveness during RV infection also had significant drops (>10%) in $FEV_1$, indicating that increased histamine responsiveness during viral infection may be related to clinically significant changes in airway obstruction. Skoner and colleagues examined effects of allergy on methacholine responsiveness in 31 subjects with allergic rhinitis and 27 normal controls experimentally infected with the same RV serotypes used by Halperin and found no effect of RV infection on airway responsiveness in either group 4 and 7 days after inoculation (62). In a third study utilizing RV2, Summers and colleagues likewise found no changes in AHR regardless of allergy status (63).

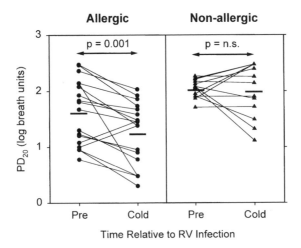

**Figure 6** Effect of allergy on RV16-induced changes in lower airway histamine responsiveness. Subjects were grouped according to the presence or absence of allergy, and histamine $PD_{20}$ was plotted precold (pre) and 2 days following RV16 inoculation (cold). Heavy horizontal lines represent group mean data. (From Ref. 59.)

The reasons for the relative lack of lower airway effects in these latter studies are unknown but may be related to differences in host factors, the inoculation technique, the timing of the histamine challenge, the viral inocula, or the severity of the induced colds. The selection criteria for study subjects are likely to greatly influence the outcome of experimental RV infections. For ethical reasons, children with a history of virus-induced exacerbations of asthma, who are the group most likely to develop lower airway changes with experimentally induced infections, are specifically excluded from such studies. It is also possible that there are differences in the pathogenicity of different RV serotypes, because lower airway changes have generally been observed with RV16 but less often with RV39 or RV2. It should be noted, however, that a large number of RV serotypes can affect the lower airway during natural infections: more than 30 serotypes have been cultured from patients with concurrent acute asthma symptoms and upper respiratory infection (10). This indicates that although some serotypes may indeed be more likely to induce wheezing in asthma, this property is not confined to a small subset of highly pathogenic serotypes.

One major difference between natural and experimental RV infection is in the use of laboratory-adapted RV isolates. Rhinoviruses have a high spontaneous mutation rate (64) and are particularly likely to become adapted to tissue culture conditions, leading to attenuation of pathogenicity. Indeed, this effect has long been recognized in other picornaviruses. For example, the trivalent oral polio vaccine contains a naturally attenuated strain of a type 2 poliovirus, but other isolates of this same virus are extremely virulent (65). Some of the RV isolates used to experimentally induce infection produce relatively mild colds and may have become attenuated by passage in cell lines. Since subclinical or very mild infections generally do not cause lower airway effects (66,67), this makes it difficult to induce lower airway effects using experimental infection.

Given these observations, it is evident that there are fundamental differences between artificially induced and naturally occurring RV infections and that these differences can influence viral effects on lower airway physiology. Under conditions that produce increased airway hyperresponsiveness, however, studies from our group and others suggest that the baseline $FEV_1$ value and the presence of atopy may be important determinants of the lower airway response to RV infection. Given the positive correlation between $PD_{20}$ and symptom scores in asthma (68), selective increases in bronchial responsiveness in allergic individuals with baseline airway obstruction could provide a mechanism for the increased lower airway symptoms experienced by asthmatic individuals during community-acquired RV infection.

## III. Possible Mechanisms for Interaction of Viral Infection and Allergy

### A. Is RV a Lower Airway Pathogen?

Why RV infections produce only upper airway symptoms in most people but frequently cause severe lower airway symptoms in patients with asthma has not yet been established. Other respiratory viruses that are associated with wheezing illnesses, such as influenza and parainfluenza infections, replicate in the lower airway and through this mechanism may cause changes in lung function. It remains to be established, however, whether or not RV infections extend into the lower airway during exacerbations of asthma and whether this is a mechanism of increased asthma severity. If RV infection does involve the lower airway, this suggests that viral replication in the lower airway could trigger a local inflammatory response and directly enhance preexisting airway inflammation. Alternatively, RV infection could be confined to the upper airway in asthma and symptoms could be increased through remote mechanisms (69).

The former scenario seems more likely, however, and this is based on several studies that support the concept that RV is a lower airway pathogen. For example, some (70–72), but not all (73,74), epidemiological studies have linked RV with lower airway syndromes such as bronchitis, bronchiolitis, and pneumonia. There are also well-documented reports of fatal RV pneumonia in children, including a case in which RV was recovered from lung tissue at autopsy (75). In addition, RV is frequently detected in the nasal secretions of elderly individuals with lower respiratory symptoms (76). Finally, although RV has proven difficult to culture from lower airway secretions obtained via bronchoalveolar lavage (BAL), we detected RV16 RNA in BAL cells from eight experimentally infected volunteers 48–96 hours after inoculation (77). These data indicate that, at least under some conditions, RV infections extend into the lower airway and suggest that replication of RV in bronchial epithelial cells and the induction of local inflammation contributes to the pathogenesis of virus-induced exacerbations of asthma.

### B. How Does RV Cause Respiratory Symptoms?

Although the precise mechanisms by which RV causes respiratory symptoms are unknown, there is an increasing body of evidence suggesting that the immune response induced by the virus plays a major role in symptom pathogenesis. First, unlike influenza or RSV infections, RV infections are not associated with extensive epithelial cell destruction (78). Second, several investigators have found that levels of mediators (kinins) or cytokines [interleukin (IL)-1, IL-8, IL-11] correlate with the severity of respiratory symptoms (79–82). Whether these factors are participating in symptom pathogenesis or are markers of inflammatory cell activation has not yet been established. Since cytokines are major regulators of inflammation associated with respiratory allergies and asthma, it seems likely that virus-induced cytokines secreted by lower airway cells could have profound effects on existing airway inflammation and consequently lung physiology.

### C. Potential Interactions Between Immune Responses to Allergens and Viruses

*Contributions of Airway Cells*

It is attractive to hypothesize that there are specific interactions between the immune responses induced by allergens and viruses, leading to amplification of preexisting airway inflammation and thus increased respiratory symptoms. The immune responses to viruses and allergens are complex, and both involve multiple airway cells and mediators. Several cells are of particular interest in the context of virus-induced exacerbations.

*Epithelial Cells*

The respiratory epithelial cell is the host cell for RV replication, and the degree of RV replication in the epithelial cell strongly influences the severity of respiratory symptoms associated with RV colds. Viral titers in nasal secretions correlate with the severity of cold symptoms (59), and during asthma exacerbations lower respiratory symptoms are worse in patients with severe URI symptoms (66,67). Moreover, the epithelial cell, once regarded as a passive host for respiratory virus infection, is now recognized as playing an active and important role in airway immune responses through secretion of a broad array of cytokines and mediators with chemotactic and inflammatory effects. Studies of epithelial cells or cell lines indicate that in vitro inoculation with RV induces secretion of IL-1, IL-6, IL-8, IL-11, RANTES, and GM-CSF (80,83–86). Several of these cytokines have profound effects on inflammatory cells that can potentiate asthma. For example, RANTES is a chemoattractant for eosinophils and memory T cells, both of which are important effector cells in asthmatic airway inflammation (87,88). Furthermore, GM-CSF is a potent activator of eosinophil survival and adhesion molecule expression and is a cofactor for eosinophil superoxide production and degranulation (89–91). IL-11 is secreted in very large amounts after epithelial cells are infected with RV or RSV in vitro and may have direct effects on bronchial hyperresponsiveness (55,80).

## T Lymphocytes

T-cell responses may be of particular importance because of their central role in orchestrating immune responses to both allergens and viruses through the regulation of effector cells that are virucidal and/or cause airway inflammation. Allergens and viral infections generally induce distinct types of T-cell immune responses. Allergy is associated with a Th2-like response with secretion of cytokines such as IL-4 and IL-5. These cytokines enhance IgE production and eosinophil activation, respectively. In contrast, viral infections typically induce IFN-$\alpha$ production by mononuclear cells and a Th1-like response characterized by secretion of IFN-$\gamma$ by activated T cells. These cytokines play an important role in the clearance of respiratory viruses: IFN-$\alpha$ inhibits viral replication in epithelial cells, which are the principal host cells for respiratory viruses, and IFN-$\gamma$ enhances the antiviral activities of a wide variety of other effector cells including the macrophage, neutrophil, and cytolytic T cell.

These two types of T-cell responses tend to be mutually antagonistic, and this increases the probability of significant interactions between allergen and virus-induced T-cell responses. For example, IL-4, which may be induced by exposure to allergen, inhibits the generation of Th1-like immunity and secretion of IFN-$\gamma$. The ability of IL-4 to modulate antiviral immunity has been demonstrated in a mouse model of RSV infection: administration of an IL-4–specific monoclonal antibody to RSV-infected mice produced greater cytotoxic T-cell activity and reduced viral replication and severity of illness (92). Experiments performed by Coyle and colleagues provide additional evidence that IL-4 and allergic responses can modify the response to viral infection (93). This group developed transgenic mice in which a large percentage of CD8[+] T cells expressed an MHC molecule specific for a viral [lymphocytic choriomeningitis virus (LCMV)] peptide. The mice were either sham-immunized or sensitized to ovalbumin, and then the LCMV glycoprotein peptide was administered intranasally. Lung T cells obtained 72 hours later were restimulated with LCMV peptide in vitro, and cytokine secretion was analyzed. Ovalbumin-sensitized mice had a very different pattern of cytokine secretion, with increased IL-5 and decreased IFN-$\gamma$ compared to control mice. Furthermore, these changes in the virus-specific immune responses were reproduced in vitro by incubating virus-specific CD8$^+$ T cells with viral peptide in the presence of IL-4. These data suggest that the immune response to viral infections can be modulated by environmental influences such as allergen sensitization and that these effects may be caused by alterations in the cytokine milieu at the time of viral infection.

### Granulocytes

Data are beginning to accumulate to suggest that the granulocyte response to viral infection in the airways of allergic or asthmatic individuals may have some distinct features. For example, neutrophil counts in peripheral blood increase during the acute phase of RV infections, and they are the first cells recruited to the airways during RV infection (94,95). Furthermore, there is evidence that quantitative changes in peripheral blood neutrophil counts parallel changes in airway biology in subjects with asthma. Grunberg and colleagues experimentally inoculated 35 subjects with atopic asthma with either RV16 or placebo and measured effects on AHR, peripheral blood leukocyte counts, and IL-8 levels in nasal secretions (82). Neutrophil counts in the peripheral blood correlated with cold and asthma symptom scores and cold-induced changes in airway hyperresponsiveness.

Although the neutrophil is the primary cell recruited to the upper airway early during the course of rhinovirus infection in normal individuals, eosinophil granular proteins have been detected in the nasal secretions of children with wheezing illnesses caused by RV or respiratory syncytial virus (RSV) (96,97). In addition, experimental RV infection induces increased eosinophils in the bronchial epithelium, and this eosinophilia persists into convalescence in subjects with asthma, but not in normal control subjects (28). Furthermore, there is evidence that the eosinophil may disturb airway physiology in an animal model of respiratory virus infection. Van Oosterhout and colleagues found that in the guinea pig, parainfluenza virus–induced airway hyperresponsiveness was blocked by an antibody specific for IL-5, a potent activator of eosinophil inflammatory functions (98). Together, these studies provide evidence that viral infections can trigger increased recruitment and activation of eosinophils and neutrophils and suggest that granulocytes contribute to virus-induced airway hyperresponsiveness and/or airway dysfunction. Additional studies will be needed to more precisely define the role of granulocytes in the pathogenesis of RV-induced respiratory symptoms.

## Macrophages

Airway macrophages are likely to be involved in antiviral immune responses because they express ICAM-1, the receptor for major group RV, have been shown to bind RV in vitro, and secrete cytokines that have antiviral (IFN-$\alpha$) and/or proinflammatory (IL-1, TNF-$\alpha$) effects (99,100). Nasal secretions of RV-infected volunteers or children with naturally acquired upper respiratory infections contain IL-1 (81,101), which can cause systemic symptoms such as fever and malaise that are commonly associated with RV colds in children. In addition, airway macrophages incubated with RV in vitro secrete TNF-$\alpha$ (99), this cytokine can increase the expression of ICAM-1 and other adhesion molecule expression on a number of different cell types (102), and its presence has been closely associated with wheezing illnesses in infancy (103) and the development of the late-phase allergic reaction and asthma (104,105). TNF-$\alpha$ also increases the susceptibility of an epithelial cell line (BEAS2B) to become infected with major group RV, and probably accomplishes this action by increasing the expression of ICAM-1 receptors (85). Thus, macrophages have the capacity to contribute to early antiviral immune responses but also could increase airway inflammation, leading to increased respiratory symptoms.

### *Contribution of Virus-Induced Cytokines to Enhanced Airway Inflammation*

Although in vitro investigations and studies of nasal secretions in patients with upper respiratory infections and/or asthma have provided a list of factors that may be involved in the pathogenesis of respiratory symptoms, there are limited data comparing the immune response to naturally acquired respiratory viral infections in normal individuals versus those with asthma. There are at least three mechanisms through which virus-induced cytokines might enhance airway inflammation and respiratory symptoms in asthma (Fig. 7). First, it is possible that viral infections induce different cytokines, with greater inflammatory effects, in patients with asthma. Second, viral infections may produce the same inflammatory cytokines in both groups, but in greater quantities in patients with asthma. Finally, the cytokine response to viral infection could be the same in patients with or without asthma, but the cytokines could have greater inflammatory effects in asthma due to existing differences in the types of cells present in the airway (i.e., more eosinophils) or differences in the activation state of airway cells.

In the first potential mechanism (Fig. 7A), T cells of allergic and nonallergic individuals secrete different cytokines in response to respiratory virus proteins, paralleling the differences in T-cell responses to allergen in allergic versus normal individuals. Viral infections are generally regarded as potent inducers of "Th1-type" cytokines such as IFN-$\gamma$ and IL-2, which enhance cell-mediated responses that clear virus from the respiratory tract. It has been proposed that

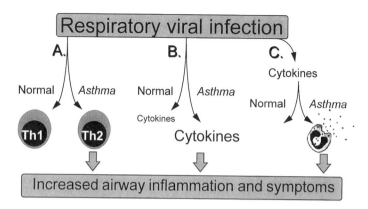

**Figure 7** Potential mechanisms for increased lower airway manifestations of viral infections in asthma (see text).

some viruses may have evolved means of stimulating "Th2-type" responses, characterized by the secretion of IL-4, IL-5, and other cytokines that inhibit antiviral responses and potentiate allergic responses. In support of this theory, Openshaw and colleagues have found that the RSV attachment protein (protein G) induces a Th2-like immune response (106). Furthermore, mice that are sequentially given protein G–specific T cells followed by an RSV infection develop pulmonary eosinophilia and more severe lung disease (107). Virus-specific Th2 cells have not yet been detected in humans, but there is indirect evidence of their existence. For example, Welliver and colleagues detected virus-specific IgE in infants with RSV and parainfluenza infections, especially in cases associated with wheezing (108,109). Although it has not been established whether virus-specific IgE contributes to airway pathology, the presence of RSV-specific IgE suggests that the viral infection induced the production of IL-4 or IL-13, since one of these cytokines must be present for IgE synthesis to occur (110,111). Furthermore, Anderson and colleagues have used RT-PCR to measure cytokine mRNA in the RSV-inoculated peripheral blood of adults and children with evidence of previous RSV infection (112). Although IFN-$\gamma$ was the predominant cytokine detected, IL-5 mRNA was found in 6 of the 22 samples analyzed.

Jackson and Scott (113) expanded on these findings by developing T-cell lines from the peripheral blood cells of adults with serological evidence of previous RSV infection. Although T-cell lines specific for either live RSV or protein F had Th1-like cytokine secretion, those lines specific for either fixed RSV or protein G secreted mainly Th2 cytokines (IL-4 and IL-10). Although these results are intriguing and have obvious implications regarding the development of antiviral vaccines, it has yet to be determined whether there are situations in vivo in which the immune system is exposed to viral proteins in the absence of live virus.

There is less information regarding the cytokine-secretion patterns of RV-specific T cells. Our group isolated T-cell clones specific for one of two RV serotypes (RV16 or RV49) from the peripheral blood of a normal individual and a subject with asthma (114). Each of the 29 clones secreted high levels of IFN-γ, although a subset of clones also secreted relatively small amounts of IL-4 and/ or IL-5. Although the cytokine responses of these clones in vitro may not be representative of the global T-cell response to RV in vivo, these results suggest that the T-cell response to RV is Th1-like.

There are recent data suggesting that there may be quantitative differences in virus-induced cytokine secretion related to asthma (Fig. 7B). Einarsson and colleagues analyzed nasal secretions from patients with either upper respiratory symptoms or wheezing associated with a viral respiratory infection (80), and IL-11 levels in nasal secretions were significantly increased in the patients with wheezing (Fig. 8). IL-11 is of particular interest in light of two recent murine studies in which IL-11 administration to normal mice caused airway hyperresponsiveness (80), and targeted airway expression of IL-11 in transgenic mice caused airway inflammation and hyperresponsiveness (55).

In addition, Grunberg and colleagues analyzed IL-8 levels in the nasal secretions of volunteers with allergic asthma after experimental inoculation with

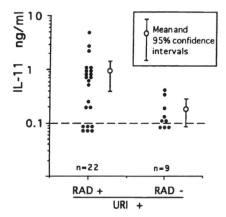

**Figure 8** IL-11 levels in the nasal aspirates from children with cold symptoms with and without clinical bronchospasm [reactive airways disease (RAD)]. The lower limit of sensitivity of the assay is illustrated with the dashed line. The means and 95% confidence intervals for each group are illustrated to the right of each column. (From Ref. 80.)

either RV16 or a placebo (82). IL-8 levels were increased in the nasal secretions of subjects that were inoculated with RV16 but not placebo. Furthermore, the quality of IL-8 detected 2 days after inoculation significantly correlated with cold and asthma symptom scores and with increases in airway hyperresponsiveness. Together with the Einarsson study, these data suggest that greater amounts of cytokines generated in respiratory viral infections are associated with adverse effects of the lower airway.

A third hypothesis to explain the association between viral infection and enhanced allergic responses is that viral infections induce similar types of cytokines in both normal and allergic or asthmatic airways, but differences in either the type of cells in the airway or the activation state of airway cells lead to enhanced airway inflammation in asthma (Fig. 7C). Although the cellular biology of asthma suggests several potential interactions, there are limited data to evaluate this hypothesis. Douglass and colleagues tested the effect of allergy on upper airway responses to topical application of recombinant IL-8 (115). IL-8 caused increased neutrophil influx and nasal symptoms in both groups, but although there were no statistically significant differences related to allergy, the data need to be interpreted with the following caveats. First, preliminary experiments revealed that IL-8 had little effect on airway physiology unless the airways were pretreated with histamine, and this was incorporated into the study design. This suggests that histamine in nasal secretions induced by mast cell or basophil degranulation in vivo may potentiate the effects of virus-induced IL-8 in the presence of acute or late-phase allergic inflammation. Second, IL-8 administration induced marked eosinophil influx in a few individuals in the atopic group, but not in the normal controls. Although the small sample size limited the interpretation of this phenomenon, this finding lends further support to the concept that inflammatory responses to virus-induced cytokines may be accentuated in the presence of allergy.

There is also in vitro evidence that the effects of cytokines may be enhanced in asthma. Although IL-8 was first reported to be a potent chemoattractant for neutrophils, IL-8 also attracts eosinophils under some conditions. For example, eosinophils from patients with asthma or those activated by preincubation with IL-5 have enhanced IL-8–induced chemotaxis (116–118). In addition, GM-CSF is also induced by respiratory viral infection (85) and has profound effects on eosinophil physiology, including enhanced mediator release and adhesion molecule expression and prolonged in vitro survival (90). It is thus reasonable to assume that virus-induced increases in GM-CSF secretion would have greater inflammatory effects in allergic or asthmatic airways that already contain eosinophils, either constitutively or following allergen-induced eosinophil recruitment. Finally, macrophages and lymphocytes from allergic and asthmatic airways are primed compared to the same cell types in nonallergic airways (119,120), thus, it is conceivable that these "activated" cells may also have enhanced inflammatory responses to virus-induced cytokines such as IL-1, IFN-$\alpha$, and IFN-$\gamma$.

## IV. Summary

Epidemiological data demonstrate that viral infections are the most important trigger for acute asthma symptoms in children, and this association persists in many adults with asthma. Studies of volunteers experimentally infected with RV suggest that atopy alone does not always predispose to unusually severe symptoms. In contrast, experimental models that combine viral infection and allergen exposure have identified potential links between virus- and allergen-induced inflammation and suggest several possible mechanisms by which virus-induced cytokines could enhance preexisting airway inflammation in asthma. While there is an increasing amount of information suggesting that cytokines may be an important part of this association, their role must be verified with additional studies comparing the upper and lower airway immune responses to viral infections in people with asthma versus normal controls.

### Acknowledgments

Supported by NIH Grants AI26609, AI40685, and HL44098.

### References

1. Martinez FD, Morgan WJ, Wright AL, Holberg CJ, Taussig LM. Diminished lung function as a predisposing factor for wheezing respiratory illness in infants. N Engl J Med 1988; 319:1112–1117.
2. Martinez FD, Wright AL, Taussig LM, et al. Asthma and wheezing in the first six years of life. N Engl J Med 1995; 332:133–138.
3. Sigurs N, Bjarnason R, Sigurbergsson F, Kjellman B, Bjorksten B. Asthma and immunoglobulin E antibodies after respiratory syncytial virus bronchiolitis: a prospective cohort study with matched controls. Pediatrics 1995; 95:500–505.
4. Cogswell JJ, Halliday DF, Alexander JR. Respiratory infections in the first year of life in children at risk of developing atopy. Br Med J 1982; 284:1011–1013.
5. Welliver RC. RSV and chronic asthma. Lancet 1995; 346:789–790.
6. Folkerts G, Busse WW, Nijkamp FP, Sorkness R, Gern JE. Virus-induced hyperresponsiveness and asthma. Am J Respir Crit Care Med 1998; 157:1708–1720.
7. Pattemore PK, Johnston SL, Bardin PG. Viruses as precipitants of asthma symptoms. I. Epidemiology. Clin Exp Allergy 1992; 22:325–336.
8. Johnston SL, Pattemore PK, Sanderson G, et al. Community study of role of viral infections in exacerbations of asthma in 9–11 year old children. Br Med J 1995; 310:1225–1229.
9. Nicholson KG, Kent J, Ireland DC. Respiratory viruses and exacerbations of asthma in adults. Br Med J 1993; 307:982–986.
10. Dick EC, Inhorn SL. Rhinoviruses. In: Feigin RD, Cherry JD, eds. Textbook of

Pediatric Infectious Diseases. 3rd ed. Philadelphia: W. B. Saunders Company, 1992:1507–1532.

11.  Gama RE, Horsnell PR, Hughes PJ, et al. Amplification of rhinovirus specific nucleic acids from clinical samples using the polymerase chain reaction. J Med Virol 1989; 28:73–77.

12.  Johnston SL, Xie P, Johnson W. Comparison of standard virology and PCR in diagnosis of rhinovirus and respiratory syncytial virus infections in nasal aspirates from children hospitalized with wheezing illness and bronchiolitis (abstr). Am J Respir Crit Care Med 1996; 153:A503.

13.  Johnston SL, Pattemore PK, Sanderson G, et al. The relationship between upper respiratory infections and hospital admissions for asthma: a time trend analysis. Am J Respir Crit Care Med 1996; 154:654–660.

14.  Duff AL, Pomeranz ES, Gelber LE, et al. Risk factors for acute wheezing in infants and children: viruses, passive smoke, and IgE antibodies to inhalant allergens. Pediatrics 1993; 92:535–540.

15.  Bardin PG, Fraenkel DJ, Sanderson G, et al. Amplified rhinovirus colds in atopic subjects. Clin Exp Allergy 1994; 24:457–464.

16.  Doyle WJ, Skoner DP, Fireman P, et al. Rhinovirus 39 infection in allergic and nonallergic subjects. J Allergy Clin Immunol 1992; 89:968–978.

17.  Doyle WJ, Skoner DP, Seroky JT, Fireman P, Gwaltney JM. Effect of experimental rhinovirus 39 infection on the nasal response to histamine and cold air challenges in allergic and nonallergic subjects. J Allergy Clin Immunol 1994; 93:534–542.

18.  Skoner DP, Doyle WJ, Tanner EP, Kiss J, Fireman P. Effect of rhinovirus 39 (RV-39) infection on immune and inflammatory parameters in allergic and non-allergic subjects. Clin Exp Allergy 1995; 25:561–567.

19.  Skoner DP, Whiteside TL, Wilson JW, Doyle WJ, Herberman RB, Fireman P. Effect of rhinovirus 39 infection on cellular immune parameters in allergic and nonallergic subjects. J Allergy Clin Immunol 1993; 92:732–743.

20.  Burrows B, Martinez FD, Halonen M, Barbee RA, Cline MG. Association of asthma with serum IgE levels and skin test reactivity to allergens. N Engl J Med 1989; 320:271–277.

21.  Sears MR, Burrows B, Flannery EM, Herbison GP, Hewitt CJ, Holdaway MD. Relation between airway responsiveness and serum IgE in children with asthma and in apparently normal children. N Engl J Med 1991; 325:1067–1071.

22.  Lemanske RF, Jr., Dick EC, Swenson CA, Vrtis RF, Busse WW. Rhinovirus upper respiratory infection increases airway hyperreactivity and late asthmatic reactions. J Clin Invest 1989; 83:1–10.

23.  Empey DW, Laitinen LA, Jacobs L, Gold WM, Nadel JA. Mechanisms of bronchial hyperreactivity in normal subjects after upper respiratory tract infection. Am Rev Respir Dis 1976; 113:131–139.

24.  Hall WJ, Hall CB, Speers DM. Respiratory syncytial virus in adults: clinical, virologic and serial pulmonary function studies. Ann Intern Med 1978; 88:203–205.

25.  Laitinen LA, Elkin RB, Empey DW, Jacobs L, Mills J, Nadel JA. Bronchial hyperresponsiveness in normal subjects during attenuated influenza virus infection. Am Rev Respir Dis 1991; 143:358–361.

26.  Blair HT, Greenberg SB, Stevens PM, Bilunos PA, Couch RB. Effects of rhinovirus

infection on pulmonary function of healthy human volunteers. Am Rev Respir Dis 1976;114:95–102.

27. Calhoun WJ, Dick EC, Schwartz LB, Busse WW. A common cold virus, rhinovirus 16, potentiates airway inflammation after segmental antigen bronchoprovocation in allergic subjects. J Clin Invest 1994; 94:2200–2208.

28. Fraenkel DJ, Bardin PG, Sanderson G, Lampe F, Johnston SL, Holgate ST. Lower airway inflammation during rhinovirus colds in normal and in asthmatic subjects. Am J Respir Crit Care Med 1995; 151:879–886.

29. Halperin SA, Eggleston PA, Hendley JO, Suratt PM, Gröschel DH, Gwaltney JMJ. Pathogenesis of lower respiratory tract symptoms in experimental rhinovirus infection. Am Rev Respir Dis 1983; 128:806–810.

30. Jenkins CR, Breslin ABX. Upper respiratory tract infections and airway reactivity in normal and asthmatic subjects. Am Rev Respir Dis 1984; 130:879–883.

31. Calhoun WJ, Swenson CA, Dick EC, Schwartz LB, Lemanske RF, Jr., Busse WW. Experimental rhinovirus 16 infection potentiates histamine release after antigen bronchoprovocation in allergic subjects. Am Rev Respir Dis 1991; 144:1267–1273.

32. Cheung D, Dick EC, Timmers MC, De Klerk EPA, Spaan WJM, Sterk PJ. Rhinovirus inhalation causes long-lasting excessive airway narrowing in response to methacholine in asthmatic subjects in vivo. Am J Respir Crit Care Med 1995; 152:1490–1496.

33. Saban R, Dick EC, Fishleder RI, Buckner CK. Enhancement by parainfluenza 3 infection of contractile responses to substance P and capsaicin in airway smooth muscle from the guinea pig. Am Rev Respir Dis 1987; 136:586–591.

34. Buckner CK, Songsiridej V, Dick EC, Busse WW. In vivo and in vitro studies on the use of the guinea pig as a model for virus-provoked airway hyperreactivity. Am Rev Respir Dis 1985; 132:305–310.

35. Dusser DJ, Jacoby DB, Djokic TD, Rubinstein I, Borson DB, Nadel JA. Virus induces airway hyperresponsiveness to tachykinins: role of neutral endopeptidase. J Appl Physiol 1989; 67:1504–1511.

36. Folkerts G, Verheyen A, Janssen M, Nijkamp FP. Virus-induced airway hyperresponsiveness in the guinea pig can be transferred by bronchoalveolar cells. J Allergy Clin Immunol 1992; 90:364–72.

37. Fryer AD, Jacoby DB. Parainfluenza virus infection damages inhibitory M2 muscarinic receptors on pulmonary parasympathetic nerves in the guinea pig. Br J Pharmacol 1991; 102:267–271.

38. Jacoby DB, Tamaoki J, Borson DB, Nadel JA. Influenza infection causes airway hyperresponsiveness by decreasing enkephalinase. J Appl Physiol 1988; 64:2653–2658.

39. Lemen RJ, Quan SF, Witten ML, Sobonya RE, Ray CG, Grad R. Canine parainfluenza type 2 bronchiolitis increases histamine responsiveness in beagle puppies. Am Rev Respir Dis 1990; 141:199–207.

40. Scarpace PJ, Bender BS. Viral pneumonia attenuates adenylate cyclase but not beta-adrenergic receptors in murine lung. Am Rev Respir Dis 1989; 140:1602–1606.

41. Allan W, Carding SR, Eichelberger M, Doherty PC. Analyzing the distribution of cells expressing mRNA for T-cell receptor gamma and delta chains in a virus-induced inflammatory process. Cell Immunol 1992; 143:55–65.

42. Scherle PA, Palladino G, Gerhard W. Mice can recover from pulmonary influenza virus infection in the absence of class I-restricted cytotoxic T cells. J Immunol 1992; 148:212–217.

43. Kimsey PB, Pecquet Goad ME, Zhi-bo Z, Brackee G, Fox JG. Methyl prednisolone acetate modulation of infection and subsequent pulmonary pathology in hamsters exposed to parainfluenza-1 virus (Sendai). Am Rev Respir Dis 1989; 140:1704–1711.

44. Hennet T, Ziltener HJ, Frei K, Peterhans E. A kinetic study of immune mediators in the lungs of mice infected with influenza-A virus. J Immunol 1992; 149:932–939.

45. Sorkness R, Lemanske RF, Jr., Castleman WL. Persistent airway hyperresponsiveness after neonatal viral bronchiolitis in rats. J Appl Physiol 1991; 70:375–383.

46. Castleman WL, Sorkness RL, Lemanske RF, Jr., McAllister PK. Viral bronchiolitis during early life induces increased numbers of bronchiolar mast cells and airway hyperresponsiveness. Am J Pathol 1990; 137:821–831.

47. Castleman WL, Sorkness RL, Lemanske RF, Jr., Grasee G, Suyemoto MM. Neonatal viral bronchiolitis and pneumonia induce bronchiolar hypoplasia and alveolar dysplasia in rats. Lab Invest 1988; 59:387–396.

48. Uhl EW, Castleman WL, Sorkness RL, Lemanske RF, McAllister PK. Parainfluenza virus-induced persistence of airway inflammation, fibrosis, and dysfunction associated with TGF-$\beta_1$ expression in Brown Norway rats. Am J Respir Crit Care Med 1996; 154:1834–1842.

49. Kumar A, Sorkness RL, Kaplan MR, Lemanske RF, Jr. Chronic, episodic, reversible airway obstruction after viral bronchiolitis in rats. Am J Respir Crit Care Med 1997; 155:130–134.

50. Sorkness R, Clough JJ, Castleman WL, Lemanske RF, Jr. Virus-induced airway obstruction and parasympathetic hyperresponsiveness in adult rats. Am J Respir Crit Care Med 1994; 150:28–34.

51. Piedimonte G, Nadel JA, Umeno E, Mcdonald DM. Sendai virus infection potentiates neurogenic inflammation in the rat trachea. J Appl Physiol 1990; 68:754–760.

52. McDonald DM. Respiratory tract infections increase susceptibility to neurogenic inflammation in the rat trachea. Am Rev Respir Dis 1988; 137:1432–1440.

53. Fryer AD, Yarkony KA, Jacoby DB. The effect of leukocyte depletion on pulmonary M(2) muscarinic receptor function in parainfluenza virus-infected guinea-pigs. Br J Pharmacol 1994; 112:588–594.

54. Oosterhout AJM, Nijkamp FP. Minireview: lymphocytes and bronchial hyperresponsiveness. Life Sci 1990; 46:1255–1264.

55. Tang W, Geba GP, Zheng T, et al. Targeted expression of IL-11 in the murine airway causes lymphocytic inflammation, bronchial remodeling, and airways obstruction. J Clin Invest 1996; 98:2845–2853.

56. Folkerts G, Vanderlinde HJ, Nijkamp FP. Virus-induced airway hyperresponsiveness in guinea rigs is related to a deficiency in nitric oxide. J Clin Invest 1995; 95:26–30.

57. Nakazawa H, Sekizawa K, Morikawa M, et al. Viral respiratory infection causes airway hyperresponsiveness and decreases histamine N-methyltransferase activity in guinea pigs. Am J Respir Crit Care Med 1994; 149:1180–1185.

58.  Trigg CJ, Nicholson KG, Wang JH, et al. Bronchial inflammation and the common cold: a comparison of atopic and non-atopic individuals. Clin Exp Allergy 1996; 26:665–676.

59.  Gern JE, Calhoun WJ, Swenson C, Shen G, Busse WW. Rhinovirus infection preferentially increases lower airway responsiveness in allergic subjects. Am J Respir Crit Care Med 1997; 155:1872–1876.

60.  Bardin PG, Sanderson G, Robinson BS, Holgate ST, Tyrrell DAJ. Experimental rhinovirus infection in volunteers. Eur Respir J 1996; 9:2250–2255.

61.  Halperin SA, Eggleston PA, Beasley P, et al. Exacerbations of asthma in adults during experimental rhinovirus infection. Am Rev Respir Dis 1985; 132:976–980.

62.  Skoner DP, Doyle WJ, Seroky J, Vandeusen MA, Fireman P. Lower airway responses to rhinovirus 39 in healthy allergic and nonallergic subjects. Eur Respir J 1996; 9:1402–1406.

63.  Summers QA, Higgins PG, Barrow IG, Tyrrell DA, Holgate ST. Bronchial reactivity to histamine and bradykinin is unchanged after rhinovirus infection in normal subjects. Eur Respir J 1992; 5:313–317.

64.  Rueckert RR. Picornaviridae and their replication. In: Fields BN, Knipe DM, Chanock RM, et al., eds. Virology. 2d ed. New York: Raven Press, 1990:507–546.

65.  Murphy BR, Chanock RM. Immunization against viruses. In: Fields BN, Knipe DM, Chanock RM, et al., eds. Virology. 2d ed. New York: Raven Press, 1990:469–506.

66.  Minor TE, Dick EC, DeMeo AN, Ouellette JJ, Cohen M, Reed CE. Viruses as precipitants of asthmatic attacks in children. JAMA 1974; 227:292–298.

67.  Minor TE, Dick EC, Baker JW, Ouellette JJ, Cohen M, Reed CE. Rhinovirus and influenza type A infections as precipitants of asthma. Am Rev Respir Dis 1976; 113:149–153.

68.  Gern JE, Eggleston PA, Schuberth KC, et al. Peak flow variation in childhood asthma: a three year analysis. J Allergy Clin Immunol 1994; 93:706–716.

69.  Bardin PG, Johnston SL, Pattemore PK. Viruses as precipitants of asthma symptoms. II. Physiology and mechanisms. Clin Exp Allergy 1992; 22:809–822.

70.  Kellner G, Popow-Kraupp T, Kundi M, Binder C, Kunz C. Clinical manifestations of respiratory tract infections due to respiratory syncytial virus and rhinoviruses in hospitalized children. Acta Paediatr Scand 1989; 78:390–394.

71.  Horn MEC, Brain E, Gregg I. Respiratory viral infections in childhood. A survey in general practice. J Hyg (Camb) 1974; 157:157–168.

72.  Monto AS, Cavallaro JJ. The Tecumseh study of respiratory illness II. Patterns of occurrence of infection with respiratory pathogens. Am J Epidemiol 1971; 94:280–289.

73.  Denny FW, Clyde WA, Jr. Acute lower respiratory tract infections in nonhospitalized children. J Pediatr 1986; 108:635–646.

74.  Henderson FW, Clyde WA, Jr., Collier AM, et al. The etiologic and epidemiologic spectrum of bronchiolitis in pediatric practice. J Pediatr 1979; 95:183–190.

75.  Las Heras J, Swanson VL. Sudden death of an infant with rhinovirus infection complicating bronchial asthma: case report. Pediatr Pathol 1983; 1:319–323.

76. Nicholson KG, Kent J, Hammersley V, Cancio E. Risk factors for lower respiratory complications of rhinovirus infections in elderly people living in the community: prospective cohort study. Br Med J 1996; 313:1119–1123.

77. Gern JE, Galagan DM, Jarjour NN, Dick EC, Busse WW. Detection of rhinovirus RNA in lower airway cells during experimentally-induced infection. Am J Respir Crit Care Med 1997; 155:1159–1161.

78. Winther B, Farr B, Thoner RB, Hendley JO, Mygrind N, Gwaltney JM. Histopathologic examination and enumeration of polymorphonuclear leukocytes in the nasal mucosa during experimental rhinovirus colds. Acta Otolaryngol (Stockh) 1984; 413(suppl):19–24.

79. Naclerio RM, Proud D, Lichtenstein LM, et al. Kinins are generated during experimental rhinovirus colds. J Infect Dis 1988; 157:133–142.

80. Einarsson O, Geba GP, Zhu Z, Landry M, Elias JA. Interleukin-11: Stimulation in vivo and in vitro by respiratory viruses and induction of airways hyperresponsiveness. J Clin Invest 1996; 97:915–924.

81. Proud D, Gwaltney JMJ, Hendley JO, Dinarello CA, Gillis S, Schleimer RP. Increased levels of interleukin-1 are detected in nasal secretions of volunteers during experimental rhinovirus colds. J Infect Dis 1994; 169:1007–1013.

82. Grunberg K, Timmers MC, Smits HH, et al. Effect of experimental rhinovirus 16 colds on airway hyperresponsiveness to histamine and interleukin-8 in nasal lavage in asthmatic subjects in vivo. Clin Exp Allergy 1997; 27:36–45.

83. Dicosmo BF, Geba GP, Picarella D, et al. Airway epithelial cell expression of interleukin-6 in transgenic mice—uncoupling of airway inflammation and bronchial hyperreactivity. J Clin Invest 1994; 94:2028–2035.

84. Garafalo R, Mei F, Espejo R, et al. Respiratory syncytial virus infection of human respiratory epithelial cells up-regulates class I MHC expression through induction of IFN-$\beta$ and IL-1$\alpha$. J Immunol 1996; 157:2506–2513.

85. Subauste MC, Jacoby DB, Richards SM, Proud D. Infection of a human respiratory epithelial cell line with rhinovirus—induction of cytokine release and modulation of susceptibility to infection by cytokine exposure. J Clin Invest 1995; 96:549–557.

86. Stellato C, Beck LA, Gorgone GA, et al. Expression of the chemokine RANTES by a human bronchial epithelial cell line. J Immunol 1995; 155:410–418.

87. Kameyoshi Y, Dorschner A, Mallet Al, Christophers E, Schroder JM. Cytokine RANTES released by thrombin-stimulated platelets is a potent attractant for human eosinophils. J Exp Med 1992; 176:587–592.

88. Zhang L, Redington AE, Holgate ST. RANTES: a novel mediator of allergic inflammation? Clin Exp Allergy 1994; 24:899–904.

89. Nagata M, Sedgwick JB, Kita H, Busse WW. Granulocyte macrophage colony stimulating factor augments ICAM-1 and VCAM-1 activation of eosinophil function. Am J Respir Crit Care Med 1998; 19:158–166.

90. Lopez AF, Williamson DJ, Gamble JR, et al. Recombinant human granulocyte-macrophage colony-stimulating factor stimulates in vitro mature human neutrophil and eosinophil function, surface receptor expression, and survival. J Clin Invest 1986; 78:1220–1228.

91. Sedgwick JB, Quan SF, Calhoun WJ, Busse WW. Effect of interleukin-5 and granu-

locyte-macrophage colony stimulating factor on in vitro eosinophil function: comparison with airway eosinophils. J Allergy Clin Immunol 1995; 96:375–385.

92. Tang YW, Graham BS. Anti-IL-4 treatment at immunization modulates cytokine expression, reduces illness, and increases cytotoxic T lymphocyte activity in mice challenged with respiratory syncytial virus. J Clin Invest 1994; 94:1953–1958.

93. Coyle AJ, Erard F, Bertrand C, Walti S, Pircher H, Legros G. Virus-specific CD8(+) cells can switch to interleukin 5 production and induce airway eosinophilia. J Exp Med 1995; 181:1229–1233.

94. Turner RB. The role of neutrophils in the pathogenesis of rhinovirus infections. Pediatr Infect Dis J 1990; 9:832–835.

95. Levandowski RA, Weaver CW, Jackson GG. Nasal secretion leukocyte populations determined by flow cytometry during acute rhinovirus infection. J Med Virol 1988; 25:423–432.

96. Heymann PW, Rakes GP, Hogan AD, Ingram JM, Hoover GE, Platts-Mills TA. Assessment of eosinophils, viruses and IgE antibody in wheezing infants and children. Int Arch Allergy Immunol 1995; 107:380–382.

97. Garofalo R, Kimpen JLL, Welliver RC, Ogra PL. Eosinophil degranulation in the respiratory tract during naturally acquired respiratory syncytial virus infection. J Pediatr 1992; 120:28–32.

98. van Oosterhout AJ, van Ark I, Folkerts G, et al. Antibody to interleukin-5 inhibits virus-induced airway hyperresponsiveness to histamine in guinea pigs. Am J Respir Crit Care Med 1995; 151:177–183.

99. Gern JE, Dick EC, Lee WM, et al. Rhinovirus enters but does not replicate inside monocytes and airway macrophages. J Immunol 1996; 156:621–627.

100. Hayden FG, Albrecht JK, Kaiser DL, Gwaltney JMJ. Prevention of natural colds by contact prophylaxis with intranasal alpha$_2$-interferon. N Engl J Med 1986; 314:71–75.

101. Noah TL, Henderson FW, Wortman IA, et al. Nasal cytokine production in viral acute upper respiratory infection of childhood. J Infect Dis 1995; 171:584–592.

102. Rothlein R, Czajkowski M, O'Neill MM, Marlin SD, Mainolfi E, Merluzzi VJ. Induction of intercellular adhesion molecule 1 on primary and continuous cell lines by pro-inflammatory cytokines. J Immunol 1988; 141:1665–1669.

103. Balfour-Lynn IM, Valman HB, Wellings R, Webster ADB, Taylor GW, Silverman M. Tumour necrosis factor-alpha and leukotriene E$_4$ production in wheezy infants. Clin Exp Allergy 1994; 24:121–126.

104. Anticevich SZ, Hughes JM, Black JL, Armour CL. Induction of human airway hyperresponsiveness by tumour necrosis factor-alpha. Eur J Pharmacol 1995; 284:221–225.

105. Gosset P, Tsicopoulos A, Wallaert B, et al. Increased secretion of tumor necrosis factor α and interleukin-6 by alveolar macrophages consecutive to the development of the late asthmatic reaction. J Allergy Clin Immunol 1991; 88:561–571.

106. Alwan WH, Record FM, Openshaw PJM. Phenotypic and functional characterization of T cell lines specific for individual respiratory syncytial virus proteins. J Immunol 1993; 150:5211–5218.

107. Alwan WH, Kozlowska WJ, Openshaw PJ. Distinct types of lung disease caused by functional subsets of antiviral T cells. J Exp Med 1994; 179:81–89.

108. Welliver RC, Wong DT, Sun M, Middleton EJ, Vaughan RS, Ogra PL. The development of respiratory syncytial virus-specific IgE and the release of histamine in nasopharyngeal secretions after infection. N Engl J Med 1981; 305:841–846.

109. Welliver RC, Wong DT, Rijnaldo D, Ogra PL. Predictive value of respiratory syncytial virus-specific IgE responses for recurrent wheezing following bronchiolitis. J Pediatr 1986; 109:776–780.

110. Punnonen J, Aversa G, Cocks BG, et al. Interleukin 13 induces interleukin 4-independent IgG4 and IgE synthesis and CD23 expression by human B cells. PNAS 1993; 90:3730–3734.

111. Vercelli D, Geha RS. Regulation of IgE synthesis in humans. J Clin Immunol 1989; 9:75–81.

112. Anderson LJ, Tsou C, Potter C, et al. Cytokine response to respiratory syncytial virus stimulation of human peripheral blood mononuclear cells. J Infect Dis 1994; 170:1201–1208.

113. Jackson M, Scott R. Different patterns of cytokine induction in cultures of respiratory syncytial (RS) virus-specific human T-H cell lines following stimulation with RS virus and RS virus proteins. J Med Virol 1996; 49:161–169.

114. Gern JE, Dick EC, Kelly EAB, Vrtis R, Klein B. Rhinovirus-specific T cells recognize both shared and serotype-restricted viral epitopes. J Infect Dis 1997; 175: 1108–1114.

115. Douglass JA, Dhami D, Gurr CE, et al. Influence of interleukin-8 challenge in the nasal musosa in atopic and nonatopic subjects. Am J Respir Crit Care Med 1994; 150:1108–1113.

116. Schweizer RC, Welmers BA, Raaijmakers JA, Zanen P, Lammers JW, Koenderman L. RANTES- and interleukin-8-induced responses in normal human eosinophils: effects of priming with interleukin-5. Blood 1994; 83:3697–3704.

117. Warringa RAJ, Mengelers HJ, Raaijmakers JA, Bruijnzeel PL, Koenderman L. Upregulation of formyl-peptide and interleukin-8-induced eosinophil chemotaxis in patients with allergic asthma. J Allergy Clin Immunol 1993; 91:1198–1205.

118. Warringa RAJ, Schweizer RC, Maikoe T, Kuijper PH, Bruijnzeel PL, Koendermann L. Modulation of eosinophil chemotaxis by interleukin-5. Am J Respir Cell Mol Biol 1992; 7:631–636.

119. Calhoun WJ, Jarjour NN. Macrophages and macrophage diversity in asthma. In: Busse WW, Holgate ST, eds. Asthma and Rhinitis. Cambridge, MA: Blackwell Scientific Publications, 1995:467–473.

120. Robinson DS, Ying S, Bentley AM, et al. Relationships among numbers of bronchoalveolar lavage cells expressing messenger ribonucleic acid for cytokines, asthma symptoms, and airway methacholine responsiveness in atopic asthma. J Allergy Clin Immunol 1993; 92:397–403.

# 9

## Limitations of Human Experimental Provocation Models for Investigating the Virus–Asthma Link

**DEBORAH A. GENTILE**

Children's Hospital of Pittsburgh
Pittsburgh, Pennsylvania

**DAVID P. SKONER**

Children's Hospital of Pittsburgh
University of Pittsburgh School of Medicine
Pittsburgh, Pennsylvania

## I. Background

Results from recent epidemiological studies suggest that respiratory viruses play a role in the development and/or expression of asthma in genetically susceptible individuals (1–3). Due to a lack of ready extrapolation of results from animal models to humans and the inherent difficulties in studying naturally acquired colds in humans, several investigators have used human experimental provocation models to explore this relationship (4–19). The methodologies used in these models and results are summarized in Table 1. Interestingly, but not surprisingly, different investigators have reported conflicting results (4–13). For example, in a number of studies, bronchial reactivity and the late-phase asthmatic responses were increased in subjects experimentally infected with either rhinovirus or influenza virus (4,5,8–14). In contrast, a few other studies failed to detect an effect of experimental infection with either of these viruses on the lower airways (6,7,15–19). Moreover, few, if any, of the viruses delivered in experimental settings has been reported to trigger acute asthma or alter routine spirometric parameters, even when the study population included subjects with allergic rhinitis and/ or asthma, and virus was cultured from the lower airways (4–19).

**Table 1** Studies Using Human Experimental Provocation Models to Investigate the Virus-Asthma Link

| Investigator (Ref.) | Date | Virus | Inoculation methods | | | | | | Infected subjects | | | | |
|---|---|---|---|---|---|---|---|---|---|---|---|---|---|
| | | | $TCID_{50}$ | Drops? | Atomizer? | Nebulizer? | #Days | Cloistered? | N | Allergic? | Asthmatic? | $\downarrow FEV_1$? | $\uparrow AHR$? |
| Laitinen (4) | 1980 | FLU A | Not reported | Yes | No | No | 1 | Not reported | 6 | Not reported | Yes | No | Yes (H) |
| | | | | | | | | | 10 | Not reported | No | No | No (H) |
| Laitinen (5) | 1991 | FLU A±B | $10^{7.5}$ | Yes | Yes | No | 1 | Not reported | 6 | No | No | No | Yes (H) |
| | | | | | | | | | 21 | Yes | No | No | No (M) |
| Skoner (6) | 1996 | FLU A | $10^7$ | Yes | No | No | 1 | Yes | 25 | No | No | No | No (M) |
| Bush (7) | 1978 | RV 16 | $5.6 \times 10^{3.5}$ | Yes | No | No | 1 | Not reported | 7 | No | No | No | No (M) |
| Lemanske (8) | 1989 | RV 16 | $3.2 \times 10^{2.3}$ | Yes | Yes | No | 2 | Not reported | 10 | Yes | No | No | Yes (H,A) |
| Calhoun (9) | 1991 | RV 16 | $3.2 \times 10^{2.3}$ | Yes | Yes | No | 2 | Not reported | 8 | Yes | No | No | Yes (H,MA) |
| Cheung (10) | 1994 | RV 16 | $3 \times 10^4$ | Yes | Yes | Yes | 2 | Not reported | 7 | Yes | Yes | No | Yes (M) |

| Study | Year | Virus | Titer (TCID$_{50}$) | | | | | n | | | | Reactivity |
|---|---|---|---|---|---|---|---|---|---|---|---|---|
| Fraenkel (11) | 1995 | RV 16 | $5\text{–}10 \times 10^4$ | Yes | No | 2 | Yes | 7 | Yes | Yes | No | Yes (H) |
| Grunberg (12) | 1996 | RV 16 | $0.5\text{–}2.9 \times 10^4$ | Yes | Yes | 2 | Not reported | 11; 19; 17 | No; Yes; Yes | No | No | No (H); Yes (H); Yes (H) |
| Bardin (13) | 1996 | RV 16 | $1.5 \times 10^{2\text{-}3}$ | Yes | No | 2 | Yes | 8 | No | Yes | No | No (H) |
| Gern (14) | 1997 | RV 16 | $3.2 \times 10^{2\text{-}3}$ | Yes | No | 2 | Not reported | 18; 13 | Yes; No | Not reported; Not reported | No | Yes (H); No (H) |
| Halperin (15) | 1983 | RV Hanks | $3$ | No | No | 2 | | 14 | Yes | No | No | No (H) |
| Halperin (16) | 1985 | RV Hanks | $3\text{–}10$ | No | No | 2 | Yes | 10 | Yes | No | No | No (H) |
| Angelini (17) | 1996 | RV Hanks | $1\text{–}3 \times 10^2$ | No | No | 1 | Yes | 40; 34 | Yes; No | No; No | No | No (M); No (M) |
| Halperin (18) | 1985 | RV 39 | $3\text{–}10$ | No | No | 2 | Yes | 9 | Yes | No | No | No (H) |
| Skoner (19) | 1996 | RV 39 | $1 \times 10^2$ | No | No | 1 | Yes | 50; 46 | Yes; No | Yes; No | No | No (M); No (M) |
| Summers (20) | 1992 | RV 2 | $1 \times 10^2$ | No | No | 1 | Yes | 11; 16 | Yes; No | No; No | No | No (H,B); No (H,B) |

H = histamine; M = methacholine; A = antigen; B = bradykinin.

**Table 2**   Limitations of Experimental Provocation Models

Mild severity of infection
Varying doses and methods for administration of inoculum
Differences in viral strains and types
Viral attenuation
Immunological, atopic, pulmonary, and psychological status of
    subjects
Effect of cloistering

Collectively, these results suggest that critical host, viral, environmental, or experimental factors may operate as variables in modifying outcomes of trials involving experimental infection. One likely source of variability is the experimental provocation model itself. Although this model can provide valuable information, which may not be available in studies of natural colds, including the timing of virus inoculation and the precise onset of and duration of symptoms and signs of infection, it does have some limitations. These limitations are summarized in Table 2 and reviewed below.

## II.  Severity of Infection

The severity of infection may be an important factor governing the development of lower airway effects during experimental provocation with respiratory viruses. Indeed, previous studies have documented an association between the development of lower airway symptomatology and pathophysiology during viral respiratory infections and the severity of infection (20,21). Since experimentally induced colds are typically less severe than naturally acquired colds, lower airway effects are less likely to be observed during the former as compared to the latter (22,23). One possible explanation to account for this observation is that the majority of experimentally induced colds are diagnosed by the modified Jackson criteria, which detect illness of very mild severity (23). Other possibilities, which relate to viral and subject characteristics and inoculation methodologies, are discussed below.

## III.  Inoculation Methodologies

The inoculation method is an important factor that may potentially influence the ability of respiratory viruses to affect the lower airways. Since the methods by which patients are naturally exposed to respiratory viruses are difficult to replicate in the laboratory setting, a number of experimental inoculation methods have evolved (see Table 1). Occasionally, such methods are laboratory-specific. These include delivery on one versus two consecutive days and nasal drop instillation with or without the addition of nasal spray from an atomizer and/or nasal inhalation from a nebulizer. Some of these methods have been designed to enhance lower airway deposition (5,8–14). Unfortunately, none of these methods has been tested for comparability or validity in controlled settings. Interestingly, it has been reported that rhinovirus 16 had no effect on lower airway reactivity to methacholine when administered by nasal drops alone, but it did have a positive effect when spray from an atomizer was added to this method (7,8).

Another important factor is the inoculum size. Varying doses of inoculum, ranging from 3 to $10^4$ TCID$_{50}$ for rhinovirus and $10^7$ to $10^{7.5}$ TCID$_{50}$ for influenza virus, have been administered by different investigative groups (see Table 1) (4–19). Since the inoculum size correlates positively with the likelihood of developing a respiratory viral infection as well as the severity of illness during infection, this factor may potentially influence the development of lower airway effects following experimental provocation with respiratory viruses (22).

## IV. Viral Characteristics

Another factor that may be important in determining the extent of lower airway involvement is differences in the pathogenicity of different virus types and strains. It has become increasingly apparent that not all of the respiratory viruses used for experimental inoculation are equally likely to induce lower airway effects (see Table 1) (4–19). For example, influenza virus has a greater likelihood of causing lower airway pathophysiology than does rhinovirus since the former has a higher predilection for infecting the lungs and causing pulmonary epithelial damage (24). Similarly, rhinovirus 16, which was originally isolated from a wheezing child, has consistently induced lower airway alterations in a number of different laboratories, while other rhinovirus strains, including, 2, 39, and Hanks, typically have not (7–19). However, the latter is not entirely without exception. Indeed, one investigator reported increased bronchial reactivity to histamine in a small subset of asthmatic subjects infected with either rhinovirus 39 or Hanks (16).

Attenuations in the pathogenicity and infectivity of laboratory-adapted viral isolates may also influence the degree of lower airway involvement during experimental provocation. Picornaviruses such as rhinovirus may attenuate quickly during tissue culture passage since they have a high rate of spontaneous mutation (25). Additionally, the infectivity of respiratory viruses may decline during prolonged periods of storage (26). The fact that some of the viral isolates used for experimental provocation produce only subclinical or mild respiratory infections suggest that they may have become attenuated during culture or storage. Since the development of lower airway pathophysiology correlates positively with the severity of infection, lower airway effects may not be observed during experimental provocation with attenuated respiratory viruses.

## V.  Subject Characteristics

Certain subject characteristics, including immunological, atopic, pulmonary, and psychological status, may also be important in determining the extent of lower airway involvement (see Table 1). For example, the presence or absence of virus-specific neutralizing antibodies may influence the likelihood of infection as well as the severity of illness if infected (22,27,28). Atopic status is also hypothesized to play a role since enhanced viral-induced bronchial reactivity has been observed in subjects with allergic rhinitis as compared to subjects without allergic rhinitis (11,13,14,29). Moreover, in subjects with allergic rhinitis, recent or concomitant allergen priming may potentially enhance virus-induced responses (9,22). In that regard, it is of interest that most of the studies that reported a lack of virus-induced lower airway dysfunction typically enrolled ''nonprimed'' atopic subjects (4,15–19). It is also conceivable that subject-specific exposure to other environmental agents, including cold air, cigarette smoke, and air pollution, could similarly enhance virus-induced effects on the lower airways.

Baseline pulmonary status may also play a role since greater changes in virus-induced bronchial reactivity have been reported in subjects with $FEV_1$ values in the lower range of normal (14) as compared to those with values in the middle to upper range of normal. The presence of underlying pulmonary disease, including asthma, is also likely to be involved. Asthma is particularly important since it is usually associated with the presence of both lower $FEV_1$ values and allergic rhinitis. Future studies need to examine the effect of viral infection on lower airway responses in subjects with asthma since this is the population with the greatest risk of developing viral-induced lower airway pathophysiology.

Certain psychological factors may also play a role in determining a subject's susceptibility to infection and subsequently influence the development of lower airway dysfunction (30,31). For example, a number of studies have shown a positive correlation between the presence of severe chronic stressful life events and an increased susceptibility to developing a viral upper respiratory infection (30). Similarly, a recent study demonstrated that the risk of developing a cold is inversely associated with the number of social ties that a subject has to friends, family, work, and community (31).

## VI.  Environmental Factors

Another factor that may be important is cloistering of subjects during the acute stage of experimental infection (see Table 1) (4–19). In a cloistered setting, environmental factors such as temperature and humidity are typically regulated and held constant. Moreover, exposure to other inflammatory stimuli, including allergens, pollutants, and tobacco smoke, could be increased or decreased for a given individual. Cloistering may also intensify a subject's perception of their illness and thereby result in an overestimation of clinical severity. Factors that may contribute to this phenomenon include the focused and intense nature of the cloister, the subject's anticipation of illness, and the subject's inability to engage in routine daily activities, which may typically distract their attention away from their symptoms.

## VII. Assessment of Outcomes

Another potential source of variability in the experimental provocation model relates to differences in methodologies used to assess outcomes (see Table 1) (4–19). For example, although many investigators have assessed the effect of experimental viral infection on bronchial reactivity, they have frequently performed the challenges with different bronchoprovocation agents, including histamine, methacholine, allergen, and bradykinin (4–19). Other variables related to the measurement of bronchial reactivity include the frequency of assessment and the timing of delivery of the bronchoprovocation challenge test.

A related consideration is the sensitivity of the methods used to assess various outcomes. Many of the studies that reported negative effects of viruses on bronchial reactivity used $FEV_1$ values to assess lower airway function (see Table 1) (6,15–19). It is possible that positive effects may have been observed in these studies if a more sensitive marker of lower airway function, such as specific airway conductance, had been used. Similarly, in some of these studies, the doses of bronchoprovocation agents may not have been high enough to produce positive results (6,15–19).

Bronchoalveolar lavage and segmental allergen challenge are being increasingly used to assess lower airway effects during experimental viral provocation; however, these procedures do have some limitations (32–35). For example, there are a number of serious risks associated with these procedures, including bronchospasm, hypoxemia, fever, laryngospasm, bleeding, and pneumothorax (33). Another concern is that these procedures may enhance lower airway effects to a greater degree in subjects with, as compared to those without, underlying airway inflammation (33). Indeed, several studies have documented more marked decreases in $FEV_1$ and oxygen saturation during both bronchoalveolar lavage and segmental allergen challenge in subjects with asthma as compared to subjects without asthma (34,35). Moreover, bronchial reactivity and markers of airway inflammation may also be enhanced to a greater degree in subjects with allergic rhinitis and/or asthma (35). Another concern relates to the fact that the bronchoscope must be passed through the upper airway in order to perform a segmental allergen challenge or obtain lavage samples from the lower airway. This procedure raises the possibility that secretions recovered from the lower airway may be contaminated with secretions from the upper airway (32). Moreover, it is conceivable that introduction of secretions from the upper airway may contribute to the development of inflammation and pathophysiology in the lower airway.

## VIII.  Conclusion

Although the experimental provocation model can provide unique and valuable information about the relationship between respiratory viral infections and the development and/or expression of asthma, it has several limitations which should be considered when designing studies and assessing the outcomes of these studies.

## References

1. Pattermore PK, Johnston SL, Bardin PG. Viruses as precipitants of asthma symptoms. Clin Exp Allergy 1992; 22:325–336.
2. Johnston SL, Pattermore PK, Sanderson G, et al. Community study of viral infections in exacerbations of asthma in 9–11 year old children. Br Med J 1995; 310: 1225–1229.
3. Nicholson KG, Kent J, Ireland DC. Respiratory viruses and exacerbations of asthma in adults. Br Med J 1993; 307:982–986.
4. Laitinen LA, Kava T. Bronchial reactivity following uncomplicated influenza A infection in healthy and asthmatic patients. Eur J Respir Dis 1980; 106:51–58.
5. Laitinen LA, Elkin RB, Empey DW, Jacobs L, Mills J, Nadel JA. Bronchial hyperresponsiveness in normal subjects during attenuated influenza virus infection. Am Rev Respir Dis 1991; 143:358–361.
5. Blair HT, Greenberg SB, Stevens PM, Bilunos PA, Couch RB. Effects of rhinovirus infection on pulmonary function of healthy human volunteers. Am Rev Respir Dis 1976; 114:95–102.
6. Calhoun WJ, Dick EC, Schwartz LB, Busse WW. A common cold virus, rhinovirus 16, potentiates airway inflammation after segmental antigen bronchoprovocation in allergic subjects. J Clin Invest 1994; 94:2200–2208.
6. Skoner DP, Doyle WJ, Seroky J, Fireman P. Lower airway responses to influenza A virus in healthy allergic and non-allergic subjects. Am J Respir Crit Care Med 1996; 154:661–664.
7. Bush RK, Busse W, Flaherty D, Warshaurer D, Dick EC, Reed CE. Effects of experimental rhinovirus 16 infection on airways and leukocyte function in normal subjects. J Allergy Clin Immunol 1978; 61:80–87.
8. Lemanske RF, Dick EC, Swenson C, Vrtis R, Busse WW. Rhinovirus upper respira-

tory infection increases airway hyperreactivity and late asthmatic reactions. J Clin Invest 1989; 83:1–10.

9. Calhoun WJ, Swenson CA, Dick EC, Schwartz LB, Lemanske RJ, Jr., Busse WW. Experimental rhinovirus 16 infection potentiates histamine release after antigen bronchoprovocation in allergic subjects. Am Rev Respir Dis 1991; 144:1267–1273.

10. Cheung D, Dick EC, Timmers MC, De Klerk EPA, Spaan WJM, Sterk PJ. Rhinovirus inhalation causes long-lasting excessive airway narrowing in response to methacholine in asthmatic subjects in vivo. Am J Respir Crit Care Med 1995; 152:1490–1496.

11. Fraenkel DJ, Bardin PG, Sanderson G, Lampe F, Johnston SL. Lower airway inflammation during rhinovirus colds in normal and in asthmatic subjects. Am J Respir Crit Care Med 1995; 151:879–886.

12. Grunberg K, Timmers MC, Smits HH, deKlerk EPA, Dick EC, Spaan WJM, Hiemstra PS, Sterk PJ. Effect of experimental rhinovirus 16 colds on airway hyperresponsiveness to histamine and interleukin-8 in nasal lavage in asthmatic subjects in vivo. Clin Exp Allergy 1997; 27:36–45.

13. Bardin PG, Sanderson G, Robinson BS, Holgate ST, Tyrrell DAJ. Experimental rhinovirus infection in volunteers. Eur Respir J 1996; 9:2250–2255.

14. Gern JE, Calhoun WJ, Swenson C, Shen G, Busse WW. Rhinovirus infection preferentially increases lower airway responsiveness in allergic subjects. Am J Respir Crit Care Med 1997; 55:1872–1876.

15. Halperin SA, Eggleston PA, Hendley JO, Suraft PM, Groschel DH, Gwaltney JMJ. Pathogenesis of lower respiratory tract symptoms in experimental rhinovirus infection. Am Rev Respir Dis 1983; 128:806–810.

16. Halperin SA, Eggleston PA, Beaseley P, et al. Exacerbations of asthma in adults during experimental rhinovirus infection. Am Rev Respir Dis 1985; 132:976–980.

17. Angelini B, Van Deusen MA, Doyle WJ, Seroky J, Cohen S, Skoner DP. Lower airway responses to rhinovirus-Hanks in health subjects with and without allergy. J Allergy Clin Immunol 1997; 99:618–619.

18. Skoner DP, Doyle WJ, Seroky J, Van Deusen MA, Fireman P. Lower airway responses to rhinovirus 39 in healthy allergic and nonallergic subjects. Eur Respir J 1996; 9:1402–1406.

19. Summers QA, Higgins PG, Barrow IG, Tyrell DAJ, Holgate ST. Bronchial reactivity to histamine and bradykinin is unchanged after rhinovirus infection in normal subjects. Eur Respir J 1992; 5:313–317.

20. Minor TE, Dick EC, DeMeo AN, Ouellefte JJ, Cohen M, Reed CE. Viruses as precipitants of asthmatic attacks in children. JAMA 1974; 227:292–298.

21. Minor TE, Dick EC, Baker JW, Ouellette JJ, Cohen M, Reed CE. Rhinovirus and influenza type A infections as precipitants of asthma. Am Rev Respir Dis 1976; 113:149–153.

22. Hendley JO, Edmondson WP, Jr., Gwaltney JM, Jr. Relations between naturally acquired immunity and infectivity of two rhinoviruses in volunteers. J Infect Dis 1972; 125:243–248.

23. Jackson GG, Dowling HF, Spiesman IG, Boand AV. Transmission of the common cold to volunteers under controlled conditions: the common cold as a clinical entity. Arch Intern Med 1958; 101:267–278.

24. Richman DD. Orthomyxoviruses: the influenza viruses. In: Braude Al, Davis CE, Fierer J, eds. Infectious Diseases and Medical Microbiology. 2d ed. Philadelphia: WB Saunders Co., 1986:507–514.

25. Murphy BR, Chanock RM. Immunization against viruses. In: Fields BN, Knipe DM, Chanock RM, et al., eds. Virology. 2d ed. New York: Raven Press, 1990:469–506.

26. Tyrrell DAJ. Common Colds and Related Diseases. Baltimore: Williams & Wilkins Co., 1965.

27. Mufson MA, Ludwig WM, James HD, Gauld LW, Rourke JA, Hopler JC, Chanock RM. Effect of neutralizing antibody on experimental rhinovirus infection. JAMA 1963; 186:578–584.

28. Alper CM, Doyle WJ, Skoner DP, Buchman CA, Seroky JT, Gwaltney JM, Cohen SA. Pre-challenge antibodies moderate infection rate, and signs and symptoms in adults experimentally challenged with rhinovirus type 39. Laryngoscope 1996; 106: 1298–1305.

29. Duff AL, Pomeranz ES, Gelber LE, et al. Risk factors for acute wheezing in infants and children: viruses, passive smoke, and IgE antibodies to inhalant allergens. Pediatrics 1993; 92:535–540.

30. Cohen S, Doyle WJ, Skoner DP, Frank E, Rabin BS, Gwaltney JM. Types of stressors that increase susceptibility to the common cold in healthy adults. Health Psychol 1998; 17:214–223.

31. Cohen S, Doyle WJ, Skoner DP, Rabin BS, Gwaltney JM. Social ties and susceptibility to the common cold. JAMA 1997; 277:1940–1944.

32. Gern JE, Galagan DM, Jarjour NN, Dick EC, Busse WW. Detection of rhinovirus RNA in lower airway cells during experimentally induced infection. Am J Respir Crit Care Med 1997; 155:1159–1161.

33. Djukanovic R, Dahl N, Jajour N, Aalbers R. Safety of biopsies and bronchoalveolar lavage. Eur Respir J 1998; 11:39S–41S.

34. Spanevello A, Migliori GB, Satta A, et al. Bronchoalveolar lavage causes decrease in $PaO_2$, increase in (A-a) gradient value and bronchoconstriction in asthmatics. Respir Med 1998; 92:191–197.

35. Krug M, Teran LM, Redington AE, Gratziou C, et al. Safety aspects of local endobronchial challenge in asthmatic patients. Am J Respir Crit Care Med 1996; 153: 1391–1397.

# 10

## Stress, Viral Respiratory Infections, and Asthma

**SHELDON COHEN**

Carnegie Mellon University
Pittsburgh, Pennsylvania

**MARIO RODRIGUEZ**

Medical College of Pennsylvania
Hahnemann University
Philadelphia, Pennsylvania

## I. Introduction

Asthma is one of the most prevalent of chronic diseases worldwide. It is a chronic inflammatory disorder of the airways associated with intermittent and reversible airway obstruction. Current thinking about the pathogenesis of asthma is that inflammatory processes in the airways result in a limitation of airflow and an increased responsiveness of the airways that causes them to narrow in reaction to certain stimuli (1). Allergens and respiratory infections are the primary contributors to airway inflammation. Allergens are also common triggers of airway constriction, but so are air pollution, cold air, exercise, odors, and certain respiratory infections. Clinical wisdom has long suggested that psychological stress and related emotional factors may also play an important part in promoting airway inflammation, airway constriction, and triggering symptoms (2). Indeed, asthma patients and the physicians who treat them often report that stress and emotional factors can initiate, trigger, or exacerbate asthma symptoms. Data to corroborate this assumption, however, are relatively scarce, and the clinical significance of psychological factors in asthma remains unclear (3).

The theory that asthma has a psychosomatic component has existed at least since the early 1920s, when classic psychoanalytic studies generated the hypothesis that asthma represented in part the psychosomatic manifestation of intense emotion (4,5). At the same time, learning theorists argued that particular emotional experiences may have reinforced pulmonary physiological responses, thus increasing the likelihood of their recurring in the same context (6). The connection between asthma and emotion was based on the observation that emotionally laden stimuli could elicit small but reliable changes in the airways of asthmatic individuals (7). Conversely, the observation that asthmatic individuals experienced improvement in their respiration following relaxation procedures provided further clinical evidence supporting the idea that emotions played an important role in asthma (reviewed in Ref. 7).

Contemporary studies of the role of stress in asthma are consistent with this view. Both adult and child asthmatics report and display more negative emotion than others (reviewed in Refs. 8, 9), and asthma exacerbations have been linked temporally to periods of heightened negative emotionality (9–11). The causal interpretation of these data is, however, muddied by the possibility that asthma was the cause of the emotional distress rather than the distress causing asthma. Experimental studies of the effects of emotional stimulation on pulmonary function and other relevant physiology of asthmatics have provided a clearer interpretation of the direction of causation. When subjected to stressful experiences such as performing mental arithmetic tasks (12), watching emotionally charged films (13,14), or listening to stressful interactions (15), 15–30% of asthmatics respond with increased bronchoconstriction (reviewed in Ref. 16). The susceptibility to stress-induced constriction is not attributable to age, gender, asthma severity, atopy, or method of pulmonary assessment (16).

This chapter examines the behavioral, neural, and immune pathways that might link psychological stress to the onset or exacerbation of asthma. This focus emphasizes the role of central nervous system (CNS) interaction with immunological and endocrinological processes in explaining the association between psychological stress and airway changes in asthma (17). It also focuses on stress-elicited increases in susceptibility to and severity of respiratory infections as a major link between psychological stress and asthma.

## II.  What Is Stress?

When confronting environmental demands, people evaluate whether the demands pose a threat and whether sufficient adaptive capacities are available to cope with them (18). Threat evaluation is based on the personal values of the individual as well as the magnitude of the threat. Evaluations of coping abilities depend on past experience, personality, and the availability of material and social resources. If environmental demands are found to be taxing or threatening, and at the same time coping resources are viewed to be inadequate, we perceive ourselves as being under stress. This perception is presumed to result in negative emotional states including fear, anger, anxiety, and depression. The perception of threat and the concomitant emotional state trigger brain-based physiological responses, which in turn result in changes in autonomic and immunological activities. Hormones and neuropeptides released into the circulation when people experience stress are thought to play roles in regulating both inflammatory and airway responses (19).

Psychological stressors have been associated with the activation of the autonomic nervous system and of the hypothalamic-pituitary-adrenocortical (HPA) axis. Both the sympathetic and parasympathetic components of the autonomic system are responsive to psychological stress. The sympathetic system reacts with increased output of epinephrine and norepinephrine from the adrenal medulla and norepinephrine from adrenergic nerve endings (20). Increased sympathetic activity is generally accompanied by withdrawal of vagal tone. Certain types of stimuli, however (e.g., those requiring heightened vigilance or outward deployment of attentional resources), cause parasympathetic nervous system activation. Individuals differ widely in the magnitude of their autonomic reactions to behavioral stimuli—both sympathetic, parasympathetic, and balance of the two.

The hormonal responses of the HPA axis have long been thought to represent a nonspecific physiological reaction to excessive stimulation (21), particularly the emotional arousal associated with appraising situations as stressful (18,22). The hypothalamus releases corticotrophic-releasing hormone (CRH), which triggers the anterior pituitary gland to secrete adrenocorticotrophic hormone (ACTH), which in turn activates the adrenal cortex to secrete corticosteroids (primarily cortisol in humans). More recent work suggests that negative emotional responses disturb the regulation of the HPA system. For example, relatively pronounced HPA activation is common in depression, with episodes of cortisol secretion being more frequent and of longer duration among depressed than among other psychiatric patients and normals (23). Shifts in the circadian rhythm of cortisol have also been found among persons in stressful situations (24).

Although hormones of the autonomic nervous system and HPA are those most often discussed as the biochemical substances involved in stress responses, alterations in a range of other hormones, neurotransmitters, and neuropeptides have also been found in response to stress and may play an important role in stress influences on asthma. Examples include stressor-associated elevations in growth hormone and prolactin secreted by the pituitary gland and in the natural opiate beta-endorphin and enkephalin released in the brain (25). These substances are also thought to play a role in immune regulation (26).

Psychological stress and its biological concomitants can last for a few minutes or for years. Chronicity is to some degree based on the ongoing presence of external stimuli that triggered the stress response (e.g., ongoing unemployment) but is also dependent on the long-term success of individual coping resources. Moreover, events that last a very short time can have very long-term stress effects. Such effects are thought to be maintained by recurrent ''intrusive'' thoughts about events (27). Elevations of circulating catecholamines and cortisol also seem to be maintained by recurrent intrusive thoughts but are thought to habituate in response to many chronic stressors. Moreover, even if the circulating levels of these hormones remain elevated, there is often a downregulation of receptors over time, resulting in a habituation of the hormone effects.

### III.  How Could Stress Affect Asthma?

Figure 1 provides a simplified picture of the pathways that might link psychological stress to asthma. Psychological stress may influence asthma through autonomic, immune, or behavioral pathways. However, the strongest suggestion from the current literature is that stress may influence the pathophysiology of asthma by increasing the risk of respiratory infections, which play important roles as both promoters of airway inflammation and triggers of asthma. We will present existing evidence suggesting the plausibility of each of these mechanisms.

Asthma, of course, can also trigger psychological stress. For example, severe shortness of breath can result in a panic response based on the patient's perception that their symptoms are a threat and are beyond their control. Such an appraisal would trigger the same behavior and biological responses discussed above and further contribute to the disease event and feelings of helplessness associated with it. Asthma medications can also increase physiological activation

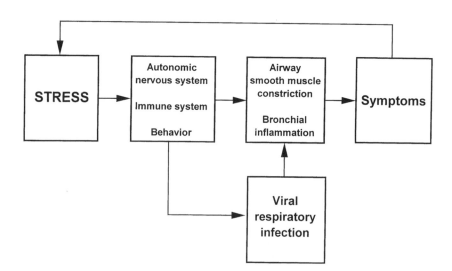

**Figure 1**   Pathways hypothesized to link psychological stress to asthma.

and concomitant emotional response, triggering the same pathways as external stressful events (9).

## A. Behavior Pathways

There are a range of behavioral responses to stress that can contribute to asthma. These include panic-type responses to acute stressful events such as crying, yelling, and hyperventilation that can trigger airway constriction by drying or irritating airway walls. Stress may also elicit deep breathing that can lead to reflex bronchoconstriction in asthmatics. Other behavioral responses include acute and chronic stress–elicited disruptions of adherence to behavioral strategies that help prevent or limit asthma events. Strategies that may be affected by stressful events include the avoidance of indoor and outdoor allergens, air pollutants, and the use of certain drugs. They also include adherence to monitoring symptoms and lung function and proper adherence to medication regimens. Stress is also associated with smokers reporting need for a cigarette, smoking more cigarettes, and being less successful at quitting or cutting down on smoking (28,29). Smoking triggers and exacerbates asthma symptoms by irritating the airways, increasing mucus production, increasing susceptibility to respiratory infections, and altering immune function (30).

## B. Autonomic Pathways

The argument that psychological stress might influence autonomic control of the airways is based primarily on the fact that many of the same autonomic mechanisms thought to play a role in asthma are involved in the activation and regulation of physiological responses to stress. These include the release of sympathetic nervous system hormones, the action of adrenergic (sympathetic) and cholinergic (parasympathetic) nerves, and the neurotransmitters and neuropeptides they produce.

The parasympathetic nervous system innervates the airways via efferent fibers that travel in the vagus nerve and synapse in small ganglia situated in the airway wall, from which short postsynaptic fibers directly supply the airway smooth muscle and submucosal glands (31). Previously, increased activity of the parasympathetic nervous system was thought to be the dominant mechanism responsible for the exaggerated reflex bronchoconstriction seen in asthmatic patients (32). More recent work, however, has shown that although parasympathetic mechanisms are involved, they are not a major cause of airflow limitation in asthma (33). In the initial phases of asthma, narrowing of the airways is thought to be attributable primarily to inflammation. However, bronchial constriction is due to some combination of vagal afference plus inflammatory product stimulation, with the relative importance of these factors depending on genetic and environmental influences.

Recent experimental studies in which asthmatic patients are exposed to stressful situations have focused on stress-induced vagal reactivity as a mediator of emotionally induced bronchoconstriction (9). This includes preliminary evidence that children with asthma who respond to stressful stimuli with high vagal activation (associated with increased cholinergic activity) have greater impairment of airway reactivity in response to methacholine (14).

Although human airway smooth muscle is not functionally innervated by adrenergic axons (34,35), studies have demonstrated adrenergic innervation of submucosal glands, bronchial blood vessels, and airway ganglia (36). Adrenergic agonists bind to adrenoceptors on the surface membrane of effector cells in the airways resulting in a variety of airway changes. Depending on the type of agonist (beta or alpha) involved, these changes can variably affect airway smooth muscle, release of inflammatory mediators, cholinergic neurotransmission, mucus secretion, and possibly mucociliary clearance, resulting in either bronchodilation or bronchoconstriction. Adrenoceptors are regulated by norepinephrine, which is released locally from sympathetic nerves and by epinephrine and norepinephrine secreted by the adrenal medulla. The regulatory effects of epinephrine and norepinephrine on adrenoceptors suggest a plausible mechanism by which stress-induced activation of the sympathetic nervous system might influence bronchomotor tone.

A glaring paradox for the argument that activation of the sympathetic nervous system by stress might contribute to bronchoconstriction is that beta agonists act to relax airway muscle and are used to treat active symptoms. Consequently, acute psychological stress, which is accompanied by a quick elevation in circulating catecholamines, might be expected to result in bronchodilation. However, after the stressor is terminated, epinephrine and norepinephrine levels quickly return to normal or below normal levels.

There are individual differences in the relative strength of sympathetic versus parasympathetic control in response to certain forms of stress, with some individuals showing a predominantly parasympathetic response (vagal tone). Such individuals might be particularly susceptible to stress-induced bronchoconstriction (9). Moreover, as noted earlier, certain types of stimuli activate a predominantly parasympathetic response. It is also possible that sympathetic activation itself might contribute to asthma symptoms. For example, elevations of circulating epinephrine and norepinephrine are known to alter a number of immune parameters that might contribute to inflammation of the airways. Prolonged elevations of these hormone levels under chronic stress might also contribute to asthma severity. For example, chronic daily use of beta agonists in mild to moderate asthmatics with a specific genetic predisposition may increase severity by downregulating beta receptors (37). It is possible that chronically elevated catecholamines could do the same for genetically susceptible subgroups.

Recent evidence suggests functional interactions between peptides released by neurons and the classic neurotransmitters that allow complex integration and regulation of functions in the airway (33). Clearly, the potential role of psychological stress and its physiological concomitants in such interactions is not understood. However, the fact that stress has been associated with modulation of many of the hormones, neurotransmitters, and neuropeptides involved in autonomic control of the airways suggests that further investigation is warranted.

### C. Immune Pathways

A focus on the inflammation of the airways in asthma has drawn attention to the possibility that stress-induced alterations in immune response might have implications for development, exacerbation, and triggering of asthma (3,8). There is now a substantial human literature demonstrating that psychological stress can influence cell trafficking, cell function including mitogen-stimulated blastogenesis and natural killer cell cytotoxicity, as well as lymphocyte production of cytokines (38). Stress can modulate immune response through nerve pathways connecting the autonomic nervous and immune systems, by triggering the release of hormones and neuropeptides that interact with immune cells, and through side effects of behaviors such as smoking and drinking alcohol that are adopted as ways of coping with stress (26,39).

Humans exposed to cognitive or social laboratory stressor tasks lasting only a few minutes show suppression of T-cell mitogenesis and increased numbers of circulating T-suppressor/cytotoxic (CD8) cells and natural killer cells (40). These effects are thought to be mediated by the autonomic nervous system because they occur quite rapidly (41), have been shown to be associated with increases in heart rate, blood pressure, and circulating catecholamines (41,42), and are blocked by administration of an adrenoceptor antagonist (43). Studies of naturalistic stressors show similar alterations of immune response (see review in Ref. 39). Living near the Three Mile Island nuclear power plant at the time of the accident, care-taking for a relative with Alzheimer's disease, and taking medical school exams have all been shown to influence both numbers and functions of various populations of lymphocytes. This includes stress-elicited alteration of the production of the cytokines IL-1β, IL-2, and IFN-γ (e.g., Refs. 44,45).

Stress is not expected to have the same effects on immune function in all people. As noted earlier, individual differences in response to stressful events are attributable to interpretation of the event and access to coping resources. However, there is also evidence of stable individual differences in immune response that occur independent of psychological response to the stressor. When exposed to multiple acute laboratory stressors over time, some subjects consistently demonstrate stress-elicited alterations in immunity, while others do not (46,47). Interestingly, these differences are not associated with their emotional response to the stressors (47).

The contemporary view of asthma pathogenesis is that a chronic inflammatory process involving the airway wall causes the development of airflow limitation and increased responsiveness that predisposes the airway to constrict in response to certain stimuli (1). Mechanisms of airway inflammation involve a cascade of events that include the release of immunological mediators triggered by both IgE-dependent and IgE-independent mechanisms (1). In more than 80% of cases, asthma is an allergic disorder and is orchestrated by antigen-triggered interactions of T and B lymphocytes, and includes B-lymphocyte synthesis of IgE induced by T-helper (TH) cell release of interleukin (IL)-4. The IgE antibody attaches to and activates basophils, mast cells, eosinophils, and platelets, resulting in the release of mediators that are thought to orchestrate the inflammatory cascade. In addition to involving IgE, appropriate antigen can trigger T lymphocytes to release cytokines, which attract and activate leukocytes, particularly eosinophils to the airway walls, and thus directly provoke the inflammatory cascade (1).

Currently, there is no evidence that the stress-altered characteristics of human immunity we have discussed contribute directly to asthma pathogenesis. However, asthmatic high school and college students respond to final examinations with the changes in cytolytic and proliferative responses characterized earlier as immune responses to stress as well as alterations that might influence the physiology of asthma including increased release of inflammatory superoxides by neutrophils (48).

It seems paradoxical that psychological stress activates the HPA resulting ultimately in the release of cortisol, which has anti-inflammatory effects. However, recent evidence suggests that CRH, which regulates the HPA response, has proinflammatory effects in the periphery. This includes triggering mast cell degranulation and increased vascular permeability (49). Moreover, acute psychological stress (by immobilization in rats) resulted in skin mast cell degranulation, and this effect was inhibited by anti-CRH serum administered prior to stress (49).

The discussion of the inflammatory response in asthma has recently emphasized the role of activated T-helper (TH) cells and the cytokines they produce, particularly IL-4 and IL-5. These cytokines are thought to initiate and orchestrate the complex cellular events in airway inflammation and hyperresponsiveness (50,51). Studies of allergic asthmatic subjects with active disease or challenged with antigen show that eosinophil recruitment to the airway is a major factor in inflammation and that IL-4 and IL-5 are instrumental in this process.

TH cells have two phenotypes: TH-1 and TH-2. TH-1 cells produce IL-2 and interferon (IFN)-$\gamma$ but little IL-4 or IL-5 and provide B-cell help for the production of protective antibodies, predominantly IgG (52). In contrast, TH-2 cells produce IL-4, IL-5, IL-6, and IL-10 but little IFN-$\gamma$ and provide B-cell help primarily for the production of IgE in response to allergens. The development of asthma may be associated with a predominance of TH-2 cytokine production (53).

Both environmental and genetic factors are thought to determine which TH cell phenotype becomes more prevalent after the first months of life (53). For example, Martinez et al. (54) provided evidence suggesting that certain lower respiratory tract infections in early life (primarily croup) enhance the production of IFN-γ by nonspecifically stimulated lymphocytes, believed to be an expression of TH-1 type behavior. However, it is possible that stress-triggered hormones in the early months of life influence TH-2 cell predominance. This could occur through a direct influence of stress hormones on the production of cytokines thought to modulate the direction of differentiation. Although there is no direct evidence for stress influencing TH phenotype differentiation in the developing immune system, there is evidence that parental reports of life stress are associated with subsequent onset of wheezing in children between birth and one year (55).

Psychological stress in adults may also alter TH-1 and TH-2 cytokine production. The administration of examinations to medical students was associated with an increase in lymphocyte production of IL-2 (45) and a decrease in the production of IFN-γ (44). A similar study of high school students, however, failed to find that exams produced differences in production of TH-1 and TH-2 cytokines (56).

Overall, there is substantial evidence for both acute and chronic stress influencing a broad range of cellular and humoral immune responses, including influences on the number of and function of cells involved in the inflammatory response. Recent work also suggests that stress might influence the production of cytokines produced by T-helper cells that are the constituents of the TH-1 versus TH-2 predominance thought to play an important role in the development and course of asthma. Hopefully, future research will clarify the potential role of stress in airway inflammation in asthma.

### D. Respiratory Infections as a Pathway

The strongest suggestion from the current literature is that psychological stress may influence the pathophysiology of asthma by increasing the risk of respiratory infections. This is based on evidence of the role of respiratory infections as both promoters of airway inflammation and triggers of asthma, for stress-induced suppression of immunity (discussed earlier), and for stress-induced risk for the development of upper respiratory infections.

As discussed earlier, some infections during childhood are thought to alter the development of the immune system in a manner that reduces the chances of subsequent allergen sensitization (53). In contrast, it has been suggested that severe infections with RSV may enhance allergy sensitization and the risk of developing asthma (57). This literature suggests that the effects of infection may depend on which pathogen infects the host early in immune development (58).

Respiratory viruses exacerbate disease among both children and adults with asthma (58). Respiratory infections can both promote airway inflammation and act as a trigger for asthma expression. Viral respiratory infections provoke wheezing in many asthma patients. Respiratory syncytial virus, parainfluenza virus, rhinovirus, and influenza virus are the most frequently identified viruses associated with increased wheezing (59–61). Rhinovirus in particular has been implicated in the majority of the exacerbations of asthma in children (62). The role of viral respiratory infections as triggers for asthma exacerbations also appears to be important in adults (63).

A number of mechanisms may be involved in explaining the exacerbation of asthma, especially wheezing and increased airway responsiveness, by viral respiratory infections. First, viral respiratory infections may cause damage to the airway epithelium causing airway inflammation. Another mechanism involves the stimulation of virus-specific IgE antibody. Respiratory syncytial virus and parainfluenza virus may potentiate the allergic response to allergens by increasing the release of inflammatory mediators from mast cells and the subsequent cascade of inflammatory events characteristic of asthma (64,65). Lastly, viral respiratory infections may also result in the appearance of a late asthmatic response to inhaled antigen (66). Thus, there is evidence that viral infections are an ''adjuvant'' to the inflammatory response and promote the development of airway injury by enhancing airway inflammation (67).

As discussed earlier, psychological stress has been shown to have a broad impact on the regulation of the human immune system. One potential consequence of stress-induced changes in immune response is suppression of host resistance to infectious agents, particularly agents that cause upper respiratory disease. The primary evidence for such effects comes from studies investigating psychological stress as a risk factor for the common cold, influenza, and other respiratory infectious diseases. Prospective epidemiological studies have demonstrated that both children and adults reporting chronic family stress have a greater subsequent incidence of serologically verified upper respiratory infections and more symptom days of respiratory illness (68–70). Similar results are reported in studies predicting the incidence of influenza during flu season (71).

Increased incidence of upper respiratory infections under stress in the epidemiological studies may be attributable to stress-induced increases in exposure to infectious agents, rather than stress-induced changes in host resistance. Control for exposure is provided by studies in which volunteers are intentionally exposed to a virus (viral-challenge trials). In these prospective studies, psychological stress is assessed before volunteers are exposed to an upper respiratory virus and monitored in quarantine for infection and illness. Using this paradigm, psychological stress has been associated with the incidence of infection and illness with increasing stress related in a dose-response manner to increasing risk (72–74). These relations were found across seven different common cold viruses including rhinoviruses types 2, 9, 14, 39, and Hanks, respiratory syncytial virus, and coronavirus 229E. Moreover, risk of infectious illness has been found to increase with increased duration of the stressful experience (73). Studies of disease severity have similarly found that psychological stress measured prior to viral exposure was associated with more severe colds and influenza as measured by both symptom reporting and by the amount of mucus produced over the course of the illness (75). These associations cannot be explained by differences in health practices among low- and high-stressed persons, and it is speculated that they are attributable to differential production of inflammatory cytokines in response to infection. Elevated levels of both epinephrine and norepinephrine in 24-hour urines are also associated with increased susceptibility in the rhinovirus trials (76).

In sum, psychological stress is associated with decreased host resistance to a wide range of respiratory infectious agents. Included are rhinoviruses and respiratory syncytial virus, both of which contribute to asthma pathophysiology. Although there is currently no direct evidence for stress influencing asthma through susceptibility to respiratory infections, existing evidence lends considerable credence to this hypothesis.

## IV. Conclusions

Both patients and clinicians have long believed that psychological stress plays an important role in the pathogenesis of asthma. Although some evidence for such a relation has accumulated over the years, there is little direct evidence of how a psychological response is translated into effects on physiological pathways that influence the course of asthma. This chapter has presented a range of pathways through which psychological stress might influence asthma pathophysiology. These include stress-elicited changes in patient behavior, in autonomic response, in immune response, and in host resistance to respiratory infections. Although all of these systems are influenced by stress, there is only scattered evidence demonstrating ties between stress, the proposed pathways, and asthma pathogenesis. Hopefully, future research will focus on directly testing the types of models proposed here and hence provide a clearer understanding of the association between stress and the onset and progression of asthma.

We view the existing evidence for stress-induced susceptibility to respiratory infections as the most promising of the proposed mechanisms. This is because of the simplicity of this model, the evidence that stress operates as a risk factor for both incidence and severity of upper respiratory infections, and evidence that respiratory infections operate as risk factors for both the onset of asthma and for the triggering of symptoms in asthmatics. This view is strengthened by growing evidence of the role of stress in modulating the inflammatory response of the immune system.

The most challenging characteristic of our current knowledge is that some but not all asthmatics respond to stress with an exacerbation of disease. It is similarly believed that only a subset of those at risk for asthma are subject to stress-induced onset (3). Susceptibility to stress may be attributable to specific kinds of asthma or specific kinds of psychological characteristics. Relevant typologies of asthma subtypes might be based on the mechanisms that play the predominant role in disease expression (8) or on lability of hyperactivity of the patient's airways (77). Psychological subtyping might be based on dispositional psychological or physiological responsivity to stressful events (14,46,47). Alternatively, it might be based on individual differences in the appraisal of threat posed by specific types of events. It is also possible that there is genetic susceptibility to stress-induced asthma onset or stress-induced exacerbation (3,8).

We have presented the emotional response to psychological stress as if it were a unitary undifferentiated response. This is an oversimplification. Different types of stressful events are thought to induce different responses, as are differences in individual interpretations of events. Intense emotional expressions that have been traditionally associated with triggering or exacerbating asthma include anger, anxiety, excitement, fear, and frustration (10,11,16). It is important to determine which emotional responses influence asthma, whether these are just airway responses or include inflammatory responses, and what the mechanisms are that link emotional response to asthma.

Finally, there is increasing evidence that interventions designed to reduce stress have palliative effects of asthma symptoms. Less clear is which patients are amenable to intervention and why and whether specific types of intervention are as effective as others.

## Acknowledgments

A Senior Scientist Award from the National Institute of Mental Health (MH00721) supported Dr. Cohen's participation. The authors are indebted to the Fetzer Institute and the Psychosocial Factors in Asthma Working Group for the intellectual stimulation and support that led to the writing of this chapter. We also are indebted to the John D. and Catherine T. MacArthur Network on Socioeconomic Status and Health for their encouragement and support. Special thanks are due to William Busse, Diane Gold, Stephen Manuck, and Scott Weiss for their comments on a preliminary draft.

## References

1.  National Heart, Lung, and Blood Institute. Global Initiative for Asthma. NIH Publication #95-3659, Bethesda, Maryland, 1995.
2.  Knapp P. Psychosomatic aspects of bronchial asthma: a review. In: Cheren S, ed. Psychosomatic Medicine: Theory, Physiology, and Practice. Vols. 1 & 2. Madison, CT: International Universities Press, Inc., 1989:503–564.
3.  Busse WW, Kiecolt-Glaser JK, Coe C, Martin RJ, Weiss ST, Parker SR. NHLBI

workshop summary: stress and asthma. Am J Respir Crit Care Med 1995; 151:249–252.

4. Weiss E. Psychoanalyse einer fallses von nervosen asthma. Int Z Psychoanal 1922; 8:440–445.
5. French TM, Alexander F. Psychogenic factors in bronchial asthma. Psychosom Med Monogr 1941; 4:2–94.
6. Fenichel O. Nature and classifications of the so-called psychosomatic phenomena. Psychoanal Q 1945; 14:287.
7. Kotses H, Hindi-Alexander M, Creer TL. A reinterpretation of psychologically induced airways changes. J Asthma 1989; 26:53–63.
8. Mrazek DA, Klinnert M. Asthma: psychoneuroimmunologic considerations. In: Ader R, Cohen N, Felten F, eds. Psychoneuroimmunology. 2d ed. New York: Academic Press, 1991:1013–1036.
9. Lehrer P, Isenberg S, Hochron SM. Asthma and emotion: a review. J Asthma 1993; 30:5–21.
10. Steptoe A. Psychological aspects of bronchial asthma. In: Rachman S, ed. Contributions to Medical Psychology. Vol. 3. Elmsford, NY: Pergamon Press, 1984:7–30.
11. Creer TL. Asthma. J Cons Clin 1982; 50:912–21.
12. Miklich DR, Rewey HH, Weiss JH, Kolton S. A preliminary investigation of psychophysiological responses to stress among different subgroups of asthmatic children. J Psychosom Res 1973; 17:1–8.
13. Levenson R. Effects of thermatically relevant and general stressors on specificity of responding in asthmatic and nonasthmatic subjects. Psychosom Med 1979; 41:28–39.
14. Miller B, Wood B. Psychophysiologic reactivity in asthmatic children: a cholinergically mediated confluence of pathways. J Am Acad Child Adolesc Psychiatry 1994; 33:1236–45.
15. Tal A, Miklich DR. Emotionally induced decreases in pulmonary flow rates in asthmatic children. Psychosom Med 1976; 38:190–200.
16. Isenberg SA, Lehrer PM, Hochron S. The effects of suggestion and emotional arousal on pulmonary function in asthma: a review and a hypothesis regarding vagal mediation. Psychosom Med 1992; 54:192–216.
17. Mrazek DA. Asthma: Psychiatric considerations, evaluation, and management. In: Middleton E, et al., eds. Allergy: Principles and Practice. 3rd ed. Mosby: St. Louis, 1988:1176–1196.
18. Lazarus RS, Folkman S. Stress, Appraisal, and Coping. New York: Springer, 1984.
19. Moran MG. Psychological factors affecting pulmonary and rheumatologic diseases. Psychosomatics 1991; 32:14–23.
20. Levi L, ed. Stress and Distress in Response to Psychosocial Stimuli. New York: Pergamon Press, 1972.
21. Selye H. The Stress of Life. New York: McGraw-Hill, 1956.
22. Mason JW. A re-evaluation of the concept of ''non-specificity'' in distress theory. J Psychiatr Res 1971; 8:323–333.
23. Stokes PE. The neuroendocrine measurement of depression. In: Marsella AJ, Hirschfeld RMA, Katz MM, eds. The Measurement of Depression. New York: Guilford Press, 1987:153–195.

24. Ockenfels MC, Porter L, Smyth J, Kirschbaum C, Hellhammer DH, Stone AA. Effect of chronic stress associated with unemployment on salivary cortisol: overall cortisol levels, diurnal rhythm and acute stress reactivity. Psychosom Med 1995; 57:460–467.

25. Baum A, Grunberg NE, Singer JE. Biochemical measurements in the study of emotion. Psychol Sci 1982; 3:56–60.

26. Rabin BS, Cohen S, Ganguli R, Lysle DT, Cunnick JE. Bidirectional interaction between the central immune system and immune system. Crit Rev Immunol 1989; 9:279–312.

27. Baum A, Cohen L, Hall M. Control and intrusive memories as possible determinants of chronic stress. Psychosom Med 1993; 55:274–286.

28. Cohen S, Lichtenstein E. Partner behaviors that support quitting smoking. J Cons Clin 1990; 58:304–309.

29. Shiffman S, Wills TA, eds. Coping and Substance Use. New York: Academic Press, 1985.

30. Holt PG. Immune and inflammatory function in cigarette smokers. Thorax 1987; 42:241–249.

31. Richardson JB. State of the art. Nerve supply to the lungs. Am Rev Respir Dis 1979; 119:785–802.

32. Nadel JA. Autonomic regulation of airway smooth muscle. In: Nadel JA, ed. Physiology and Pharmacology of the Airways. New York: Marcel Dekker, 1980:215–257.

33. Barnes PJ, Baraniuk JN, Belvisi MG. Neuropeptides in the respiratory tract. Am Rev Respir Dis 1991; 144:1187–1198, 1391–1399.

34. Ind PW, Scriven AJI, Dollery CT. Use of tyramine to probe pulmonary noradrenaline release in asthma (abstr). Clin Sci 1983; 64:9P.

35. Nadel JA, Barnes PJ. Autonomic regulation of the airways. Annu Rev Med 1984; 35:451–467.

36. Sheppard MN, Kurian SS, Kenzen Logmans SC, Michetti F, Cocchia D, et al. Neuron-specific enolase and S-100. New markers for delineating the innervation of the respiratory tract in man and other animals. Thorax 1983; 38:333–340.

37. Drazen JM, Israel E, Boushey HA, Chinchilli VM, Fahy JV, et al. Comparison of regularly scheduled with as-needed use of albuterol in mild asthma. N Engl J Med 1996; 335:841–847.

38. Herbert TB, Cohen S. Depression and immunity; a meta-analytic review. Psychol Bull 1993; 113:472–486.

39. Cohen S, Herbert T. Health psychology: psychological factors and physical disease from the perspective of human psychoneuroimmunology. Annu Rev Psychol 1996; 47:113–142.

40. Kiecolt-Glaser JK, Cacioppo JT, Malarkey WB, Glaser R. Acute psychological stressors and short-term immune changes; what, why, for whom, and to what extent? Psychosom Med 1992; 54:680–685.

41. Herbert TB, Cohen S, Marsland AL, Bachen EA, Muldoon MF, Rabin BS, Manuck, SB. Cardiovascular reactivity and the course of immune response to an acute psychological stressor. Psychosom Med 1994; 56:337–344.

42. Manuck SB, Cohen S, Rabin BS, Muldoon M, Bachen E. Individual differences in cellular immune response to stress. Psychol Sci 1991; 2:111–115.

43. Bachen EA, Manuck SB, Cohen S, Muldoon MF, Raibel R, et al. Adrenergic blockage ameliorates cellular immune responses to mental stress in humans. Psychosom Med 1995; 57:366–372.

44. Dobbin JP, Harth M, McCain GA, Martin RA, Cousins K. Cytokine production and lymphocyte transformation during stress. Brain Behav Immun 1991; 5:339–348.

45. Glaser R, Kennedy S, Lafuse WP, Bonneau RH, Speicher C, Hillhouse J, Kiecolt-Glaser JK. Psychological stress-induced modulation of interleukin 2 receptor gene expression and interleukin 2 production in peripheral blood leukocytes. Arch Gen Psychiatry 1990; 47:707–712.

46. Marsland AL, Manuck SB, Fazzari TV, Steward CJ, Rabin BS. Stability of individual differences in cellular immune responses to acute psychological stress. Psychosom Med 1995; 57:295–298.

47. Cohen S, Hamrick N, Rodriguez M, Rabin B, Manuck B. The stability of and interrelations between cardiovascular, immune, endocrine, and psychological reactivity to an acute stressor. Unpublished manuscript, Department of Psychology, Carnegie Mellon University, Pittsburgh, 1997.

48. Kang D-H, Coe CL, McCarthy DO, Nizar NJ, Kelly EA, Rodriguez RR, Busse WW. Cytokine profiles of stimulated blood lymphocytes in asthmatic and healthy adolescents across the school year. J Interferon Cytokine Res 1997; 17:481–487.

49. Singh L, Boucher W, Pang X, Theoharides TC. Corticotropin-releasing hormone and immobilization stress induce skin mast cell degranulation and increased vascular permeability. New Orleans, LA: Society for Neuroscience, 1997.

50. Barnes PJ. Cytokines as mediators of chronic asthma. Am J Respir Crit Care Med 1994; 150:S42–49.

51. Bittleman DB, Casale TB. Allergic models and cytokines. Am J Respir Crit Care Med 1994; 150:S72–76.

52. Romagnani S. Induction of TH1 and TH2 responses: a key role for the natural immune response? Immunol Today 1992; 13:379–381.

53. Martinez FD. Role of viral infection in the inception of asthma and allergies during childhood: Could they be protective? Thorax 1994; 49:1189–1191.

54. Martinez FD, Stern DA, Wright AL, Taussig LM, Halonen M, and the Group Health Medical Association. Association of non-wheezing lower respiratory tract illness in early life with persistently diminished serum IgE levels. Thorax 1995; 50:1067–1072.

55. Wright RJ, Weiss ST, Cohen S, Hawthorne M, Gold DR. Life events, perceived stress, home characteristics and wheeze in asthmatic/allergic families. Am J Respir Crit Care Med 1996; 153:A420.

56. Kang D, Coe CL, McCarthy D, Ershler WB. Immune alterations in healthy and asthmatic adolescents induced by final examinations. Nurs Res 1997; 46:12–19.

57. Sigurs N, Bjarnason R, Sigurbergsson F, Kjellman B, Bjorksten B. Asthma and immunoglobulin E antibodies after respiratory syncytial virus bronchiolitis: a prospective cohort study with matched controls. Pediatrics 1995; 95:500–505.

58. Folkerts DG, Gern JE, Nijkamp FP, Sorkness R, Busse WW. State-of-the-art virus-induced airway hyperresponsiveness and asthma. Am J Respir Crit Care Med 1998; 157:1708–1720.

59. Busse WW, et al. The role of respiratory infections in asthma. In Holgate ST, et al., eds. Asthma: Physiology, Immunopharmacology, and Treatment. London: Academic Press, 1993:345–352.
60. Lemanske RF Jr, et al. Rhinovirus upper respiratory infection increases airway hyperreactivity and late asthmatic reactions. J Clin Invest 1989; 83:1–10.
61. Martinez FD, et al. Diminished lung function as a predisposing factor for wheezing respiratory illness in infants. N Engl J Med 1988; 319:1112–1117.
62. Johnston S, et al. Viral infections in exacerbations in schoolchildren with cough or wheeze: a longitudinal study. Am Rev Respir Dis 1992; 145:A546.
63. Nicholson KG, Kent J, Ireland DC. Respiratory viruses and exacerbations of asthma in adults. Br Med J 1993; 307:982–986.
64. Welliver RC, et al. The development of respiratory syncytial virus specific IgE and the release of histamine in nasopharyngeal secretions after infection. N Engl J Med 1981; 305:841–846.
65. Castleman WL, et al. Viral bronchiolitis during early life induces increased numbers of bronchiolar mast cells and airway hyperresponsiveness. Am J Pathol 1990; 137: 821–831.
66. Weiss ST, Tager IB, Munzo A, Speizer FE. The relationship of respiratory infections in early childhood to the occurrence of increased levels of bronchial responsiveness and atopy. Am Rev Respir Dis 1985; 131:573–578.
67. Busse WW. Respiratory infections: their role in airway responsiveness and the pathogenesis of asthma. J Allergy Clin 1990; 85:671–683.
68. Boyce WT, Chesney M, Alkin A, et al. Psychobiologic reactivity to stress and childhood respiratory illness: results of two prospective studies. Psychosom Med 1995; 57:411–422.
69. Graham NMH, Douglas RB, Ryan P. Stress and acute respiratory infection. Am J Epidemiol 1986; 124:389–401.
70. Meyer RJ, Haggerty RJ. Streptococcal infections in families. Pediatrics 1962; 29: 539–549.
71. Clover RD, Abell T, Becker LA, Crawford S, Ramsey JC. Family functioning and stress as predictors of influenza B infection. J Fam Pract 1989; 28:535–539.
72. Cohen S, Tyrrell DAJ, Smith AP. Psychological stress and susceptibility to the common cold. N Engl J Med 1991; 325:606–612.
73. Cohen S, Frank E, Doyle WJ, Skoner DP, Rabin BS, Gwaltney JM. Types of stressors that increase susceptibility to the common cold. Health Psychol 1998; 17:214–223.
74. Stone AA, Bovbjerg DH, Neale JM, Napoli A, Valdimarsdottir H, et al. Development of common cold symptoms following rhinovirus infection is related to prior stressful events. Behav Med 1992; 8:115–120.
75. Cohen S, Doyle WJ, Skoner DP, Fireman P, Gwaltney J, Newsom J. State and trait negative affect as predictors of objective and subjective symptoms of respiratory viral infections. JPSP 1995; 68:159–169.
76. Cohen S, Doyle WJ, Skoner DP, Rabin BS, Gwaltney JM. Social ties and susceptibility to the common cold. JAMA 1997; 277:1940–1944.
77. Avner SE, Kinsman RA. Psychologic factors and allergic diseases. In: Bierman CW, Pearlman DS, eds. Allergic disease from infancy to adulthood. Philadelphia: W.B. Saunders, 1988:300–317.

# 11

## General Virology and Targets for Therapy

DAVID TYRRELL

Common Cold Unit
Salisbury, Wiltshire, England

## I. Introduction

There have been many important advances in our understanding of the role played by viruses in the clinical problems of asthma and related diseases. The purpose of this essay is to look again at some general features of the biology and behavior of viruses in order to see how they fit into what we know of the condition and to look for guidance as to where significant new advances might be made.

A huge number of viruses are now known to science, and their structure and behavior are amazingly diverse, although we shall ignore the viruses of insects, plants, and bacteria and consider only those of warm-blooded vertebrates (Table 1). Fortunately, although we need to think of some of the viruses that affect farm animals, those involved in asthma all belong to the group commonly called respiratory viruses of humans. To molecular biologists this is an unsatisfactory classification, for it brings together viruses with profound differences in their genome. Some encode genes in DNA, but many more use RNA, and in many the particle contains a positive sense strand while in some it is negative stranded; profound differences in the strategy of virus replication result from this. Proteins, some of which are enzymes, are encoded by the genes and synthesized with the ribosomes of the host cell. In some cases they condense around nucleic acid and

**Table 1**  Classification and Basic Structure of Viruses Causing Human
Respiratory Infections

| Family | Name | Genome | Size (nm) | Lipid envelope | Serotypes |
|---|---|---|---|---|---|
| Picornaviridae | Rhinovirus | RNA ss+ | 20–30 | 0 | 100+ |
| Picornaviridae (enterovirus) | Coxsackie viruses A & B Echovirus | RNA ss+ | 20–30 | 0 | 70+ |
| Orthomyxoviridae | Influenza virus | RNA ss− | 80–120 | + | Types A, B, and C Many strain differences |
| Paramyxoviridae (paramyxovirus) | Human parainfluenza virus | RNA ss− | 150–300 | + | 4 |
| Paramyxoviridae (pneumovirus) | Respiratory syncytial virus | RNA ss− | 150–300 | + | 2 |
| Paramyxoviridae (morbillivirus) | Measles virus | RNA ss− | 150–300 | + | 1 |
| Coronaviridae | Human coronavirus | RNA ss+ | 80–160 | + | 2 |
| Adenoviridae (mastadenovirus) | Human adenovirus | DNA ds± | 70–90 | 0 | 35+ |

ss = single stranded; ds = double stranded; + and − indicate polarity of nucleic acid in particle.

in others they are aligned in a cell membrane and fold around the nucleic acid
as it buds out of the membrane surface. What brings these organisms together
is their common attribute of being able to reach the respiratory tract of their host
and to initiate infection and replicate efficiently there, usually in the cells lining
the nose or lower airways. A major reason for their occupying this particular
biological niche is that they are shed into respiratory secretions or onto the surface
of the membranes and are then shed into the environment, often with the assistance of reflex mechanisms such as coughing or sneezing. They generally resist
drying long enough to land on respiratory epithelium, to bind to and infect surface
cells and then spread across the mucosa provided that they are not neutralized
by antibody directed against proteins of the virus particle.

Some of their properties can be linked to their pathogenic role. In most
cases they are toxic to cells and cause the cells in which they replicate to degener-
ate. However, they are mostly adapted to growth at temperatures below that of
the body core. This probably explains, at least in part, why they often infect only
the upper airways and do not descend into the lower respiratory tract or produce

generalized systemic infections. In recent years more attention has been given to the mechanisms by which they induce widespread signs and symptoms, both in the airways and systemically. At one time it was thought that this would prove to be analogous to that produced by antigen inhaled into the airway of an allergic subject. However, this has not proved to be so; at least the nasal symptoms of a cold that are so like those of hay fever are virtually unaffected by potent antihistamine drugs. It has recently been found that there may be general nasal symptoms even when only a limited number of cells are infected (1). It appears that respiratory viruses, which can infect cells without killing them, may induce them to produce cytokines, but whether this occurs in natural disease is not known (2).

## II. Virus Diagnosis

A major contribution to the subject has been the gradual development over the past 40 years of a range of novel methods for cultivating and detecting common respiratory viruses (see Ref. 3). During the 1950s it was shown that inoculating tissue cultures of monkey kidney cells showed the presence of parainfluenza viruses, which could cause acute lower airway illnesses in children and common colds in adults. In the same way respiratory syncytial virus (RSV) was discovered in the secretions of cases of bronchiolitis of infants using cultures of transformed human epithelial cells that developed characteristic syncytia. Later on these viruses were detected more rapidly in the nasal secretions of children by immunofluorescence. During the 1960s human embryo kidney cells or fibroblasts were shown to detect rhinoviruses in about one in four individuals with common colds, and then coronaviruses were detected using fibroblasts or organ cultures of human embryo tracheal or nasal cells. These methods began to be applied to patients with asthma or relapses of chronic bronchitis, but the results were largely negative at first until research workers began to go out into the community to test for viruses at the very onset of an episode. However, the positive results were outnumbered by the negative, which was not surprising since it was only with difficulty that these methods would detect a virus in normal subjects with an acute virus-type respiratory illness.

In the 1980s new sensitive antibody-binding tests were being developed and variants, such as the ELISA, were applied to detecting virus antigens and antibodies. Indeed they made it relatively easy to detect coronavirus infections serologically, but they were not successful in detecting respiratory virus antigens except in the case of infections in early childhood, and improved methods developed using europium were prohibitively expensive (4). However, methods were also being developed to detect virus nucleic acid. One by one they were evaluated, in our case using rhinoviruses (5). Probes for hybridization tests produced from

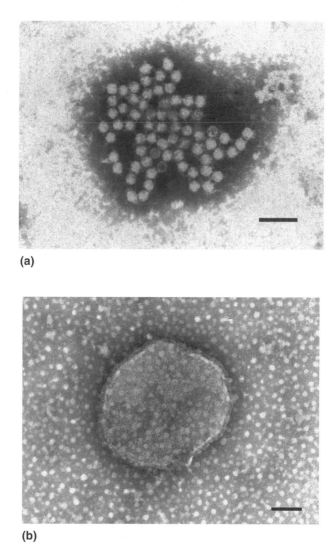

**(a)**

**(b)**

**Figure 1** Negative contrast electron micrographs of virus particles. The bars in each panel represent 100 nm. Note the great variation in particle size. (a) A cluster of rhinovirus particles. Some are "empty," i.e., lacking internal RNA. (b) A single particle of respiratory syncytial virus (RSV). Note the outer membrane with projections. (c) A group of coronavirus particles. Note the great variability in shape and the large club-shaped projections of the surface virus protein. (d) A single adenovirus particle and some debris. The individual capsomeres of the particle can be seen arranged to form the triangular faces of an icosahedron. (Figure 1a courtesy of Barry Dowsett; Figures 1b–1d courtesy of Heather Davies.)

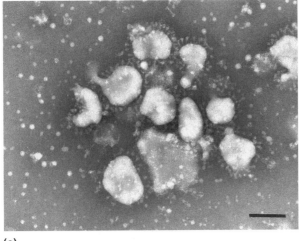

**(c)**

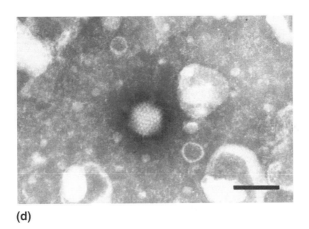

**(d)**

cDNA in bacteria were useful but not sufficiently sensitive for use as diagnostic tests on clinical material, and neither were oligonucleotides designed to detect well-conserved sequences in virus nucleic acids. However, after some years of refining it was shown that polymerase chain reaction (PCR) can be used to detect respiratory virus infections in clinical material, such as nasal aspirates, from patients acquiring infection with these viruses in the community (6). They have been applied to children and adults with wheezy tendency or diagnosed asthma and show that a virus can now be detected in about four out of five episodes of upper respiratory and lower respiratory illness (6).

Thus, as described elsewhere in this volume, we now have the results of quite reliable and repeatable estimates of the frequency and type of virus infections associated with wheezing and asthma in different categories of disease. These can be summarized by saying that virus infections can be demonstrated in a high proportion of cases and that the viruses found reflect those found in normal subjects with mild acute respiratory diseases—rhinoviruses and coronaviruses—and influenza viruses in epidemic years. RSV and parainfluenza viruses are relatively important in infants and young children. The evidence strongly suggests that infection with these viruses plays a causative role, but a prepared host is certainly necessary for disease to develop, although the details of the pathogenesis have yet to be worked out.

## III.  Prevention or Treatment of Virus Infection

### A.  Hygiene

The simplest and most direct way to apply this knowlege would be to prevent or treat the virus infection. Good hygiene has greatly reduced the burden of gastrointestinal illness by preventing infection with both bacteria and viruses in well-developed societies.

However, the level of hygiene at present employed does not prevent frequent acute respiratory infections. This is probably because airborne transmission is not as easy to interrupt as that by food and water. This view has been challenged over many years, but early attempts to reduce colds in schoolchildren by ultraviolet irradiation of classroom air failed, though it had some effect on the transmission of measles. More recent work was based on the hypothesis that colds are frequently transmitted by fingers and fomites. Effective methods of inactivating viruses on these surfaces were devised, but controlled trials showed a barely detectable effect on the transmission rate in families (7). It is customary in certain societies, particularly in the Far East, to wear a surgical mask to prevent the spread of colds and influenza. I know of no formal studies to validate their efficacy in the field. Experience in the control of allergic and other health problems due to the inhalation of respirable dusts has shown that well-designed and well-fitted masks can be effective, as can air filtration and extraction plants. However, it is often found that healthy employees are very resistant to wearing or using such equipment, though the resistance can be overcome. Nevertheless, such ideas have not yet been applied and shown to be effective in westernized communities particularly to prevent the spread of infection from or to young people in the home. Perhaps the problem should be addressed again among individuals for whom a respiratory virus infection is not a trivial matter, especially patients with asthma.

## B. Vaccines

Vaccination has been shown to be one of the most successful and cost-effective ways of preventing virus infections. However, it works best against infections in which there is a crucial viremic phase, such as poliomyelitis, measles, or hepatitis and is not as satisfactory in combating infections in which the key steps in pathogenesis occur at a mucosal surface; this applies to all the respiratory viruses. Of course, influenza vaccination has been part of clinical practice for decades. It is usually found to be about 70% effective, and this may be because vaccines administered parenterally induce mainly circulating antibodies, which are less effective in protecting mucosal surfaces than secretory antibodies, although these can be induced by live vaccines administered to the mucosae. It is therefore an attractive idea to make vaccines against RSV and parainfluenza viruses, as these can be covered by a few serotypes. Early attempts to make inactivated vaccines failed, but there are continuing detailed studies of the immune mechanisms that protect people from natural infection and of candidate vaccine products to protect both children and animals. If useful products are developed, they should be tried for the prevention of asthma, but it is important to realize that although there may be local flurries of cases of influenza, these other viruses on average produce only a small percentage of infections.

It was generally thought in the 1930s and 1940s that there was a single common cold virus that, when cultured, could be made into a vaccine that would prevent colds. It is generally accepted now that this is not so. The largest species of common cold virus is the rhinovirus, which exists in at least 100 distinct serotypes, and it would be impractical to include so many serotypes in a single vaccine to be used to partially control a single syndrome. It was hoped that it would turn out that a few serotypes cause most of the clinical effects, but the problem could not be simplified by selecting a few strains that were clinically important—or even by selecting a small set of strains that induced immunity against a range of serotypes. Coronaviruses seem to be less varied antigenically, as there are only two major serotypes, but natural immunity seems to decline quite quickly and no serious efforts to develop a human vaccine are reported. Because coronaviruses cause serious problems in the health of farm animals, vaccines may be developed for these, which might serve as a starting point for developing a product for humans. If any possible vaccines are developed they should be evaluated in patients with asthma or chronic bronchitis, but it is worth remembering that the influenza vaccines that are already available are not always used for asthma or related conditions.

## C. Antiviral Drugs

There has not been research targeted at producing antiviral drugs for the treatment of asthma, but a considerable amount has been aimed at treating or preventing influenza or colds, and as we have seen, success in these fields might readily be applied to the relief of asthma. Early work was done by giving candidate molecules to animals infected with viruses. But on occasion false hopes were raised. Compounds that were too toxic damaged cells, and these cells produced less virus. Pessimists asserted that truly selective drugs would never be found. Nevertheless, in this way it was shown that amantadine was active against influenza virus infection in mice. After its discovery amantadine made slow progress towards clinical use, but when interferon was identified in the course of basic research on the biology of influenza virus hopes rose again.

The importance of interferon was that it showed that it was possible to treat a cell with a protein that produced no damage or obvious metabolic change and yet inhibited very strongly the replication of a virus such as influenza. There were, however, frustrations. One was that interferons made by cells from different animals were often active only in those or closely related species. Another was that the molecule could be very difficult to produce and purify. After a great deal of effort, enough human leukocyte interferon was produced to show that if sprayed up the nose repeatedly it would prevent experimental rhinovirus colds in a few volunteers. Proper field trials on colds in families had to wait until, in entirely unrelated developments, the first techniques for cloning human DNA and expressing it in bacteria were discovered. As a result, milligram amounts of pure interferons could be obtained, and it was shown that natural rhinovirus colds could be prevented by spraying the nose of contacts of cases (8). But even with these large amounts it was not possible to influence a cold once it had started to become clinically evident, and if one continued treatment of normal subjects beyond a matter of days, they developed nasal inflammation and symptoms rather like the cold one wanted to prevent. Indeed, it is now known that interferons have so much to do with the mediation of inflammatory and immunological effects that they must be considered along with cytokines and not simply for their directly antiviral effects. As described elsewhere, gamma interferons are deeply involved in the networks of communication between T lymphocytes, macrophages, and so on.

### Antirhinovirus Drugs

While interferons were being investigated various pharmaceutical laboratories around the world began to use the newly developed tissue culture methods to search for antiviral activity in various materials in their screening programs. One of the first of these was the Wellcome Research Laboratories, who screened natural products for their ability to prevent the growth of rhinoviruses in tissue cultures. They found such activity and modified the active molecule to enhance it. The final outcome was dichloroflavan, which at the time of its discovery was one of the most active antiviral molecules known. Another was Nippon Roche, a branch of Hoffmann LaRoche, which found activity in a traditional Chinese herbal tea used for minor respiratory diseases. This led to a highly active chalcone. Third, Janssen in Belgium set up a screening program with a series of compounds that had been synthesized as targets or as intermediates in a previous search for improved drugs with central nervous system (CNS) activity. Out of this came several very active molecules. Thus, these molecules had very diverse origins and considerable differences in structure, but they all had certain common features. They inactivated virus particles (rather than blocking virus replication) and bound to the protein, preventing the release of virus nucleic acid into the cell. They were also very insoluble in aqueous solutions. As a result there were problems in formulating them for administration to volunteers. Dichloroflavan was made up in oil, and a prodrug of the chalcone was synthesized that could be absorbed when given by mouth. Although the drug reached the circulation, it did not enter the nasal secretions, and unfortunately when then given as a nasal spray, as interferon had been, it did not prevent rhinovirus infections. Finally the Janssen drug, which was more active, was formulated with cyclodextrin and had a clear-cut effect on colds, but again only if given during the latent period (9–11).

While this work was continuing, Sterling Winthrop Laboratories in the United States had started from the observation that fermentation liquors might have antiviral activity against poliovirus. On this basis they synthesized a number of derivatives of the active molecule actidione, varying the length of the carbon chain in the middle and the size and composition of the bulky groups at both ends. They showed that these changes produced a wide variety of changes in the antiviral activity. Rather than testing whether they could be used to prevent or treat human disease, they tried to find out how the most active compound, disoxaril, worked. The crystallographic structure of picornaviruses had just been solved by M. Rossmann and his group at Purdue University, and by soaking crystals of viruses in the drug and examining them by x-ray crystallography they were able to show that the active molecules became inserted into a hydrophobic cleft in one of the proteins of the outer coat of the virus, the so-called capsid shell. Subsequent research showed that the antirhinovirus drugs bound to a similar cleft in rhinoviruses (12), and mutations that made viruses drug resistant often led to amino acid substitutions in the cleft so that the drug molecule could not ''dock'' properly.

Thus, although none of these drugs is influencing clinical practice, it is clear that we can find nontoxic molecules and begin to understand how they behave in molecular terms. It is critical that potent antiviral molecules also have properties that enable them to reach infected sites effectively if they are to be successfully exploited as useful drugs.

### Molecularly Designed Antivirals

We are now moving into the era of designing drugs to interact with specific molecules or active sites within molecules. The antirhinovirus drugs just mentioned were selected as a result of screening for their capacity to prevent the replication of the whole virus, and only in retrospect was it discovered that the structure of picornaviruses has a vulnerable point with which all the molecules chosen were interacting. Drugs are now being introduced that have been developed by a "reversed" process. For instance, using respiratory viruses as an example, new anti-influenza drugs are now in view, which were found by deciding to block the neuraminidase enzyme because it plays a key part in the entry of viruses into cells and their release from the cell surface. Rather than screening compounds for their ability to reduce enzyme activity in vitro, the recent work started from the results of crystallographic research on the structure of the pure virus protein. This showed that it has a "propellerlike" shape, within which lies the active center of the enzyme. Working from this, an algorithm was constructed to define the size, shape, charge, and so on of a molecule, which would bind specifically and could be expected to inactivate the enzyme function. This led to a relatively small number of molecules, and it has already been shown in the Glaxo-Wellcome Laboratories that at least one is nontoxic and prevents virus replication and disease in animals and humans at very low concentration. It is significant that its use will still be constrained by the fact that it does not reach the respiratory tract if given by mouth and so has to be used as an intranasal spray. Another compound is being developed in a collaboration between Gilead and Roche, and this may be effective if given by mouth.

## IV. Further Prospects

This is just a snapshot of research on antivirals for respiratory viruses but it does indicate that there are powerful new techniques that could be applied to developing new drugs on the basis of our increased understanding of the molecular details of virus growth. For example, it is now known that rhinoviruses enter cells by interacting with the terminal two domains of the ICAM-1 molecule on the cell surface. A specific monoclonal antibody against this site prevents virus particles from initiating infection. This would not be a realistic therapeutic agent in humans, but a small synthetic molecule might be developed to have the same effect (reviewed in Ref. 3). As in the case of all drugs directed at cellular components, there is a chance that molecules directed at such a target might have effects on other biological functions such as inflammatory and immune responses, and these would need to be evaluated as well as antiviral activity. Thus, the use of these new methods will have to be backed up with many of the older techniques used in drug development in the past. The entry of coronaviruses might also be blocked. There is scope too for targeting enzymes late in the growth cycle, as has been done so successfully with retroviruses such as human immunodeficiency virus (HIV). Rhinoviruses have a specific protease, which is used to cleave the virus proteins, and this is better conserved than capsid proteins so it is likely that there would be fewer differences in the sensitivity of different serotypes than have been found with the capsid-binding drugs. The polymerase of RNA viruses does not copy as accurately as DNA polymerase, and there is no editing mechanism for RNA copies. As a result, in any sample of virus there are variants that may be resistant to a drug directed at a specific site. Thus drug-resistant mutants can rapidly emerge. However, it seems to be a general principle that in such situations the problem can be largely overcome by combining drugs that are directed at different targets, that is, different molecules or different sites on the same molecule. Therefore, our experience with tuberculosis and AIDS teaches us that although some respiratory viruses are variable, we may be able to find effective ways of employing specific antivirals against them.

## V. General Comments

This chapter has covered some aspects of the study of virology that are relevant to the therapy of virus infection in asthma. This is, however, a partial view, and whether one approach or another will actually benefit patients will be made clear by research on the pathogenesis of disease, the clinical responses of patients in practice, and formal trials. Whether specific antiviral drugs can be used may depend on how well PCR or other novel techniques can be incorporated into routine diagnostic procedures to make rapid virus diagnosis a practical possibility.

Finally, we may decide that the best treatment may still focus on what follows the virus infection. After all, in many gastrointestinal infections we leave the body to deal with the infection and assist by giving fluid and electrolytes. It may be that it is more important to understand and correct the changes in the release of cytokines and lymphokines induced by viruses and the immune responses to their antigens and leave the body to control the infections, as it does so well in persons without an asthmatic tendency. We started on this road by testing an early partial antagonist of kinins in the treatment of experimental colds on the grounds that kinins might be responsible for many of the nasal symptoms. It was not successful, but then neither were many early experiments on interferon.

An even more speculative approach would be to apply the studies showing that personal stress may substantially increase susceptibility to respiratory virus infection, although the mechanism of this effect is quite obscure (13). We have been taught for decades that it may be beneficial to consider the role of psychosomatic effects in asthma attacks. The usual hypothesis is that the mental state might alter the reactivity of the bronchial tree or the intensity of an allergic response. Perhaps it can also alter resistance to viral infections and influence the syndrome in that way.

## References

1.  Turner RB, Winther B, Hendley JO, Mygind N, Gwaltney JMJ. Sites of virus recovery and antigen detection in epithelial cells during experimental rhinovirus infection. Acta Otolaryngol Suppl Stockh 1984; 413:9–14.
2.  Becker S, Quay J, Soukup J. Cytokine (tumour necrosis factor, IL 6 and IL 8) production by respiratory syncytial virus infected human alveolar macrophages. J Immunol 1991; 147:430.
3.  Diagnostic Procedures for Viral, Rickettsial and Chlamydial Infections. 7th ed. Washington, DC: American Public Health Association, 1995:1–633.
4.  Hierholzer JC, Bingham PG, Coombs RA, Johansson KH, Anderson LJ, Halonen PE. Comparison of monoclonal antibody time-resolved fluoroimmunoassay with monoclonal antibody capture-biotinylated detector enzyme immunoassay for respiratory syncytial virus and parainfluenzavirus antigen detection. J Clin Microbiol 1989; 27:1243–1249.
5.  Gama RE, Horsnell PR, Hughes PJ, et al. Amplification of rhinovirus specific nucleic acids from clinical samples using the polymerase chain reaction. J Med Virol 1989; 28:73–77.
6.  Johnston SL, Sanderson G, Pattemore PK, et al. Use of polymerase chain reaction for diagnosis of picornavirus infection in subjects with and without respiratory symptoms. J Clin Microbiol 1993; 31:111–117.
7.  Hendley JO, Gwaltney JM. Mechanisms of transmission of rhinovirus infections. Epidemiol Rev 1988; 10:242–258.
8.  Scott GM, Tyrrell DAJ. In vivo and clinical studies. In: Finter NB, Oldham RK, eds. Interferon. Vol. 4. Amsterdam: Elsevier, 1985:181–215.
9.  Al-Nakib W, Willman J, Higgins PG, Tyrrell DAJ, Shepherd W, Freestone DS. Failure of intranasally administered 4′-6-dichloroflavan to protect against rhinovirus infection in man. Arch Virol 1987; 92:255–260.
10. Al-Nakib W, Higgins PG, Barrow GI, Tyrrell DAJ, Lenox-Smith I, Ishitsuka H. Intranasal chalcone Ro 9-o410 as prophylaxis against rhinovirus infection in volunteers. J Antimicrob Chemother 1987; 20:887–892.
11. Al-Nakib W, Higgins PG, Barrow GI, et al. Suppression of colds in human volunteers challenged with rhinovirus by a new synthetic drug (R61837). Antimicrob Agents Chemother 1989; 33:522–525.
12. Chapman MS, Minor I, Rossmann MG, Diana GD, Andries K. Human rhinovirus 14 complexed with antiviral compound R 61837. J Mol Biol 1991; 217:455–463.
13. Cohen S, Tyrrell DA, Smith AP. Psychological stress and susceptibility to the common cold [see comments]. N Engl J Med 1991; 325:606–612.

# 12

## Advances in the Diagnosis of Respiratory Virus Infections

**A. J. CHAUHAN and SEBASTIAN L. JOHNSTON**

University of Southampton
Southampton, England

## I. Introduction

Advances in the diagnosis of respiratory viruses have led to a reexamination of the role of virus infections in asthma (1,2) and a range of other clinical conditions. Rapid diagnostic methods are of particular importance. Because of the short incubation periods of respiratory viruses, they have the potential to rapidly lead to epidemics (3,4). The availability of specific pharmacological therapy for some of the viruses, if detected early enough in the course of an illness, adds particular importance to the rapidity required in the identification of respiratory infections (5). The diagnosis of respiratory viruses broadly falls into the categories of detecting the virus by electron microscopy (EM), detection of viral antigens, detection of antibody to the virus, detection of the toxic effects of the virus, and, most recently, detection of the viral genome in clinical samples. The most noteworthy advances in the diagnosis of respiratory viruses have been made in the selection of particularly sensitive cell lines for virus culture, the early detection of antigens in these cultures (otherwise referred to as rapid culture assays) by monoclonal antibodies using immunoperoxidase (IP) staining, immunofluorescence (IF), enzyme immunoassay (EIA) and time-resolved fluoroimmunoassay (TR-FIA), and, perhaps most importantly, the use of polymerase chain reaction (PCR) methods to detect virus RNA or DNA in clinical samples. This chapter focuses on the principles of the advances in viral diagnostic methods as applied to respiratory viruses but is not intended to be an exhaustive catalog of all published reports or detection techniques.

## II. Specimens

The respiratory tract can be directly sampled by nasal or throat swabs, nasal washings, nasal aspirates, nasopharyngeal aspirates, sputum, transtracheal aspirates, bronchoalveolar lavage, or biopsy. The method used to collect the specimen is chosen on the technique to be used to identify the virus. A nasal swab is usually taken from the inferior turbinates for maximum virus recovery but usually involves some discomfort to the patient. Similarly, nasal washings [requiring solutions such as phosphate-buffered saline (PBS)] may also be uncomfortable for the patient. Compared to nasal and throat swabs, nasal washings are a more reliable method of recovering virus but are less convenient for both operator and patient. Both methods are suitable for virus culture. Nasopharyngeal aspirates (NPAs) are particularly suitable for virus culture, antigen detection, and PCR and are collected using a mucus extractor using disposable suction catheters that are commercially available (Vygon Laboratories, Ecouen, France). In the authors' experience, the diagnosis of common cold viruses can be made using nasal aspirates (NAs) in preference to NPAs, particularly as acute infections are accompanied by rhinorrhea, the same equipment can be used with less discomfort, and are more suitable for use in infants, children, and neonates. Sputum is rarely used for respiratory viruses because the clinical syndrome of viral pneumonia is usually accompanied by upper and lower respiratory tract symptoms and the diagnosis can be made on either a NA or NPA. In terms of diagnosis in severely ill patients, whether intubated or not, or for research purposes, the diagnosis can be made using bronchoalveolar lavage (BAL) samples (6,7) or in biopsy specimens (8,9), which reduce the risk of contamination by respiratory pathogens in the upper airways.

Irrespective of the type of sample collected, it is imperative for maximum virus recovery that specimens are collected when symptomatic, usually in the first 2–3 days of infection, because virus titers can fall rapidly following this period. The advantages of detecting viral genomes by PCR in clinical samples is that viruses may be detected in the recovery phase of acute illnesses even when conventional antigen-detection techniques may not detect the virus, thus allowing a larger window of opportunity in which virus infection can be identified. Respiratory viruses are particularly labile and are best transported to the laboratory at 4°C and, if not processed immediately, then frozen at −70°C. Multiple freeze-thawing should be avoided because some viruses, e.g., respiratory syncytial (RS) virus, are particularly vulnerable to multiple freeze-thawing. If multiple testing is necessary, aliquots of the specimen should be made prior to storage. For antigen detection assays such as TR-FIA and EIA, transportation and storage are less critical, and a storage temperature of 4°C (or −20°C for longer periods) is often sufficient.

## III. Detection of Virus by Electron Microscopy

For the diagnosis of respiratory virus infections, electron microscopy is usually used to confirm the causes of a particular cytopathic effect in cell culture rather than a first-line diagnostic tool. Although the primary reason for this is because of low virus titers in clinical samples, EM has been used for the detection of coronaviruses and influenza viruses. Despite advances in the sensitivity of EM using specific immunological enhancement, few diagnostic laboratories use this tool for detection of respiratory viruses (10).

## IV. Detection of Virus by Cell Culture

The cell monolayer culture remains the gold standard for detection of respiratory viruses and remains the reference to which other methods such as genomic amplification are compared. Although cell culture may not be as sensitive as PCR techniques in many instances, most hospital laboratories use cell culture as a reliable screening method for respiratory viruses. Furthermore, it is often impractical for most laboratories to carry all cell lines, and in this respect a broad practical coverage of viruses can be obtained by using a continuous human epithelial line (HEp-2, A-549, HeLa), a human fibroblast cell strain (HLF, HELF, MRC-5, WI-38), and primary rhesus monkey kidney (PMK) cells for most applications. The inoculum is adsorbed on the monolayers at room temperature and the cultures washed with maintenance medium and incubated at 33–36°C for up to 3 weeks, with subpassaging as required. Roller culture tubes are often used to enhance the cytopathic effects (CPE). All tubes are examined at least twice weekly, and virus growth is detected by the characteristic CPE under light microscopy or by other methods such as hemadsorption (11).

Adenoviruses replicate readily in HEp-2, MRC-5, and A-549 cells, with or without rolling (12). They are easier to identify than other respiratory viruses because they produce large quantities of soluble antigens and are differentiated from other viruses (which may grow in the same cells and with similar CPE) by various methods including EM, IF, and EIA. Parainfluenza viruses replicate well in roller cultures of PMK cells under a fortified medium without trypsin. The CPE induced by these viruses can develop in 4–7 days, but the cultures often require further "blind" passage to ensure viral growth, as they may sometimes not show obvious CPE at all. Cultures for these viruses therefore often require hemadsorption with guinea pig, human, or monkey erythrocytes at the end of the culture period (13,14). Influenza A, B, and C viruses are best recovered in roller cultures of PMK cells and in embryonated eggs (chick embryo, MDCK, and other cells require a fortified medium containing trypsin for optimal sensitivity). Again, these viruses are detected in PMK cells by hemadsorption (15,16). Picornaviruses produce CPE in PMK, Hep-2, HeLa, and MRC-5 cell lines often in roller cultures (17,18). Enteroviruses are distinguished from rhinoviruses by the former's acid stability. Coronaviruses can be identified directly in nasal and throat specimens by antigen detection using methods such as IF and EIA (because the viruses are extremely labile and difficult to recover in the laboratory) or by serological tests. Clone 16 cells can be used to culture coronavirus 229E specifically. The important cell lines for the culture of the main respiratory viruses have been reviewed elsewhere (19).

## V.  Additional Test for Cell Culture (Rapid Culture Assays)

Cell culture tests often provide results after several days and are therefore of limited use in the acute management of patients. However, the use of centrifugation followed by immunological staining as an adjunct to cell culture, otherwise referred to as rapid culture assay, enhances the speed of diagnosis. Rapid culture assays combine the high sensitivity of standard virus isolation with the speed of viral antigen–detection methods in clinical specimens. Viral antigens are detected in cell cultures by immunofluorescence 16–48 hours after inoculation, usually before a distinct, virus-induced CPE is visible. Cells are grown in shell vials or in 24-well cell culture dishes. Clinical specimens are inoculated into an adequate number of vials or wells, and the cultures centrifuged at approximately $700 \times g$ at room temperature for an hour. Viral antigens in the cultured cells are detected by IF or by IP staining (20). For IF, cultures are usually grown on coverslips in shell vials, and after staining the coverslips are mounted on microscope slides. IP staining is performed in the 24-well plates.

   This technique has been applied to the detection of a range of respiratory viruses including RS virus, adenovirus, and influenza and parainfluenza viruses (20–24), although the results have often been inconsistent. Although the theoretical sensitivity of rapid culture assays is one infectious virus per inoculation volume, the sensitivity has varied (10–80%) when applied to clinical samples, probably as a result of a lack of standardization. Although rapid culture assays do not yield an isolate for further analysis, positive samples can be reinoculated into standard cultures without significant loss of infectivity once the result of the rapid culture is known. Alternatively, the culture supernatant can be stored and used for reinoculation.

## VI. Detection of Viral Antigen

### A. Immunofluorescence

The detection of viruses in nasopharyngeal aspirates of patients with acute respiratory disease by IF was developed in 1968 using rabbit antisera and antispecies conjugates and was considered one of the original rapid diagnostic methods. Commercial polyclonal sera are available for most respiratory viruses, but these are being replaced by monoclonal antibodies (mAbs), which have more consistent specificity and therefore are less likely to require absorption before use (25–28). Furthermore, the use of mAbs (now commercially available) increases the intensity of specific fluorescence and reduces nonspecific fluorescence. Immunofluorescence can be divided into direct and indirect assays; in the direct IF assay, the sample (usually a cell deposit by cytospin) is fixed on a microscope, and virus-specific serum labeled with a fluorescent dye is added and any unbound antibody washed away. Bound antibody is then detected by fluorescent microscopy (16). In the indirect method, specific unlabeled antiviral antibody is first bound to any antigen and then a second labeled antiantibody from another species is used to detect the presence of the first (29). This increases the number of bound antibodies and, therefore, increases sensitivity. The prior use of cyto-centrifugation increases the sensitivity of the assay (30,31). The results of IF assays are usually available within 2–3 hours of taking the sample. Although simple in principle, IF assays have drawbacks in that the specimen needs to contain an adequate number of cells, the antibodies need to be specific, and background fluorescence occurs frequently. Recently, an indirect IF assay containing a pool of mAbs screening for the panel of influenza A, B, RS virus, parainfluenza viruses 1–3, and adenovirus has been described, with a reported sensitivity of 89% (32).

### B. Other Immunoassays

More sensitive immunoassays have now been developed for the detection of respiratory viruses based broadly on the principles of immunofluorescence. The principle of the enzyme-linked immunosorbent assay (ELISA) is that any virus or viral antigen present in a sample is added to specific antibody bound to a solid phase. Any bound or unbound material is then washed away and a second antiviral antibody of another species labeled with an enzyme is added, which binds to any antigen now present. The addition of a substrate for the enzyme then produces a color reaction, which can be read colorimetrically (33). As with IF assays, polyclonal sera have been used but are being replaced by more specific mAbs (34). Recently, ELISA kits that allow the detection of RS virus or influenza virus type A in clinical specimens within 20 minutes have become commercially available (4). These tests are sufficiently sensitive and have the advantage of being able to be performed at the bedside or in a clinic (35).

Immunoperoxidase (IP) staining is the enzymatic equivalent of immuno-fluorescence and instead of a fluorochrome dye being conjugated to antibody, the latter is labeled with peroxidase enzyme, which in the presence of a substrate produces a color reaction. As with IF assays, both direct and indirect methods have been described. Although they have the inherent advantage that only light microscopy is needed, these tests have been more commonly used in conjunction with rapid culture assays (20,24). The use of TR-FIA has recently gained popularity in some diagnostic and research laboratories. The TR-FIA method is similar in format to the ELISA assay, except that the detector antibody has a fluorescent label, Europium-chelate, which is activated by the addition of an "enhancer" solution. Fluorescence is measured immediately by a single photon fluorimeter. A variant of the TR-FIA technique is the biotin-enzyme immunosorbent assay. In this method, the fluorescent label is biotin, and peroxidase labeled avidin is used in place of the enhancement solution. Sensitivities up to 0.1 ng/ml of antigen have been described with mAb incubation TR-FIAs. Monoclonal TR-FIAs have been described for the main respiratory viruses including parainfluenza virus (36), adenovirus (37), influenza virus (38), and RS virus (39).

Although the final interpretation of the test results often requires expertise, the immunoassays described have several advantages over standard IF assays. Specimens can be transported more robustly since intact cells are not required, bulk testing of specimens is possible, and reading the printout of the results is more objective than reading immunofluorescence (40).

## VII.  Detection of Viral Nucleic Acids

Respiratory viruses can be detected in clinical samples by direct or indirect identification of the virus-specific genome. Direct detection comprises the isolation of nucleic acid and then visualization in agarose or polyacrylamide gels by staining with a suitable dye such as ethidium bromide. For respiratory virus infections the amount of virus and hence nucleic acid tends to be too small for direct detection. Hence either indirect detection of nucleic acid with probes is necessary, or direct detection can still be used but after multiplying copies of the viral genome over a millionfold by amplification techniques, principally the polymerase chain reaction. The principles involved in these new techniques are discussed in the following sections.

### A.  Nucleic Acid Hybridization

This technique is based on simple biological principles; all organisms including prokaryotes or eukaryotes contain deoxyribonucleic acid (DNA) or ribonucleic acid (RNA) or both. These nucleic acids comprise the four nucleosides: adenosine (A), cytidine (C), guanosine (G), and either thymidine (T) in DNA or uridine

(U) in RNA. DNA usually exists as a double strand with one chain being complementary to the other, which arises from the specific binding that exists between A and T (or U) and C and G nucleotides. RNA is, with few exceptions, made up of a single chain of nucleotides. Viral nucleic acids are usually double-stranded (ds) DNA or single-stranded (ss) molecules (the majority are RNA viruses). DNA can be dissociated or denatured into single-strand form by heating or by chemical treatment (e.g., NaOH). On removing these physical and chemical agents, the two ssDNAs or RNAs will return to the double-strand form, binding according to their sequence complementarity, referred to as annealing. Hybridization is the process of two different ssDNAs or RNAs with sufficient homology (matching of base pairs) annealing to form a hybrid under controlled physical and chemical reaction conditions (stringency). An integral part of the hybridization assay is the target-specific probe, a short piece of DNA or RNA complementary to a specific region of the viral genome. The probe can be labeled directly with enzymes or other reporter molecules or with linker molecules such as biotin or digoxigenin that serve as a bridge to which reporter molecules can be attached.

### General Principles

All hybridization reactions share the same general principles: the target viral nucleic acid is first denatured and bound to a liquid-phase or solid-phase support such as nylon membrane. The probe, which is also denatured, is incubated with the target DNA under a controlled reaction, after which the unbound probe is removed by thorough washing and a reporter molecule is added to the membrane. After another incubation, excess unbound reporter molecule is removed by washing and a specific substrate solution is added that, when catalyzed by the enzyme, generates a signal that can be detected by a variety of means—visually, fluorometrically, or luminometrically, or a combination of these depending on the substrate used (41).

### Probes, Hybridization Conditions, and Test Formats

Probes are designed from known viral target nucleic acid sequences, and the specificity varies according to the length. The most useful oligonucleotide probes are 20–30 bases in length, have 40–60% G+C content (which affects the melting and annealing temperatures), are without ''within-probe'' complementary regions, and have less than 70% homology with ''nontarget'' regions. Computer software is now readily available in the design of oligonucleotide probes. The stringency of the hybridization reaction is dependent on several parameters, including the temperature, salt concentration, and the presence or absence of inert substances that can serve to accelerate the hybridization reaction. These are reviewed more fully elsewhere (41).

The test format used in the hybridization assay may require modifications depending on the specific method used to detect the virus. In general, there are two formats in use: single-phase hybridization comprises a liquid environment, and dual-phase (or mixed phase) hybridization has either the probe or target bound to a solid matrix. Single-phase hybridization is rarely used in viral diagnostics because they are tedious, time consuming, and cannot be readily automated. Most non–amplification-based probe methods use a dual-phase system. The two most commonly used types of solid phase are nitrocellulose and nylon membranes, followed by magnetic beads and polystyrene microtiter plates. The reasons for using a solid phase is that bound strands of nucleic acid will not self-anneal, the time for hybridization is reduced, multiple targets or probes can be incorporated into a single hybridization reaction, the solid phase can be recovered to enable detection of hybrids, and hybridization reactions using different probes can often be repeated on the same solid phase (19). The main problem—that of nonspecific binding to the solid phase producing "background" interference— can be reduced by prehybridizing the solid phase with components such as nontarget nucleic acid (e.g., salmon sperm) and using blocking agents and detergents such as sodium dodecyl sulfate (SDS). A posthybridization washing step with a detergent is also usually used to remove nonspecifically bound components. The stringency of the hybridization reaction is controlled by the washing step following hybridization and by varying both the temperature of the wash and the amount of detergent used.

### Labeling and Detection Systems

Probes can be labeled by isotopic (radioactive) or nonisotopic (nonradioactive) methods. Isotopes such as $^{32}P$ and $^{35}S$ have been used to label probes, which have allowed sensitive detection by autoradiography. Because of the hazards associated with isotopic methods, the routine use of radioactivity to detect viruses has been superseded by a number of nonradioactive methods without loss of sensitivity of the former methods. The first of these utilized biotin-avidin whereby biotinylated nucleotides are incorporated into the probe and then avidin coupled to an enzyme, such as alkaline phosphatase, is used as a secondary detector molecule. After the addition of an appropriate substrate for the enzyme, a colorimetric or chemiluminescence reaction can be detected as described earlier. Chemiluminescent labels have the added advantage that the results can be conveniently recorded on light-sensitive film. Oligonucleotide probes can be labeled by a variety of techniques including nick translation (42), random priming (43), or from plasmid vectors (44).

Several assays have now been described to detect signals in hybridization assays and are based on the general principles first described by Southern. In this method, the target DNA is separated by gel electrophoresis and transferred to a solid phase (membrane) by capillary action. The membrane is then hybridized to probes in solution. Target nucleic acid can be applied directly to a membrane or filter as either a ''dot'' or a ''slot'' for subsequent probing. This slot-blot hybridization method has the added advantage of being semi-quantitative if a densitometer is used. Several manufacturers produce manifolds that allow nucleic acids in solution to be applied under vacuum to a membrane, thus ensuring uniformity of size of dots or slots (e.g., Schleicher and Schuell, Dassel, Germany). A further development of hybridization is the in situ hybridization assay, which allows the localization of nucleic acids within cells and tissues. Intact cells are fixed on a solid phase, either a membrane or microscope slide, hybridized and probed, and examined under a microscope for signal. These nonisotopic methods allow direct visualization of target sites.

### B. Nucleic Acid Amplification

The amplification of nucleic acids, particularly by the polymerase chain reaction, has led to great advances in the molecular science of genetic diseases, oncology, and forensic medicine. Although other nucleic acid amplification methods have been described, PCR techniques are the most widely used because of their simplicity and flexibility. PCR is directly applicable in diagnostic virology due to the presence of unique sequences found in all viral genomes and the accessibility of nucleotide sequence information for many viruses. PCR has transformed nucleic acid analysis from a research tool to a clinical diagnostic discipline and has been applied to the detection of respiratory viruses in clinical samples (9,18, 37,45–49).

PCR is based on the repetition of three successive reactions outlined in Figure 1. First, double-stranded DNA (dsDNA) is denatured into single-stranded DNA (ssDNA) at high temperature, usually 94–95°C. Second, two specific primers (synthetic oligonucleotides usually 18–22 bases long) anneal (hybridize) to each ssDNA at the 5′ and 3′ termini at 37–72°C. Finally, a thermostable DNA polymerase enzyme extends the primers by always adding nucleotides at the 3′ end of the primers to synthesize new complementary DNA strands at 72°C. These three steps represent a single cycle, and the number of DNA molecules doubles at the end of each cycle and repeated cycles result in the exponential accumulation of specific DNA products whose termini are defined by the 5′ ends of the primers. After the first cycle, the DNA target and newly synthesized DNA strands also become templates for amplification. The length of the newly synthesized DNA is equal to the sum of the length of two primers plus the distance separating the two primers on the original DNA template. Typically 30–50 cycles are used and the entire process is usually automated on specialized thermal cyclers. The products of a PCR reaction are then visualized by gel electrophoresis, and the size of the product corresponds to that of the two

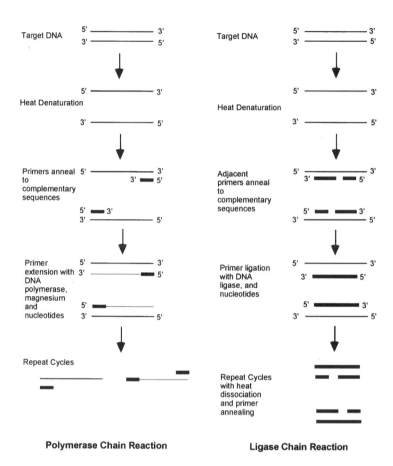

**Figure 1**    Principles of the polymerase chain reaction (PCR) and the ligase chain reaction (LCR).

primers plus the intervening region. To ensure specificity, and often to increase sensitivity, it is then usual to confirm these products as being the required target region by probing with an oligonucleotide probe or alternatively by sequencing (confirming the nucleotide sequence).

There are many factors that influence the quality and sensitivity of a PCR reaction, including the nature of the target sequence and sample preparation, primer, deoxynucleotide triphosphate (dNTP) and magnesium concentrations, and the cycle temperature, number, and hold times. These parameters are discussed in more detail in other reviews (19,41).

### C. Variations of PCR and Other Nucleic Acid Amplification Methods

The principles of the PCR assay have been varied according to the application in diagnostic virology, and the main variations of this theme applicable to the diagnosis of respiratory viruses are discussed. Nested PCR involves a second round of 15–30 cycles of PCR performed on the first-round PCR product using a new set of internal or "nested" primers. This secondary amplification produces a shorter, high-yield DNA product and can improve sensitivity and specificity, which is particularly important in respiratory samples containing inhibitors. Multiplex PCR uses multiple primer pairs that allow the simultaneous amplification of several sites on the target DNA. This method has been used to test for several subgroups of viruses (particularly coronaviruses 229E and OC43, influenza viruses A, B, and C, and parainfluenza viruses 1–3) using a single PCR reaction and the different groups separated by product size on gel electrophoresis or probe hybridization. The multiplex method requires that the annealing temperatures of the primers and the lengths of the PCR amplification products are very similar to ensure balance in the amplification of the different PCR products. For example, differences in the length of the primers will favor the extension of the shorter target over the longer one.

Asymmetrical PCR involves the use of unequal, or asymmetrical concentrations of primers. During the initial phase of the amplification, most of the product generated exponentially is double-stranded and as the limiting primer becomes depleted, further cycles generate excess copies of the opposite or complementary strand. This technique is used if the amplification products are to be sequenced but has recently been applied to improve the quality of subsequent probe hybridization in the diagnosis of adenovirus infections in clinical samples. Quantitative PCR is based on the observation that, under carefully controlled conditions, the concentration of PCR product correlates directly with the number of template molecules, providing a rapid and reliable way to quantitate the amount of viral DNA in a sample. This method does not have many applications in the diagnosis of respiratory virus infections and only assumes importance in circumstances where a measure of the viral load may be useful, such as in retrovirus infections.

Because of the legal restrictions on PCR technology and the expanding interest in nucleic acid–based diagnostic tests, commercial companies have developed alternative methods of nucleic acid amplification. Nucleic acid amplification is achieved in two main ways: by target (viral genome) amplification, where a specific sequence of interest is amplified to detectable levels, or by probe amplification, where the nucleic acid probe itself is amplified to detectable levels. Target amplification systems, including PCR, self-sustained sequence replication (3SR), and strand displacement amplification (SDA) incorporate target-specific sequences into the amplification product that are distinct from the sequences of the primers used to promote the reactions. Alternatively, probe amplification systems such as ligase chain reaction (LCR) and Q-beta replicase amplify the probe itself without incorporating target information different from that used to start the reaction. The differences in reaction cycles between PCR and LCR are shown in Figure 1. Different amplification methods have been reviewed by Forghani and Erdman (41). To date, the majority of methods describing the detection of respiratory viruses by nucleic acid amplification have used PCR, and rapid developments using LCR for viral diagnostics or a combination of PCR and LCR are awaited.

### D. Application of PCR to Detection of Respiratory Viruses

Most respiratory viruses causing common cold–like symptoms have RNA genomes with the notable exceptions of adenoviruses and the atypical bacteria *Mycoplasma pneumoniae* and *Chlamydia pneumoniae*. Amplification of RNA target sequences by PCR therefore requires the prior step of making cDNA copies, and for the viruses with DNA genomes the nucleic acid is amplified directly without prior reverse transcription. A major requirement of PCR diagnostics is uniformity of reagents and standardization of PCR protocols if rapid multiple testing of all the major respiratory viruses is required, and the method of nucleic acid extraction (whether DNA or RNA) is important in the success of the assay. A major problem with using PCR directly on clinical samples is the presence of inhibitors in some clinical specimens, and although there are numerous published reports on the extraction of nucleic acids from clinical samples for PCR, different methods of sample preparation and extraction may lead to inconsistent results. Because the mRNA of prokaryotic and most eukaryotic cells contains a long tract of 20 or more A residues (the polyA tail) at the 3' end, multiple copies of single-strand cDNA can be made from the total RNA extracted from clinical specimens using commercially available poly-dT or random primers (Fig. 2). The single step of RNA extraction and cDNA synthesis per clinical sample (which can then be used to test for multiple viruses) has obvious labor and cost advantages to using multiple extractions and cDNA synthesis based on using virus-specific primers for reverse transcription. Commercially available RNA extraction kits are now used to extract total RNA from clinical samples based on the guanidium isothiocyanate method described by Chomczynski and Sacchi (50). In most instances the total RNA will be comprised of about 90% ribosomal RNA and the rest by nuclear RNA (mainly mRNA). The advantage of using primers complementary to viral mRNA not only supports the observation that any positive virus samples represent active virus replication, but also that if primers complementary to an abundant mRNA are selected for PCR, then even viruses and atypical bacteria with primary DNA genomes can be reverse transcribed. In this respect, the authors' have developed reverse transcription–based PCRs for adenoviruses, *M. pneumoniae*, and *C. pneumoniae*.

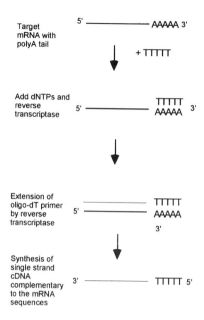

Target
mRNA with
polyA tail
5' —————— AAAAA 3'

↓ + TTTTT

Add dNTPs and
reverse
transcriptase
5' —————— TTTTT
AAAAA 3'

↓

Extension of
oligo-dT primer
by reverse
transcriptase
5' ——————— TTTTT
AAAAA
3'

↓

Synthesis of
single strand
cDNA
complementary
to the mRNA
sequences
3' —————— TTTTT 5'

**Figure 2**   Principles of reverse transcription to synthesize single-strand cDNA from the viral target mRNA.

### A Typical Protocol for RNA Extraction, cDNA Synthesis, PCR, and Probe Hybridization

The following description is of a PCR method for the detection of rhinoviruses and enteroviruses currently used in the University Medicine Laboratories at the University of Southampton. The method is typical of other PCR protocols that have been developed for testing of all the major respiratory viruses, using novel sets of primers or optimizing primers from previously published studies, and serves to illustrate the principles of nucleic acid extraction, PCR, and probe hybridization described earlier. The protocols have been established to test for infection in nasal aspirates.

### RNA Extraction

RNA is extracted in a single stage using a modification of the guanidium isothiocyanate-phenol-chloroform method. Briefly, 10 µl of sample is diluted 1:5 with ultra-high-quality water (UHQ) followed by the addition of an equal volume of Trizol™ (Gibco BRL, Paisley, Scotland) and 1/10 volume of chloroform and precipitated with glycogen (20 mg/ml, Boehringer Mannheim, Lewes, England) and isopropyl alcohol overnight at −20°C. Dilution of sample is required to reduce the amount of inhibitors present in nasal mucus. The RNA pellet is purified by washing with 80% ethanol and dried under vacuum. Each pellet is then dissolved in 5 µl warm UHQ with 20 units of RNAase inhibitor (RNAguard™, Pharmacia Biotech, Uppsala, Sweden). Relevant positive controls from cell culture lysates with known 50% tissue culture infective doses ($TCID_{50}$) and negative controls are prepared from noninfected viral transport medium.

## Primers

The oligonucleotide primers are synthesized using isocyanoethyl phosphoramidite chemistry. The primers used for picornavirus amplification are OL 26 (5′ GCA CTT CTG TTC CC 3′) and OL27 (5′ CGG ACA CCC AAA GTA G 3′), which are complementary to the RNA at positions 169–185 and 542–557 in the 5′ noncoding region of rhinovirus-1B (18,51,52). This primer pair generates an amplification product (amplicon) that does not differentiate between rhinovirus and enterovirus.

## Reverse Transcription

For cDNA synthesis using random primers, each RNA pellet is made up to a 10-µl volume with UHQ containing 50 µg/ml concentration of random hexamers (Promega Corp., Southampton, England). After heating the mixture to 70°C for 10 minutes and cooling on ice, the total volume is made up to 20 µl containing final concentrations of the following reagents: 50 mM Tris-HCl (pH 8.3 at room temperature), 75 mM KCl, 15 mM $MgCl_2$, 20 mM DTT, 0.5 mM dNTPs, and 200 U of reverse transcriptase (Superscript™ RNAase H⁻, Gibco BRL, Paisley, Scotland). The mix is incubated to 37°C for 60 minutes to yield 20 µl of single-strand cDNA and then stored at −70°C as appropriate.

## PCR

The PCR is performed on 10 µl of cDNA in a reaction volume of 50 µl made up with UHQ water containing final concentrations of the following reagents: 1 × PCR buffer (50 mM KCl, 10 mM Tris-HCl [pH 9 at 25°C], 0.1% Triton X-100), 0.2 mM dNTPs, 1.5 µM both primers, 1.5 mM $Mg^{2+}$, and 4.25 U Taq DNA polymerase (Promega Corp., Southampton, England). The reaction cycle consists of 32 cycles of denaturation at 94°C for 30 seconds, annealing at 50°C for 30 seconds, and extension at 72°C for 2 minutes, including a post-PCR extension step at 72°C for 4 minutes.

## Gel Electrophoresis

The OL26-OL27 primers generate a picornavirus product size of 380 bp visualized by gel electrophoresis on an ethidium bromide–stained 1.5% gel. Serial 10-fold dilutions of the positive controls to the appropriate detection limits are also run on the gel to confirm that each PCR run was successfully completed prior to probe hybridization.

## Oligonucleotide Probes

Oligonucleotide probes are synthesized by the same method described for primers. The probe JWA-1b (5′ CAT TCA GGG GCC GGA GGA 3′) is used to confirm the picornavirus-specific OL26-OL27 amplicons, while the probe PR8 complementary to the 5′ noncoding/VP4 antisense RNA between positions 457 and 478, derived from a previously published sequence (53), is used to confirm rhinovirus-specific sequences in the same amplicons.

## Probe Hybridization

Ten microliters of PCR product are mixed with an equal volume of 3:2 mix of 20 × SSC and 37% formaldehyde and incubated at 65°C for 15 minutes. The samples are applied to nitrocellulose membranes (63 by 288 mm; pore size 0.45 μm; Schleicher and Schuell, Dassel, Germany) with the aid of a vacuum slot-blot manifold (Minifold II; Schleicher and Schuell). The products are then cross-linked to the membranes by UV light at 120,000 J/m$^2$. The membrane is prehybridized individually in glass bottles (Hybaid, Teddington, England) containing 30 ml of prehybridization buffer; 5 × SSC, 0.02% SDS, buffer component (NIP547; Amersham Int., Bucks, England) and a 20-fold dilution of liquid block (RPN3601; Amersham) for a minimum of 1 hour to reduce nonspecific probe hybridization. The membranes are hybridized overnight with the fluorescin-11-dUTP–labeled oligonucleotide probes JWA-1b at 45°C (or PR8 at 42°C) at a final concentration of 10 ng/ml and signal detected by using an antibody-based, chemiluminescent slot-blot system (ECL, Amersham, England). Briefly, after hybridization the membranes are washed twice with 5 × SSC at room temperature for 5 minutes and twice with 1 × SSC at the hybridization temperature for 15. The membranes are then rinsed for 1 minute in buffer 1 (NaCl 0.15 M and Tris 0.1 M at pH 7.5) before incubation in a 20-fold dilution of liquid block (RPN3022, Amersham) at room temperature. The membranes are again rinsed in buffer 1 for 1 minute before a final 30-minute incubation in a 1000-fold dilution of anti-fluorescein HRP conjugate in buffer 2 (NaCl 0.4 M and Tris 0.1 M at pH 7.5) containing 0.5% bovine serum albumin. Membranes are then rinsed four times for 5 minutes each with an excess of buffer 2. Chemiluminescent signal generation is achieved by adding equal volumes of ECL-detection reagents (RPN2105, Amersham) to the membranes, which are then exposed to light-sensitive film (Hyperfilm ECL, RPN 2103H, Amersham) for 10 minutes at room temperature. Any visible signal in the clinical samples are taken as positive if consistent signals are present in the serial dilutions of the positive controls while absent in the negative controls. A typical film detecting chemiluminescent signals from rhinovirus amplification products (using the slot-blot technique) is shown in Figure 3. The lower limit of detection of the assay is 10 TCID$_{50}$ of virus, and this technique has been shown to detect three times as many rhinovirus- and enterovirus-positive samples in nasal aspirates as virus culture alone (18).

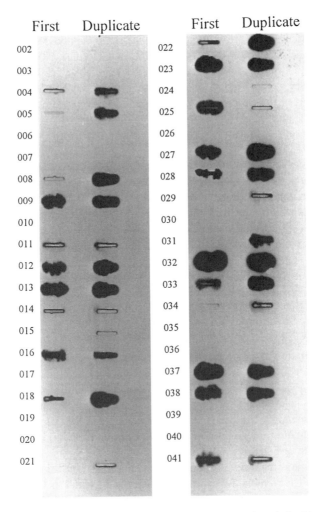

**Figure 3** Chemiluminescent signal detected on an antibody-based slot-blot film of pi-cornavirus-specific amplicons using the probe JWA-1b. Forty samples are shown. Only signal present on duplicate testing was taken as positive, which included lanes 4, 5, 8, 9, 11–14, 16, 18, 21–23, 25, 27, 28, and 32–34. Lanes 37 ($2 \times 10^3$ TCID$_{50}$), 38 ($2 \times 10^2$ TCID$_{50}$), and 41 (20 TCID$_{50}$) are rhinovirus 16 positive controls and lanes 39 and 40 are VTM negative controls. Sample lanes 9, 12, 13, 16, 18, 23, 27, 32, and 33 were also positive by cell culture. (Reproduced courtesy of Dr X. Ping.)

The type of PCR method, the target virus genome, and detection limits of the assays currently in use for the main respiratory viruses and atypical bacteria in the authors' laboratory are shown in Table 1.

### PCR as a Diagnostic Tool

Many studies in the past 8 years have used the PCR assay to detect respiratory virus infections. Many of the earlier studies used the assay to detect virus in laboratory cell cultures, and a few tested for virus infections in large numbers of clinical samples. The sensitivity of in vitro amplification of viral nucleic acid generally compares favorably with virus cell culture and other methods of antigen detection such as IF assays for many respiratory viruses. Nucleic acid amplification does not require virus viability, whereas many viruses cannot be grown in cell culture or may grow slowly, requiring days or weeks for identification. In the long run, in vitro amplification by PCR is cost effective and has recently been shown to reduce overall health costs in detecting RS virus in children admitted to hospital with acute respiratory illnesses (54). Genomic sequence variation, detectable because of the specificity of nucleotide base pairing during hybridization, can provide useful information about virus strain specificity, useful for both early diagnosis and epidemiological surveillance. DNA is generally resistant to organic solvents and other extreme physical conditions and can therefore be used to test for infection in stored samples several years after they are first collected.

Despite all these advantages, the role of detecting respiratory virus infections by PCR remains to be firmly established, primarily because of the costs, lack of standardization, and uncertainties about whether the presence of virus genome in clinical samples represent true infections or are false positives. Because of the exquisite sensitivity of these assays, the use of sensitivity testing of PCR assays by serial dilutions of stock laboratory virus does not necessarily relate to the sensitivity in detecting viruses in clinical samples; newly developed PCR assays require careful testing against panels of symptomatic and asymptomatic samples and need to be evaluated alongside samples that have been tested concurrently with conventional cell culture and antigen-detection methods. For example, using the picornavirus PCR and rhinovirus-specific probe hybridization described earlier, rhinoviruses were detected in 52% of acute samples by PCR compared to 29% by cell culture and in 12% of asymptomatic samples by PCR and none by cell culture (18). Using the panels of RT-PCRs available in the authors' laboratories, viruses were similarly detected in approximately 80% of acute samples taken from children aged 9–11 years in a community-based longitudinal study, compared to 18% in asymptomatic samples (collected throughout autumn, winter, and spring, thus allowing for seasonal effects) taken from the same subjects. In another study testing for a panel of RS virus, parainfluenza virus, and picornavirus, the RT-PCR methods had a sensitivity of 94% in comparison with virus

**Table 1** Applications of PCR Assays for Detection of Respiratory Virus Nucleic Acids in Clinical Samples

| Virus | Target genome | RT | Type of PCR | $TCID_{50}$ by 1st/single round gel | $TCID_{50}$ by PH | $TCID_{50}$ by 2nd round gel |
|---|---|---|---|---|---|---|
| Picornavirus | 5' Noncoding RNA | Yes | S, PH | 200 | 20 | — |
| RS virus | 22K protein mRNA | Yes | N | — | — | <5 |
| Coronaviruses | Nucleocapsid protein RNA | Yes | S or N, M, PH | | | |
|   OC43 | | | | 5000 | 500 | 50 |
|   229E | | | | 5000 | 500 | 50 |
| Influenza A and B | N and NS protein mRNAs | Yes | N, M | | | |
|   Type AH1 | | | | — | — | 1 |
|   Type AH3 | | | | — | — | 1 |
|   Type B | | | | — | — | 20 |
| Parainfluenza | HN + NP protein RNA | Yes | S, M, PH | | | |
|   Type 1 | | | | 500 | 50 | — |
|   Type 2 | | | | 50 | 5 | — |
|   Type 3 | | | | 500 | 50 | — |
| Adenovirus | Ad2 Hexon mRNA | Yes | S, PH | <1 | 1 | — |
| *M. pneumoniae* | 16s RNA | Yes | S, PH | — | — | — |
| *C. pneumoniae* | OMP-1 mRNA | Yes | N | 4.5 ng | — | 4.5 fg |

All limits are $TCID_{50}$ per/ml of virus.
S = Single round; M = multiplex; N = nested; PH = probe hybridization.

culture and showed evidence of a dual infection in 20% by RT-PCR compared to 3.8% by culture. Clearly with the increasing availability of commercial extraction and PCR kits, automation of the PCR processes, and accessibility to virus genomic sequences by computer, more information will be gathered and PCR will be more widely used as a diagnostic rather than simply as a research tool. Before this becomes a reality, the problems of standardizing the methods (e.g., in extraction of nucleic acids), the costs, and reproducibility of the assays between different operators and laboratories need to be addressed.

## VIII. Conclusions

It is clear from current evidence that rapid diagnostic methods using direct antigen and genomic amplification methods are becoming more common for diagnosing respiratory virus infections. Depending on the virus to be detected, the type of respiratory sample, and the target viral genome, PCR and often antigen-detection methods can be more sensitive than cell culture. Furthermore, although cell culture and antigen-detection methods may be cheaper and have specificity, they either do not provide a result early enough or lack appropriate sensitivity compared to PCR. Despite these potential advantages, until more is known about the viability of virus detected in asymptomatic samples by PCR between different age groups, seasons, and disease states, cell culture methods (supported by antigen detection and PCR when appropriate) remain the front-line investigation for most respiratory viruses in many general diagnostic laboratories.

## References

1. Nicholson KG, Kent J, Ireland DC. Respiratory viruses and exacerbations of asthma in adults [see comments]. Br Med J 1993; 307:982–986.
2. Johnston SL, Pattemore PK, Sanderson G, Smith S, Lampe F, Josephs L, Symington P, O'Toole S, Myint SH, Tyrrell DA, et al. Community study of role of viral infections in exacerbations of asthma in 9–11 year old children [see comments]. Br Med J 1995; 310:1225–1229.
3. Atmar RL, Baxter BD, Dominguez EA, Taber LH. Comparison of reverse transcription-PCR with tissue culture and other rapid diagnostic assays for detection of type A influenza virus. J Clin Microbiol 1996; 34:2604–2606.
4. Dominguez EA, Taber LH, Couch RB. Comparison of rapid diagnostic techniques for respiratory syncytial and influenza A virus respiratory infections in young children. J Clin Microbiol 1993; 31:2286–2290.
5. McIntosh K, Halonen P, Ruuskanen O. Report of a workshop on respiratory viral infections: epidemiology, diagnosis, treatment, and prevention. Clin Infect Dis 1993; 16:151–164.

6. de Barbeyrac B, Bernet-Poggi C, Febrer F, Renaudin H, Dupon M, Bebear C. Detection of *Mycoplasma pneumoniae* and *Mycoplasma genitalium* in clinical samples by polymerase chain reaction. Clin Infect Dis 1993; 17:S83–S89.

7. Gern JE, Galagan DM, Jarjour NJ, Dick EC, Busse WW. Detection of rhinovirus RNA in lower airway cells during experimentally induced infection. Am J Respir Crit Care Med 1997; 155:1159–1161.

8. Gleaves CA, Smith TF, Wold AD, Wilson WR. Detection of viral and chlamydial antigens in open-lung biopsy specimens. Am J Clin Pathol 1985; 83:371–374.

9. Bates PJ, Sanderson G, Holgate ST, Johnston SL. A comparison of RT-PCR, in-situ hybridisation and in-situ RT-PCR for the detection of rhinovirus infection in paraffin sections. J Virol Methods 1997, in press.

10. Miller SE. Diagnosis of viral infections by electron microscopy. In: Lennette EH, Lennette DA, Lennette ET, eds. Diagnostic Procedures for Viral, Rickettsial, and Chlamydial Infections. 7th ed. Washington, DC: American Public Health Association, 1995:

11. Lennette DA. General principles for laboratory diagnosis of viral, rickettsial, and chlamydial infections. In: Lennette EH, Lennette DA, Lennette ET, eds. Diagnostic Procedures for Viral, Rickettsial, and Chlamydial Infections. 7th ed. Washington, DC: American Public Health Association, 1995.

12. O'Neill HJ, Russell JD, Wyatt DE, McCaughey C, Coyle PV. Isolation of viruses from clinical specimens in microtitre plates with cells inoculated in suspension. J Virol Methods 1996; 62:169–178.

13. Minnich LL, Ray CG. Early testing of cell cultures for detection of hemadsorbing viruses. J Clin Microbiol 1987; 25:421–422.

14. Henrickson KJ, Kuhn SM, Savatski LL, Sedmak J. Recovery of human parainfluenza virus types one and two. J Virol Methods 1994; 46:189–205.

15. Baxter BD, Couch RB, Greenberg SB, Kasel JA. Maintenance of viability and comparison of identification methods for influenza and other respiratory viruses of humans. J Clin Microbiol 1977; 6:19–22.

16. Hijazi Z, Pacsa A, Eisa S, el Shazli A, abd el-Salam RA. Laboratory diagnosis of acute lower respiratory tract viral infections in children. J Trop Ped 1996; 42:276–280.

17. Kellner G, Popow-Kraupp T, Kundi M, Binder C, Wallner H, Kunz C. Contribution of rhinoviruses to respiratory viral infections in childhood: a prospective study in a mainly hospitalized infant population. J Med Virol 1988; 25:455–469.

18. Johnston SL, Sanderson G, Pattemore PK, Smith S, Bardin PG, Bruce CB, Lambden PR, Tyrrell DA, Holgate ST. Use of polymerase chain reaction for diagnosis of picornavirus infection in subjects with and without respiratory symptoms. J Clin Microbiol 1993; 31:111–117.

19. Myint S. Diagnosis of viral respiratory tract infections. In: Myint S, Taylor-Robinson D, eds. Viral and Other Infections of the Human Respiratory Tract. London: Chapman and Hall, 1996:61–82.

20. Swenson PD, Kaplan MH. Rapid detection of influenza virus in cell culture by indirect immunoperoxidase staining with type-specific monoclonal antibodies. Diag Microbiol Infect Dis 1987; 7:265–268.

21. Lee SH, Boutilier JE, MacDonald MA, Forward KR. Enhanced detection of respira-

tory viruses using the shell vial technique and monoclonal antibodies. J Virol Methods 1992; 39:39–46.

22. Rabalais GP, Stout GG, Ladd KL, Cost KM. Rapid diagnosis of respiratory viral infections by using a shell vial assay and monoclonal antibody pool. J Clin Microbiol 1992; 30:1505–1508.

23. Schirm J, Luijt DS, Pastoor GW, Mandema JM, Schroder FP. Rapid detection of respiratory viruses using mixtures of monoclonal antibodies on shell vial cultures. J Med Virol 1992; 38:147–151.

24. Waris M, Ziegler T, Kivivirta M, Ruuskanen O. Rapid detection of respiratory syncytial virus and influenza A virus in cell cultures by immunoperoxidase staining with monoclonal antibodies. J Clin Microbiol 1990; 28:1159–1162.

25. Stout C, Murphy MD, Lawrence S, Julian S. Evaluation of a monoclonal antibody pool for rapid diagnosis of respiratory viral infections. J Clin Microbiol 1989; 27: 448–452.

26. Pattyn SR, Provinciael D, Lambrechts R, Ceuppens P. Rapid diagnosis of viral respiratory infections. Comparison between immunofluorescence on clinical samples and immunofluorescence on centrifuged cell cultures. Acta Clin Belg 1991; 46:7–12.

27. Minnich LL, Shehab ZM, Ray CG. Application of pooled monoclonal antibodies for 1-hr detection of respiratory syncytial virus antigen in clinical specimens. Diag Microbiol Infect Dis 1987; 7:137–141.

28. Freymuth F, Quibriac M, Petitjean J, Amiel ML, Pothier P, Denis A, Duhamel JF. Comparison of two new tests for rapid diagnosis of respiratory syncytial virus infections by enzyme-linked immunosorbent assay and immunofluorescence techniques. J Clin Microbiol 1986; 24:1013–1016.

29. Bromberg K, Tannis G, Daidone B. Early use of indirect immunofluorescence for the detection of respiratory syncytial virus in HEp-2 cell culture. Am J Clin Pathol 1991; 96:127–129.

30. Ukkonen P, Julkunen I. Preparation of nasopharyngeal secretions for immunofluorescence by one-step centrifugation through Percoll. J Virol Methods 1987; 15:291–301.

31. Cubie HA, Winter GF, Leslie EE, Inglis JM. Rapid detection of respiratory syncytial virus antigens in nasopharyngeal secretions. J Virol Methods 1990; 27:121–124.

32. Shen K, Zhaori G, Zweygberg-Wirgart B, Ying M, Grandien M, Wahren B, Linde A. Detection of viruses in nasopharyngeal secretions with immunofluorescence technique for multiplex screening—an evaluation of the Chemicon assay. Clin Diag Virol 1996; 6:147–154.

33. Takimoto S, Grandien M, Ishida MA, Pereira MS, Paiva TM, Ishimaru T, Makita EM, Martinez CH. Comparison of enzyme-linked immunosorbent assay, indirect immunofluorescence assay, and virus isolation for detection of respiratory viruses in nasopharyngeal secretions. J Clin Microbiol 1991; 29:470–474.

34. Reina J, Munar M, Blanco I. Evaluation of a direct immunofluorescence assay, dot-blot enzyme immunoassay, and shell vial culture in the diagnosis of lower respiratory tract infections caused by influenza A virus. Diag Microbiol Infect Dis 1996; 25: 143–145.

35. Obel N, Andersen HK, Jensen IP, Mordhorst CH. Evaluation of Abbott TestPack

RSV and an in-house RSV ELISA for detection of respiratory syncytial virus in respiratory tract aspirates. Apmis 1995; 103:416–418.

36. Hierholzer JC, Bingham PG, Coombs RA, Johansson KH, Anderson LJ, Halonen PE. Comparison of monoclonal antibody time-resolved fluoroimmunoassay with monoclonal antibody capture-biotinylated detector enzyme immunoassay for respiratory syncytial virus and parainfluenza virus antigen detection. J Clin Microbiol 1989; 27:1243–1249.

37. Hierholzer JC, Halonen PE, Dahlen PO, Bingham PG, McDonough MM. Detection of adenovirus in clinical specimens by polymerase chain reaction and liquid phase hybridisation quantitated by time resolved fluorometry. J Clin Microbiol 1993; 31: 1886–1891.

38. Nikkari S, Halonen P, Kharitonenkov I, Kivivirta M, Khristova M, Waris M, Kendal A. One-incubation time-resolved fluoroimmunoassay based on monoclonal antibodies in detection of influenza A and B viruses directly in clinical specimens. J Virol Methods 1989; 23:29–40.

39. Waris M, Halonen P, Ziegler T, Nikkari S, Obert G. Time-resolved fluoroimmunoassay compared with virus isolation for rapid detection of respiratory syncytial virus in nasopharyngeal aspirates. J Clin Microbiol 1988; 26:2581–2585.

40. Halonen P, Herholzer J, Ziegler T. Advances in the diagnosis of respiratory virus infections. Clin Diag Virol 1996; 5:91–100.

41. Forghani B, Erdman DD. Amplification and detection of viral nucleic acids. In: Lennette EH, Lennette DA, Lennette ET, eds. Diagnostic Procedures for Viral, Rickettsial, and Chlamydial Infections. 7th ed. Washington, DC: American Public Health Association, 1995:97–120.

42. Rigby PWS, Dieckmann M, Rhodes C, Berg P. Labelling deoxyribonucleic acid to high specific activity *in-vitro* by nick translation with DNA polymerase I. J Mol Biol 1977; 113:237–251.

43. Feinberg FP, Vogelstein B. A technique for radiolabelling DNA restriction endonuclease fragments to high specific activity. Anal Biochem 1983; 132:6–13.

44. Melton DA, Krieg PA, Rebagliati MR, Maniatis T, Zinn K, Gren MR, Efficient *in-vitro* synthesis of biologically active RNA and RNA hybridisation probes from plasmids containing a bacteriophage SP6 promoter. Nucl Acids Res 1984; 12:7035–7056.

45. Claas EC, van Milaan AJ, Sprenger MJ, Ruiten-Stuiver M, Arron GI, Rothbarth PH, Masurel N. Prospective application of reverse transcriptase polymerase chain reaction for diagnosing influenza infections in respiratory samples from a children's hospital. J Clin Microbiol 1993; 31:2218–2221.

46. Myint S, Johnston SL, Sanderson G, Simpson H. Evaluation of nested polymerase chain reaction methods for the detection of human coronaviruses 229E and OC43. Mol Cell Probes 1994; 8:357–364.

47. Paton AW, Paton JC, Lawrence AJ, Goldwater PN, Harris RJ. Rapid detection of respiratory syncytial virus in nasopharyngeal aspirates by reverse transcription and polymerase chain reaction amplification. J Clin Microbiol 1992; 30:901–904.

48. van Kuppeveld FJ, Johansson KE, Galama JM, Kissing J, Bolske G, Hjelm E, van der Logt JT, Melchers WJ. 16S rRNA based polymerase chain reaction compared

with culture and serological methods for diagnosis of Mycoplasma pneumoniae infection. Eur J Clin Microbiol Infect Dis 1994; 13:401–405.

49. van Milaan AJ, Sprenger MJ, Rothbarth PH, Brandenburg AH, Masurel N, Claas EC. Detection of respiratory syncytial virus by RNA-polymerase chain reaction and differentiation of subgroups with oligonucleotide probes. J Med Virol 1994; 44:80–87.

50. Chomczynski P, Sacchi N. Single-step method of RNA isolation by acid guanidium thiocyanate-phenol-chloroform extraction. Anal Biochem 1987; 162:156–159.

51. Bruce CB, Al-Nakib W, Almond JW, Tyrrell DAJ. Use of synthetic oligonucleotide probes to detect rhinovirus RNA. Arch Virol 1989; 105:179–187.

52. Gama RE, Horsnell PJ, Hughes PJ, North CB, Bruce W, Al-Nakib W, Stanway G. Amplification of rhinovirus specific nucleic acids from clinical samples using the polymerase chain reaction. J Med Virol 1989; 28:73–77.

53. Mori J, Clewley JP. Polymerase chain reaction and sequencing for typing rhinovirus RNA. J Med Virol 1994; 44:323–329.

54. Woo PY, Chiu SS, Seto W-H, Peiris M. Cost-effectiveness of rapid diagnosis of viral respiratory tract infections in pediatric patients. J Clin Microbiol 1997; 35:1579–1581.

# 13

## Current Modalities for Treatment of Respiratory Viruses and Virus-Induced Asthma

**ELLIOT F. ELLIS**

MURO Pharmaceutical
Tewksbury, Massachusetts

During the past two decades there has been substantial progress in the development of chemotherapeutic agents and vaccines for the treatment of human viral infections. As important as these advances have been in the management of certain infections, e.g., the wide variety of herpes simplex virus (HSV) infections, pharmaceutical research laboratories have been, with two notable exceptions, ribavirin for respiratory syncytial virus (RSV) infection, and amantidine/rimantidine for influenza A infections, notably unsuccessful in bringing to market new agents effective against the common respiratory viruses. The ideal characteristics of an antiviral agent for treatment or prevention of respiratory virus infection are seen in Table 1.

It has become abundantly clear, over the past 20 years, that respiratory viruses have a major role as provocateurs of exacerbations of symptoms in known asthmatics in both children and, to a lesser extent, adults (1–5). The question of whether virus respiratory infection leads to the development of atopy (6) or protects against it has not been resolved (7,8). The principal respiratory viral agents involved in asthma are RSV, parainfluenza virus (I–III), coronaviruses, rhinoviruses, and, to a lesser extent, influenza virus (1,2). Adenoviruses, which may cause serious lower respiratory tract illness in infants and epidemic upper respiratory and gastrointestinal illness in community settings, are rarely associated with

**Table 1**  Ideal Characteristics of an Antiviral Agent for Treatment
or Prevention of Respiratory Virus Infection

---

Broad spectrum of antiviral inhibitory activity against respiratory
   syncytial virus, rhinoviruses, coronaviruses, parainfluenza type
   I–IV, influenza A and B viruses
Effective by oral or intranasal administration
Relatively inexpensive to synthesize
Chemical structure modification possible in the event of emergence
   of drug-resistant viruses
Good stability with shelf life of at least 18–24 months
Free of significant adverse effects

---

exacerbations of asthma. During early life RSV, parainfluenza, and coronaviruses
are most important, with influenza only rarely being implicated (1). Later in life,
rhinoviruses by far are the most common agents associated with flare-ups of
asthma (2). This chapter will focus on the chemotherapy of respiratory viruses
implicated in exacerbations or possible causation of asthma and on controlled
clinical trials conducted in patients with virus-induced asthma. Currently marketed products as well as those under development will be discussed.

## I.  Chemotherapy of Rhinovirus Infection

In school-age children and adults, rhinovirus infections account for 60% of cases
of respiratory viruses associated with exacerbations of asthma. Clinically, rhinovirus infection manifests itself as a common cold and is responsible for 40–50%
of cold cases. Because there are approximately 100 serotypes of rhinovirus (9)
and immunity is serotype specific, prevention of rhinovirus infection by immunization has not been feasible. However, during the past 20 years there has been
considerable interest in the use of interferon (IFN-$\alpha$) for prophylaxis of rhinovirus
infection (10–16).

   Interferon was discovered 40 years ago by Isaacs and Lindenmann, who
found that fluids from virus-infected cell cultures possessed a protein that could
confer on cells resistance to infection by many viruses (17). It is now known
that interferons are a family of glycoprotein molecules with antiviral effects. The
interferons designated IFN-$\alpha$, IFN-$\beta$, and IFN-$\gamma$ differ physicochemically, antigenically, and in terms of cellular source and function (18). The interferon genes
have been cloned, and recombinant IFN-$\alpha$, IFN-$\beta$, and IFN-$\gamma$ have been produced
by genetically engineered bacteria and in cell culture for therapeutic use. As a
group, in addition to possessing potent antiviral activity, the interferons have
metabolic, growth, immunomodulatory, and antitumor properties. Effective

against both RNA and DNA viruses, they do not directly inactivate the virus but induce resistance in host cells by acting on different parts of the various viral-replication cycles. With specific reference to viral respiratory disease, work on prophylaxis of rhinovirus colds was initiated by Tyrrell and associates in the early 1970s and extended by Gwaltney and associates in the 1980s (10–12). Using intranasal IFN-α2 well-controlled short-term clinical studies with rhinovirus-infected volunteers showed approximately 80% effectiveness in *prevention* of rhinovirus-induced colds (13–16). Daily long-term (28 days) prophylaxis during the respiratory disease season, although demonstrating an antiviral effect, caused an unacceptable degree of local nasal irritation, and therefore this approach was abandoned. Attention was then directed toward testing the efficacy of IFN-α2 for *treatment* of rhinovirus-caused common colds. While the treatment was well tolerated and a good antiviral effect was shown, symptoms were only marginally reduced. Continued investigation of the common cold by Gwaltney led to the conclusion that the symptoms were due to release of inflammatory mediators rather than simply viral destruction of the cells lining the nasal and upper airway. Therefore, in addition to terminating the stimulus to inflammation by interrupting viral replication, Gwaltney hypothesized that adding drugs to block the various inflammatory pathways responsible for symptoms might be useful. During the past several years various combinations of naproxen, ipratropium, and several antihistamines plus intranasal IFN-α2 have given encouraging results in terms of reduced viral shedding and amelioration of common cold symptoms (19). Further development of this combined antiviral-antimediator approach is being pursued. The potential of reducing the communicability of the common cold due to rhinovirus infections would be of substantial value to families of asthmatic children or adults. The combination could be used on a prn basis administered intranasally as either a nasal spray or drops shortly before or after exposure and prophylactically to contacts in family outbreaks. According to Gwaltney, interferon has a long-lasting antiviral effect in the nose after a single application, permitting infrequent dosing. Furthermore, the cost of IFN-α2 production has been substantially reduced to the point where the product could be reasonably priced.

Intercellular adhesion molecule-1 (ICAM-1) has been recognized as the cellular receptor for 90% of the rhinoviruses (major group) (20). In addition to several inflammatory cytokines (IL-4, IL1-β, IFN-γ, and TNF-α), parainfluenza virus, one of the respiratory viruses known to precipitate asthma, also has the capability of upregulating expression of ICAM-1 on respiratory epithelium (21). As the cellular receptor for the great majority of rhinovirus strains, upregulation of ICAM-1 could lead to increased susceptibility to rhinovirus infection and precipitation of asthma. There has therefore been an interest in developing therapies directed against ICAM-1, e.g., monoclonal antibodies to ICAM-1 that block the receptor site on the cells (22) or blockade of the receptor-binding site on the virus with soluble ICAM-1 (23). These agents would be administered as a nasal spray. Unfortunately, the problem of assuring adequate residence time on the nasal mucosa has yet to be resolved.

## II.  Chemotherapy of Coronaviruses

Although primarily studied for prevention of rhinovirus infections, IFN-α2 has also been used as a therapeutic agent in experimental coronavirus infections. Coronaviruses, well-known veterinary infectious agents, belong to two serogroups, A and B, present as upper respiratory illnesses, typically as common colds, and are responsible for up to 30% of the latter. In the United States and England, coronaviruses are second only to rhinoviruses as causes of the common cold. As provocateurs of asthma symptoms in asthmatic children, up to 30% of acute wheezing episodes may be due to coronavirus infection. Two controlled clinical trials of experimentally induced coronavirus colds have reported reduction in duration of viral shedding and lessening of clinical symptoms in subjects treated with intranasal recombinant IFN-α2 given for 4 days in one study (3.53 $\times$ 10$^7$ IU t.i.d.) (24) and 15 days (2 $\times$ 10$^6$ IU/day) (25) in the other. The interferon was well tolerated in both trials except for some mild nasal irritation with bleeding in some instances.

## III.  Chemotherapy of Influenza A

Influenza virus infection has a marked cytopathic effect on the upper and lower airway epithelial lining. While infection causes relatively mild symptoms in prepubertal children with asthma, influenza can be a significant problem in asthmatic adults. Fortunately, since the mid-1960s, chemotherapy for both prophylaxis and treatment of influenza A infection has been available but is underused. The original compound amantadine and its analog rimantadine are both acyclic amines, which differ structurally only in the presence of a methyl group in the latter. This change in the rimantadine molecule prevents it from crossing the blood-brain barrier and significantly reduces central nervous system adverse effects compared to amantadine, without altering its antiviral activity. Both drugs exert their therapeutic effect by interfering with viral uncoating and inhibiting the function of the M2 membrane protein. Drug resistance readily occurs to both compounds and involves a single amino acid change in one of four amino acid residues in the M2 membrane protein. Curiously, in spite of the emergence of drug resistance, no reduction in drug efficacy has been demonstrated in epidemic situations (26). Pharmacokinetic studies have shown that both amantadine and rimantadine have excellent oral bioavailability, which is unaffected by food with peak serum concentrations of 0.4–0.8 μg/ml 2–6 hours after a 100-mg oral dose. Both drugs may be detected in respiratory tract secretions in therapeutic concentrations. There is a significant difference in the metabolism of amantadine and rimantadine. Amantadine is virtually completely (90%) eliminated unchanged in the urine, while rimantadine is extensively (>80%) metabolized. This has important implications when the drugs are administered to individuals with either advanced renal or liver disease. In particular, patients with any degree of renal insufficiency need to be monitored carefully for adverse effects to amantadine and the dose adjusted downward as indicated. Toxicity manifests principally as excitatory central nervous system and gastrointestinal effects and is dose related. Rimantadine has a significantly better adverse effect (AE) profile than amantadine (5–10% vs. 30%), and for this reason rimantadine is the drug of choice. Both drugs are marketed in the United States for prevention and treatment of H1N1, H2N2, and H3N2 strains of influenza type A virus. Controlled clinical trials have shown the drugs to be about 50% effective in preventing infection in epidemic situations but are 70–90% effective in the prevention or amelioration of clinical symptoms. The recommended usage of both drugs for prophylaxis and therapy is seen in Table 2. Dosing recommendations are presented in Table 3. Amantadine and rimantadine are not FDA approved for use in children under 1 year. Rimantadine is FDA approved for prophylaxis, but not for treatment, of children.

Neuraminidase (NA) is one of the two major surface glycoproteins expressed by influenza A and B viruses. In addition to its role in elution of new-formed viruses from infected cells, NA may also promote the movement of virus

**Table 2** Recommended Usage of Amantadine and Rimantadine in Prophylaxis and Therapy

1. There should be clear epidemiological and virological evidence of influenza A virus in the community.
2. Individuals immunized less than 2 weeks before virus appears in the community should be treated.
3. Amantadine or rimantadine should be used prophylactically each day for 4–8 weeks.
4. Drug prophylaxis should not replace immunization because amantadine does not inhibit influenza B virus.
5. Groups recommended for special consideration for prophylactic treatment:
   a. High-risk persons, such as the elderly and those with chronic heart, respiratory, or circulatory disease, and those with compromised immunity, whether immunized or not.
   b. Special community groups such as people in institutional settings, caretakers of high-risk individuals, physicians, nurses, hospital employees.
6. Therapy should be initiated within 24–48 hours of first symptoms and given for 10 subsequent days.

**Table 3** Dosage Recommendations for Amantadine (Symmetrel®) and Rimantadine (Flumadine®)

|  | Age (yrs) | | |
| --- | --- | --- | --- |
|  | | >10 | |
|  | 1–9 | Weight < 40 kg | Weight ≥ 40 kg |
| Treatment | 5 mg/kg/day, maximum 150 mg/day, in 1 or 2 divided doses | 5 mg/kg/day in 1 or 2 divided doses | 200 mg/day in 1 or 2 divided doses |
| Prophylaxis | Dosages may be the same as those for treatment. An alternative and equally acceptable dosage is 100 mg/day for children weighing >20 kg and adults. For either regimen, the total daily dosage may be given in 1 or 2 divided doses. | | |

*Source*: Modified from American Academy of Pediatrics Report of the Committee on Infectious Diseases, 24th Edition, 1997 Red Book.

through respiratory tract mucus, thereby enhancing infectivity of the virus. Novel compounds have recently been designed, synthesized, and evaluated by in vitro methods for their inhibitory action on NA. These compounds, known as carbocyclics, have potent in vitro and in vivo activity with good oral bioavailability at least in several animal models (mice, rats, and dogs). One of these compounds, designated GS4104, is being developed for the oral treatment and prophylaxis of influenza infection (27).

## IV. Chemotherapy of Paramyxoviruses (RSV and Parainfluenza)

Of all respiratory viruses that precipitate asthma during early life, RSV appears to be the most "asthmagenic." In the first large epidemiological prospective study of asthmatic children 1–5 years of age, hospitalized at the National Jewish Hospital in Denver, which investigated the relationship between viral agents and exacerbation of disease, RSV was implicated as a cause of symptoms 24 out of 25 times that it was identified by culture or serology (1). Since it is often difficult to distinguish between RSV bronchiolitis and the first attack of asthma precipitated by RSV, undoubtedly some infants with severe acute obstructive airway disease subsequently shown to have asthma have been treated with ribavirin on the premise that they had RSV bronchiolitis. Ribavirin is a synthetic nucleoside analog whose structure closely resembles the guanine-ribose combination guanosine. Its in vivo properties depend upon the activity of phosphorylated derivatives.

Ribavirin is active against a wide variety of RNA and DNA viruses. The initial enthusiasm for its use in infants and young children with underlying diseases as well as otherwise healthy infants suffering with severe RSV disease has waned as a result of recent reports (28,29). In fact, in one of these reports, a prospective cohort study of otherwise healthy infants under one year of age with RSV-precipitated respiratory failure, the use of ribavirin during mechanical ventilation was strongly associated with prolonged duration of ventilation, intensive care, and hospitalization (29). Because of concerns about costs, benefit, safety, and conflicting results of efficacy trials, the recommendations of American Academy of Pediatrics, Committee on Infectious Disease for use of ribavirin have become more restrictive (30).

In recognition of the importance of RSV as a cause of hospitalization of infants and children, the lack of a safe and effective RSV vaccine, and problems with ribavirin therapy, an investigation of passive immunization of high-risk infants with intravenous immunoglobulin was undertaken. In the initial trials in which nonhyperimmune standard intravenous immunoglobulin was used, reduction in hospitalization rates was not observed (31). Subsequently, trials with a high-titered RSV-neutralizing antibody preparation (RSV-IGIV) given prophylactically have been more encouraging in reducing the severity of the illness. The PREVENT trial was a 54-center, 510-patient, randomized, placebo-controlled study of the safety and effectiveness of RespiGAM™ 750 mg/kg given monthly from November through April for prophylaxis of RSV disease in infants with and without bronchopulmonary dysplasia (BPD) ≤24 months of age or prematurity (≤35 weeks gestation) ≤6 months of age at study entry. RespiGAM™ reduced the incidence of RSV hospitalization by 41%, total days of RSV hospitalization by 53%, total RSV hospital days with increased supplemental oxygen requirement by 60%, and total RSV hospital days with a moderate or severe lower respiratory tract infection by 54%. There was also a 46% reduction in the total days of hospitalization for respiratory illness per 100 randomized children for the RespiGAM™ recipients (32). Subsequent trials have essentially confirmed the results observed in the PREVENT trial except in children with congenital heart disease less than 48 months of age at the time of enrollment. In this group, efficacy was not established. Unfortunately, clinical trials with RSV-IGIV have not shown any beneficial effect in the treatment of established RSV disease. The mechanism of attenuation of the expression of RSV in passively immunized infants may not be due to the presence of RSV-neutralizing antibody alone. Standard IGIV has a number of well-established immunomodulatory activities, some of which may be responsible for the beneficial effect observed (33). Although not mentioned as one of the indications in a recently published consensus statement on the guidelines for selection of patients eligible to receive RSV-IGIV (34), there may be an occasional infant up to 24 months of age with severe asthma who would benefit from prophylactic therapy given on a monthly basis during the RSV season. The cost of such treatment with RSV-IGIV (RespiGAM™) over one respiratory disease season is approximately $5,000 (35).

At present, there are no antiviral chemotherapeutic agents known to be effective for treatment of parainfluenza induced upper or lower respiratory tract disease.

## V.  Prevention/Treatment of Virus-Induced Asthma

Expert opinion on the prevention and management of acute exacerbations of asthma emphasizes the importance of early intervention with corticosteroids (36). While many mild exacerbations may be managed with bronchodilator therapy alone, attacks characterized as moderate to severe with incomplete response to bronchodilator therapy should be treated with corticosteroids (37). Especially in young children in whom a great majority of exacerbations are triggered by viral respiratory tract infections, early intervention with glucocorticoids is indicated. In a study of preschool children with a history of severe asthma attacks precipitated by viral upper respiratory infections, frequently necessitating hospitalization, the addition of oral glucocorticoids to the conventional bronchodilator regimen at the first sign of a "cold" had remarkable results (38). The control group showed no change in morbidity during the 2-year observation period; however, in the prednisone-treated group, the number of wheezing days decreased by 65%, attacks of asthma by 56%, emergency department visits by 61%, and hospitalizations by 90% (Fig. 1). It should be noted that the study was not well controlled with subjects not randomly assigned to steroid versus control groups. However, the results were impressive enough to suggest validity of the observations. Although not specifically targeted to virus-precipitated asthma exacerbations, there are a number of other studies, mostly in children but in adults as well, supporting the use of corticosteroids in early-intervention treatment of acute asthma (39,40).

The risk of adverse effects associated with the use of systemic corticosteroids in the treatment of virus-induced asthma are dose and dosing interval related (41). Both children and adults who receive HPA axis–suppressive doses of corticosteroids in daily regimens may be at risk of the various complications of glucocorticoid therapy. In the context of viral-induced asthma, the course of therapy typically lasts no longer than 7–10 days, and while the doses used may be considered high (1–2 mg/kg/day for children and up to 80 mg/day for adults), significant adverse effects are rarely seen—especially those of an infectious nature (42). In fact, glucocorticoids have been used to treat several viral infections including acute hepatitis and herpes zoster with no adverse effects observed (43). Additionally there is a report of modulation of infection and subsequent pulmonary pathology in hamsters exposed to parainfluenza I (Sendai) virus by treatment with meth-

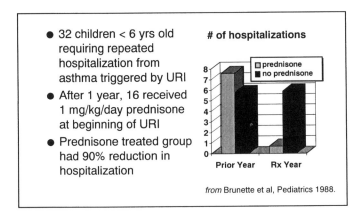

- 32 children < 6 yrs old requiring repeated hospitalization from asthma triggered by URI
- After 1 year, 16 received 1 mg/kg/day prednisone at beginning of URI
- Prednisone treated group had 90% reduction in hospitalization

# of hospitalizations

*from* Brunette et al, Pediatrics 1988.

**Figure 1** In addition to a remarkable reduction in the number of hospitalizations, the number of wheezing days, emergency visits, and acute attacks of asthma were also substantially reduced in the steroid-treated children as compared to the control group during a 2-year observation period.

ylprednisolone (44). The most widely publicized association of glucocorticoid adverse effects and viral disease is with varicella. This association was first noted in the 1950s (45). Even then the risk of disseminated varicella occurred primarily in children whose immunity was compromised by their underlying disease, e.g., leukemia. Reports since then have concluded that the risk of this occurrence in an otherwise normal child is extremely rare and dose dependent (46). Children with asthma and no history of prior clinical varicella or varicella immunization whose immunity is compromised by malignant disease or drug therapy (immunosuppressive agents or TAO-Medrol combination prescribed for severe asthma) (47) who require systemic steroids should be treated with zoster immune globulin (VZIG) if exposed to varicella. The dose is 125 U (1.25 ml) per 10 kg body weight given intramuscularly. Protection lasts for 3 weeks. In the event of clinical varicella, acyclovir in a dose of 1500 mg/m$^2$/day should be given intravenously in three divided doses for 7–10 days (36).

In addition to the early use of systemic steroids for exacerbation of asthma, the successful use of high-dose inhaled beclomethasone (750 μg three times a day for 5 days) at the first sign of virus-induced acute asthma in children has been reported (48). A more recent study using inhaled budesonide supported this initial observation (49). On the other hand, a subsequent study in preschool children with virus-precipitated asthma using relatively low-dose beclomethasone (400 mg daily) failed to show any improvement (50). In a more recent study, regular beclomethasone treatment (400 μg/day) for 6 months offered no clinically significant benefit in school-age children with wheezing episodes associated with viral infection, despite improvements in lung function (51). From the above, one might conclude that high-dose inhaled steroids may be of some value in the treatment of acute asthma but that low-dose therapy is ineffective. For this reason the use of oral steroids is preferred for treatment.

Inhaled and intranasal cromolyn and intranasal nedocromil have been reported to reduce the symptoms of the common cold in two studies (52,53). In addition, nebulized nedocromil has been found to be useful in the prophylaxis of presumed wintertime viral respiratory infection–precipitated asthma in children who were treated daily over 6 months. In a recently reported study (54), there was a decrease in the number of symptomatic days, asthma scores, cough, and albuterol rescue therapy. When the children appeared clinically to have an upper respiratory infection, asthma symptoms resolved more rapidly in the nedocromil-treated group compared to the placebo group.

## VI.  Note Added in Proof

Two important experimental studies on the treatment of respiratory virus infections have been recently published. The first reported the results of four randomized, double-blind, placebo-controlled trials of tremacamra (formerly BIRR), a recombinant soluble form of the membrane-bound ICAM-1 glycoprotein (the cellular receptor for most rhinovirus serotypes). Tremacamra, as a nasal spray or powder, or placebo were administered 7 h before or 12 h after nasal challenge with type 39 rhinovirus. The results of the studies showed that both formulations of tremacamra, by blockade of the ICAM-receptor on respiratory tract epithelial cells were effective in reducing the symptoms of experimental common colds. Other than some nasal irritation with the powder formulation, adverse effects were minimal (55).

The second study, conducted at two clinical sites, reported the results of trials of the neuraminidase inhibitor zanamivir (GG167), a sialic acid analog, on naturally acquired influenza infection in healthy adults. Zanamivir was administered prophylactically shortly before the influenza season for a 28-day period. The drug or placebo was given by oral inhalation once daily in a dose of 10 mg, using a self-actuated inhalation device (Diskhaler-Glaxo Wellcome). The results showed that zanamivir was effective in the prevention of influenza for a 4-week period in the subjects studied. The drug was well tolerated. Of interest was the finding that, like amantadine or rimantadine, zanamivir was more effective in preventing disease (especially severe disease) than preventing infection. While only type A influenza circulated during the clinical trials, data exist that support similar effectiveness against type B infections, an obvious advantage over the two older drugs. Additionally, viral resistance to zanamivir, which develops rapidly with amantadine or rimantadine, has not yet been observed (56).

## References

1. McIntosh K, Ellis EF, Hoffman LS, Lybass TG, Eller JJ, Fulginiti VA. The association of viral and bacterial respiratory infections with exacerbations of wheezing in young asthmatic children. J Pediatr 1973; 82:578–590.
2. Pattemore PK, Johnston SL, Bardin PG. Viruses as precipitants of asthma symptoms I. Epidemiology. Clin Exp Allergy 1992; 22:325–326.
3. Potter P, Weinberg E, Shore S. Acute severe asthma: a prospective study of the precipitating factors in 40 children. S Afr Med J 1984; 66:397–402.
4. Storr J, Lenney W. School holidays and admissions with asthma. Arch Dis Child 1989; 64:103–107.
5. Nicholson KG, Kent J, Ireland DC. Respiratory viruses and exacerbations of asthma in adults. Br Med J 1993; 307:982–986.
6. Frick OL, German DF, Mills J. Development of allergy in children. J Allergy Clin Immunol 1979; 63:228–241.
7. von Mutius E, Fritsch C, Weiland S, Roll G, Magnussen H. Prevalence of asthma and allergic disorders among children in united Germany. Br Med J 1992; 305: 1395–1399.
8. von Mutius E, Martinez F, Fritsch C, Nicolai T, Reitner P, Thieman H. Skin test reactivity and number of siblings. Br Med J 1994; 308:692–695.
9. Hamparian VV, Colonno RJ, Cooney MK. A collaborative report: rhinoviruses-extension of the numbering system 89–100. J Virol 1987; 159:191–192.
10. Merigan TC, Reed SE, Hall TS, Tyrrell DAJ. Inhibition of respiratory virus infection by locally applied interferon. J Lancet 1973; 1:563–567.
11. Scott GM, Phillpotts RJ, Gauci CL, Greiner J, Tyrrell DAJ. Purified interferon as protection against rhinovirus infection. Br Med J 1982; 284:1822–1825.
12. Scott GM, Phillpotts RJ, Gauci CL, Greiner J, Tyrrell DAJ. Prevention of rhinovirus colds by human interferon α-2 from *Escherichia coli*. J Lancet 1982; 2:186–188.
13. Hayden FG, Albrecht JK, Kaiser DL, Gwaltney JM Jr. Prevention of natural colds by contact prophylaxis with intranasal $\alpha_2$ interferon. N Engl J Med 1986; 314:71–75.
14. Hayden FG, Gwaltney JM Jr. Intranasal interferon-$\alpha_2\beta$ for prevention of rhinovirus infection and illness. J Infect Dis 1983; 148:543–550.
15. Monto AS, Shope TC, Schwartz SA, Albrecht JK. Intranasal interferon-$\alpha_2\beta$ for seasonal prophylaxis of respiratory infection. J Infect Dis 1986; 154:128–133.
16. Hayden FG, Gwaltney JM Jr. Intranasal interferon-$\alpha_2$ treatment of experimental rhinoviral colds. J Infect Dis 1984; 150:174–180.
17. Isaacs A, Lindenmann J. Virus interference. I. The interferon. J Proc R Soc Lond 1957; 147:258–267.

18. Baron S, Dianzani F. Interferons: a biological system with therapeutic potential in viral infections. Anti Viral Res 1994; 24:97–110.
19. Gwaltney JM Jr. Combined antiviral and antimediator treatment of rhinovirus colds. J Infect Dis 1992; 166:776–782.
20. Greve JM, Davis G, Myer AM, Forte CP, Yost SC, Martor CW, Kamarck ME, McClellan A. The major human rhinovirus receptor is ICAM-1. Cell 1989; 56:839–847.
21. Papi A. Epithelial ICAM-1 regulation and its role in allergy. Clin Exp Allergy 1997; 27:721–724.
22. Colonno RJ, Callahan PL, Long WJ. Isolation of a monoclonal antibody that blocks attachment of the major group of human rhinoviruses. J Virol 1986; 57:7–12.
23. Crump CE, Arruda E, Hayden FG. In vitro inhibitory activity of soluble ICAM-1 for the numbered serotypes of human rhinovirus. Antiviral Chem Chemother 1993; 4:323–327.
24. Higgins PG, Phillpotts RJ, Scott GM, Wallace J, Bernhardt LL, Tyrrell DAJ. Intranasal interferon as protection against experimental respiratory coronavirus infection in volunteers. Antimicrob Agents Chemother 1983; 24:713–715.
25. Turner RB, Felton A, Kosak K, Kelsey DK, Meschievitz CK. Prevention of experimental coronavirus colds with intransasal α-2β interferon. J Infect Dis 1986; 154:443–447.
26. Kubar OI, Brjantseva EA, Nikitina LE, Zlydnikov DM. The importance of drug resistance in the treatment of influenza with rimantadine. Antiviral Res 1989; 11:313–316.
27. Kim CU, Lew W, Williams MA, Liu H, Zhang L, Swaminathan S, Bischofberger N, Chen MS, Mendel DB, Tai CY, Laver WG, Stevens RC. Influenza neuraminidase inhibitors possessing a novel hydrophobic interaction in the enzyme active site: design, synthesis, and structural analysis of carbocyclic sialic acid analogues with potent anti-influenza activity. J Am Chem Soc 1997; 119:681–690.
28. Meert KL, Sarnaik AP, Gelmini MJ, Lieh Lai MW. Aerosolized ribovirin in mechanically ventilated children with respiratory syncytial tract lower respiratory tract disease: a prospective, double blind, randomized trial. Crit Care Med 1994; 22:566–572.
29. Moler FW, Steinhart CM, Ohmit SE, Sidham GL. The Pediatric Critical Care Study Group. Effectiveness of ribavirin in otherwise well infants with respiratory syncytial virus associated respiratory failure. J Pediatr 1996; 128:422–428.
30. American Academy of Pediatrics Committee on Infectious Diseases. Reassessment of the implications for ribavirin therapy in respiratory syncytial virus infections. Pediatrics 1996; 97:137–149.
31. Meissner HC, Fulton DR, Groothuis JR, Geggel RL, Marx GR, Hemming VG, Houghen T, Snyderman DR. Controlled trial to evaluate protection of higher-risk infants against respiratory syncytial virus disease by using standard intravenous immunglobulin. Antimicrob Agents Chemother 1993; 37:1655–1658.
32. The Prevent Study Group. Reduction of RSV hospitalization and among premature infants with bronchopulmonary dysplasia using respiratory syncytial virus immunoglobulin prophylaxis. Pediatrics 1997; 99:93–99.
33. Meissner HC, Groothuis JR. Immunoprophylaxis and the control of RSV disease. Pediatrics 1997; 100:260–262.

34. Meissner HC, Welliver RC, Chartrand SA, Fulton DR, Rodriguez WJA, Groothuis JR. Prevention of respiratory virus infection in high risk infants: consensus opinion on the role of immunoprophylaxis with respiratory syncytial virus hyper-immunoglobulin. Pediatr Infect Dis J 1996; 15:1059–1068.

35. Hay JW, Ernst RL, Meissner HC. Respiratory immunoglobulin: a cost effective analysis. Am J Man Care 1996; 2:851.

36. National Asthma Education and Prevention Program. Expert Panel Report 2 Guidelines for the Diagnosis and Management of Asthma. Bethesda, MD: National Heart, Lung and Blood Institute, 1997. NIH Publication No. 97-4053.

37. Harris JB, Weinberger MM, Nassif E, Smith G, Milavetz G, Stillerman A. Early intervention with short courses of prednisone to prevent progression of asthma in ambulatory patients incompletely responsive to bronchodilators. J Pediatr 1987; 110: 627–633.

38. Brunette MG, Lands L, Thibodeau LP. Childhood asthma: prevention of attacks with short-term corticosteroid treatment of upper respiratory tract infection. J Pediatr 1988; 81:624–628.

39. Tal A, Levy N, Bearman JE. Methylprednisolone therapy for acute asthma in infants and toddlers: a controlled clinical trial. J Pediatr 1990; 86:350–356.

40. Chapman KR, Verbeek PR, White JG, Rebuck AS. Effect of a short course of prednisone in the prevention of early relapse after the emergency room treatment of acute asthma. N Engl J Med 1991; 324:788–894.

41. Mukwaya G. Immunosuppressive effects and infections associated with corticosteroid therapy. Pediatr Infect Dis 1988; 7:499–504.

42. Grant CG, Duggan AK, Santosham M, De Angelis C. Oral prednisone as a risk factor for infections in children with asthma. Arch Pediatr Adolesc Med 1996; 150: 58–63.

43. Englstein WH, Katz R, Brown JA. The effects of early corticosteroid therapy on the skin eruption and pain of herpes zoster. JAMA 1970; 211:1681–1683.

44. Kimsey PB, Goad MEP, Zhi-Bo Z, Brackee G, Fox JG. Methylprednisolone acetate modulation of infection and subsequent pulmonary pathology in hamsters exposed to parainfluenza-1 (Sendai) virus. Am Rev Respir Dis 1989; 140:1704–1711.

45. Cheatham WJ, Weller TH, Dolan TF. Varicella: report of two fatal cases with necropsy, virus isolation and serologic studies. Am J Pathol 1956; 32:1015–1028.

46. Falliers CJ, Ellis EF. Corticosteroids and varicella: six year experience in an asthmatic population. Arch Dis Child 1965; 40:593–599.

47. Lantner RA, Rockoff J, DeMasi J, Boran-Ragotzy R, Middleton E Jr. Fatal varicella in a corticosteroid dependent asthmatic receiving troleandomycin. J Allergy Proc 1990; 11:83–87.

48. Wilson NW, Silverman M. Treatment of acute, episodic asthma in preschool children using intermittent high dose inhaled steroids at home. Arch Dis Child 1990; 65: 407–410.

49. Connett G, Lenney W. Prevention of viral induced asthma attacks using inhaled budesonide. Arch Dis Child 1993; 68:85–87.

50. Wilson N, Sloper K, Silverman M. Effect of continuous treatment with topical corticosteroid on episodic viral wheeze in preschool children. Arch Dis Child 1995; 72: 17–20.

51. Doull IJM, Lampe FC, Smith S, Schreiber J, Freezer NJ, Holgate ST. Effect of inhaled corticosteroids on episodes of wheezing associated with viral infection in school age children: Randomized double blind placebo controlled trial. Br Med J 1997; 315:858–862.

52  Åberg N, Åberg B, Ålestig K. The effect of inhaled and intransasal sodium cromoglycate on symptoms of upper respiratory tract infections. Clin Exp Allergy 1996; 26:1045–1050.

53. Barrow GI, Higgins PG, Al-Nakib W, Smith AP, Winham RBM, Tyrell DAJ. The effect of intranasal nedocromil sodium on viral upper respiratory tract infections in human volunteers. Clin Exp Allergy 1990; 20:45–51.

54. Konig P, Eigen H, Ellis M, Ellis E. The effect of nedocromil sodium on childhood asthma during the viral season. Am J Respir Crit Care Med 1995; 152:1879–1886.

55. Turner RB, Wecker MT, Pohl G, Witek TJ, McNally E, St. George R, Winther B, Hayden FG. Efficacy of tremacamra, a soluble intercellular adhesion molecule 1, for experimental rhinovirus infection. JAMA 1999; 281:1797–1804.

56. Monto AS, Robinsons DP, Healocher ML, Hinson JM, Jr, Elliott MJ, Crisp A. Zanamivir in the prevention of influenza among healthy adults. JAMA 1999; 282: 31–35.

# 14

# Previously Conducted Trials to Evaluate New Avenues of Therapy

**ROBERT L. ATMAR**

Baylor College of Medicine
Houston, Texas

**RONALD B. TURNER**

Medical University of South Carolina
Charleston, South Carolina

## I. Experimental Models for the Study of Viral Respiratory Pathogens

The relatively benign and self-limited illnesses associated with most of the viral respiratory pathogens present both unique opportunities and formidable challenges for the design of clinical trials. In contrast to most other pathogens, these organisms lend themselves to experimentally induced infections for studies of both pathogenesis and treatment. Clinical trials conducted in both the experimental infection model and in natural infections have contributed to our understanding of these illnesses and the evaluation of effective treatments.

The study of naturally acquired viral respiratory infections in human subjects presents several challenges. One problem is the selection of subjects who are infected with the same pathogen. The clinical syndromes produced by the various respiratory viruses are similar, and accurate differentiation on the basis of clinical findings is not possible. Furthermore, diagnostic studies are generally neither sensitive enough nor rapid enough to permit enrollment of subjects with a known pathogen into a clinical trial of natural infections. A second difficulty is the relatively rapid development and subsequent resolution of the symptoms associated with these illnesses. The time from first recognition of symptoms to the peak of the symptom burden is generally only 1–2 days. Institution of experimental treatments after the peak of illness reduces the potential for a treatment effect and makes it more difficult to detect a true ''signal'' against the background noise inherent in any human volunteer study (1). Study of natural infections may also introduce bias with regard to symptom severity. Subjects who present for treatment in trials of natural infections may have more severe illnesses than those who do not participate. The modification of the natural infection model by enrolling subjects from a surveillance panel has proven useful for providing a broader spectrum of illness severity and allowing earlier therapeutic intervention.

The use of experimentally induced infections for clinical trials addresses some of these difficulties (Table 1) (1). In the experimental model, infection is induced with a known pathogen under controlled conditions. The knowledge of the precise time of infection allows heightened surveillance for the onset of symptoms and ensures early treatment. The disadvantages of the experimental infection model are that the mechanism of infection is usually (although not necessarily) unnatural, the ability to treat symptoms early has the potential disadvantage of including subjects in the analysis who have minimal symptoms, and the artificial nature of the experimental model raises questions about the generalizability of the results to the natural setting.

The best approach to evaluation of therapies for viral respiratory infection is a combination of the two clinical trial models. Preliminary studies of efficacy and dosing can be done more cheaply and with greater sensitivity in the experimental model. The ultimate impact of a treatment in the general population, however, can only be determined by clinical trials using the natural model.

**Table 1** Comparison of the Natural and Experimentally Induced Cold Models for Clinical Trials of Treatments for Viral Respiratory Infections

| Characteristic of trial | Natural model | Induced model |
|---|---|---|
| Known pathogen | | X |
| Natural route of inoculation | X | |
| Known time of virus infection | | X |
| Controlled environment | | X |
| Consistent recovery of viral isolates | | X |
| Immediate therapeutic intervention | | X |
| Potential bias in symptom severity | X | X |
| Results readily generalized to the natural setting | X | |
| Reliance on subjective symptom reporting | X | X |

## II. Rhinoviruses

### A. Clinical Trials of Antiviral Agents for the Prevention or Treatment of Rhinovirus Infections

The prevention or treatment of rhinovirus infections has been attempted in many clinical trials since the discovery of the virus in 1956. In spite of the effort and resources that have been expended in this endeavor, no antiviral drugs are currently marketed for the prevention or treatment of rhinovirus infection. Recent studies of the pathogenesis of rhinovirus infections suggest that the host response contributes to the symptom complex associated with these infections (2–5). Inhibition of both the inflammatory response and viral replication may be required for a clinically significant effect on the rhinovirus colds.

### Capsid-Binding Agents

The capsid-binding agents are a diverse group of compounds that inhibit virus replication by altering the ability of the virus to attach to the host cell or by preventing uncoating of the virus. The flavonoids, chalcones, RMI 15,731, and oxazolines (WIN compounds) have excellent activity against a broad spectrum of rhinovirus serotypes in vitro. However, prophylactic administration of these compounds has no effect on either infection or illness in the experimental challenge model (6–11). Another capsid-binding agent, R 61837 (3-methoxy-6 [4-methylphenyl-1-piperazinyl]pyridazine), when given by the intranasal route, was effective for prevention of rhinovirus associated illness but had no effect on infection (12,13). A similar but more potent agent, pirodavir (R 77975), was also effective for prevention of illness and at high doses had a modest effect on virus shedding (14). Pirodavir was ineffective when treatment was initiated 24 hours after virus challenge.

### Zinc Salts

In the mid-1970s, it was reported that zinc ions inhibit rhinovirus replication (15). As a result of this observation there have been numerous studies of the efficacy of zinc, given as oral lozenges, for the treatment of common cold symptoms. In spite of the in vitro effect of zinc on virus replication, there has been no detectable effect of zinc lozenges on virus replication in vivo (16,17). The effect of zinc on symptoms has been inconsistent; some studies have reported dramatic effects on the duration of cold symptoms, and other studies have found no effect (16–20). There is no correlation between the dose of zinc given and the clinical efficacy, although different formulations of zinc lozenge were used in the various studies and the studies may not be directly comparable. A major problem with the interpretation of these studies is the very high frequency (50–

90%) of side effects in subjects who receive zinc and the difficulty in producing an adequately matched placebo.

### Interferons

The first successful clinical trial of interferon for treatment of rhinovirus infection was done in the early 1970s (21). However, definitive evaluation of the interferons was delayed until large quantities of material were made available by the development of recombinant DNA techniques. The effectiveness of intranasal administration of α-interferon for prevention of rhinovirus infections was established in a number of studies both in the experimental and natural rhinovirus infection models (22–31). The cost and the side effects of α-interferon preclude its use as an agent for the prevention of rhinovirus colds (26,27,29,32,33). In spite of the clear effect of α-interferon for prevention of rhinovirus infection, little effect was seen when interferon was administered as treatment (24,34). In limited studies, β-interferon was found to have fewer side effects but was also less effective than α-interferon for prevention of rhinovirus colds (35,36). Also in limited studies, γ-interferon was ineffective as an antiviral agent for rhinovirus (37).

### Miscellaneous Agents

A number of other antiviral agents with in vitro activity against the rhinoviruses have had limited testing in clinical trials. These agents—enviroxime, 44081 RP, DIQA, isoquinolone UK2054, SKF 40491, GL R9-338, and RP 19326—had no effect on either symptom severity or viral infection, and no further testing was done (38–44).

## B. Studies of Receptor Blockade for Prevention and Treatment of Rhinovirus Infections

In 1984, Abraham and Colonno reported that different rhinovirus serotypes shared the same cellular receptor (45). Subsequent studies have shown that all rhinoviruses but one attach to cells via only two different receptors (45,46). The majority of serotypes bind by a single receptor that has subsequently been identified as intercellular adhesion molecule 1 (ICAM-1) (47,48). Blockade of the receptor site on the cells with antibody to ICAM-1 or of the receptor-binding site on the virus with soluble ICAM-1 have both been shown to inhibit viral infection in vitro and are potential treatments for the common cold (46,49–52). The logistics of maintaining an appropriate concentration of either of these proteins in the nasal cavity for prolonged periods of time present formidable obstacles to the effective use of these agents, however.

Clinical trials of both anti-ICAM antibody and soluble ICAM for the prevention or treatment of rhinovirus infection have been done using the experimental rhinovirus infection model. Prophylaxis with intranasal monoclonal antibody to ICAM-1 was attempted by Hayden et al. in experimental colds in volunteers (53). In the most successful of these studies, a total of 1 mg/subject of anti-ICAM antibody was given over a period beginning 3 hours before and ending 36 hours after virus challenge. This treatment regimen reduced symptoms and viral shedding during the time the medication was being administered; however, when the medication was discontinued the amount of virus shedding increased and symptoms became more severe.

The efficacy of soluble ICAM-1 for prevention of rhinovirus colds in the experimental model has been recently reported (54). In this study, soluble ICAM-1 given intranasally either shortly before or shortly after virus challenge reduced symptoms and viral shedding but had no effect on the incidence of viral infection. Additional studies will be needed to assess the potential utility of soluble ICAM-1 for prevention or treatment of rhinovirus colds.

### C.  Clinical Trials of Symptomatic Treatments for Rhinovirus Colds

Symptomatic therapy remains the mainstay of treatment for rhinovirus colds. The use of symptomatic therapies available over the counter and directed at specific symptoms of colds has been the subject of some controversy (55). Many of the clinical trials of symptomatic treatments for the common cold have been done in subjects with natural colds where no attempt was made to define the viral agent responsible for the illness.

#### Adrenergic Agents

Both topical and oral adrenergic agents are effective nasal decongestants; however, there are relatively few reports of clinical trials in rhinovirus infections or in subjects with natural colds (56–58). A beneficial effect of an adrenergic agent administered in combination with an antihistamine has been found in a single study to reduce the severity of cough (59).

#### Antihistamines

First-generation antihistamines have been used for many years for treatment of rhinorrhea associated with the common cold. A modest, but statistically significant, effect on rhinorrhea has been found in several small studies, although other studies have failed to detect any therapeutic effect (60–63). A large study in experimental rhinovirus colds found that clemastine fumarate, a first-generation antihistamine, reduced rhinorrhea by approximately 27% compared to placebo (64). This observation was subsequently confirmed in a natural cold trial. A more recent study of brompheniramine in the rhinovirus experimental model found similar results (65). In each of these studies the antihistamine had a significant effect on sneezing, and in the brompheniramine study it also appeared that the antihistamine may have a beneficial effect on cough. The second-generation or ''nonsedating'' antihistamines have had no effect on common cold symptoms in a limited number of studies (66,67).

### Anticholinergic Agents

Treatment with ipratropium bromide has consistently resulted in an effect on rhinorrhea and nasal mucus weights. In a small study in experimental rhinovirus colds, nasal mucus weights were reduced by approximately 40% by ipratropium; however, these results were not statistically significant (68). In subsequent larger studies of subjects with natural colds, ipratropium produced a 22–31% decrease in rhinorrhea compared to placebo (69–71). A single small study of atropine in the rhinovirus experimental model found no significant effect on nasal mucus weights (72).

### Anti-Inflammatory/Antimediator Therapy

The observation that inflammatory mediators, particularly the kinins, may play a role in the pathogenesis of rhinovirus colds has resulted in several clinical trials of anti-inflammatory therapy directed at inhibiting these mediators. The effect of steroids on rhinovirus colds has been evaluated in two separate trials using the experimental colds model (73,74). Although in one of these trials steroid treatment significantly reduced the levels of kinins in nasal lavage fluid, there was no significant effect on symptoms in either study. Similarly, the cyclooxygenase inhibitor naproxen had no effect on the nasal symptoms associated with rhinovirus although there was an effect on some systemic symptoms (75). A specific bradykinin antagonist, NPC 567, also was ineffective for treatment of rhinovirus colds (76).

### Cromolyn

The cromolyns have a variety of effects that result in decreased release of inflammatory mediators. Cromolyns have been used in two studies: a study of prophylaxis in experimental rhinovirus colds and a study of treatment in natural colds of unknown etiology (77,78). In both of these studies, treatment had a statistically significant effect on the total symptom score toward the end of the cold. Scores for individual symptoms were not reported in these studies; however, the effect the cromolyns appears to be due primarily to amelioration of nonnasal symptoms.

### Dextromethorphan and Codeine

Although these preparations are commonly used for the treatment of cough in colds, there are no controlled clinical trials of these agents in this illness.

### Vitamin C

Vitamin C was perhaps the earliest subject of a controlled clinical trial for treatment of the common cold. More than 50 years and many studies later, there is still no consensus on the effect of vitamin C for the prevention or treatment of common cold symptoms. In general, proponents of vitamin C therapy have argued that studies in which no effect was detected used an insufficient dose of vitamin C, while those who doubt the effect of vitamin C suggest that studies in which a positive effect was found were poorly designed or improperly blinded (79–81). A review of the studies in which vitamin C was given in doses of at least 1 g/day concluded that there was no effect on incidence of colds but that there was a consistent but highly variable effect on severity of illness (81). In this analysis, which largely discounts concerns about blinding and study design, only half of the studies cited demonstrated a decrease in duration of illness of at least 20%.

### Combination Therapy

Gwaltney reported effective treatment of established rhinovirus infections with a combination of naproxen, ipratropium bromide, and interferon-$\alpha$2b (82). The effect of this combination appeared to be greater than the effects usually seen with available common cold therapies.

## III.  Coronavirus Infections

There are few studies of coronavirus respiratory infections that involve human subjects. An experimental model of coronavirus colds has been used for studies of the natural history of infection. However, this model has been infrequently used for studies of treatment for coronavirus colds. Two studies examined the effect of prophylactic $\alpha$-interferon on coronavirus colds (83,84). Both studies found a significant effect on illness; however, the incidence of viral infection was reduced in only one of the studies. The study of symptomatic treatment of coronavirus colds found no effect of nedocromil sodium on coronavirus cold symptoms (78). Additional studies using the coronavirus experimental challenge model are unlikely in light of recent observations that suggest that coronavirus infection may be associated with multiple sclerosis (85,86).

The study of natural coronavirus colds has been hampered by the difficulty of isolating coronavirus in standard cell cultures. The recent development of sensitive detection methods may permit studies in natural colds; however, the relatively low incidence of infection and the lack of a clearly defined epidemic season will continue to be an obstacle to the study of coronavirus infections using the natural model (87).

## References

1. Gwaltney JM Jr, Buier RM, Rogers JL. The influence of signal variation, bias, noise, and effect size on statistical significance in treatment studies of the common cold. Antiviral Res 1996; 29:287–295.
2. Naclerio RM, Proud D, Lichtenstein LM, Kagey-Sobotka A, Hendley JO, Sorentino J, Gwaltney JM Jr. Kinins are generated during experimental rhinovirus colds. J Infect Dis 1988; 157:133–142.
3. Turner RB, Weingand KW, Yeh C-H, Leedy D. Association between nasal secretion interleukin-8 concentration and symptom severity in experimental rhinovirus colds. Clin Infect Dis 1998; 26.
4. Zhu Z, Tang W, Ray A, Wu Y, Einarsson O, Landry ML, Gwaltney JM, Jr., Elias JA. Rhinovirus stimulation of interleukin-6 in vivo and in vitro: evidence for nuclear factor kB-dependent transcriptional activation. J Clin Invest 1996; 97:421–430.
5. Zhu Z, Tang WL, Gwaltney JM, Elias JA. Rhinovirus stimulation of interleukin-8 in vivo and in vitro- role of NF-kappa-β. Am J Physiol 1997; 17:L814–L824.
6. Phillpotts RJ, Wallace J, Tyrrell DA, Freestone DS, Shepherd WM. Failure of oral 4′, 6-dichloroflavan to protect against rhinovirus infection in man. Arch Virol 1983; 75:115–121.
7. Al-Nakib W, Willman J, Higgins PG, Tyrrell DA, Shepherd WM, Freestone DS. Failure of intranasally administered 4′, 6-dichloroflavan to protect against rhinovirus infection in man. Arch Virol 1987; 92:255–260.
8. Al-Nakib W, Higgins PG, Barrow I, Tyrrell DA, Lenox-Smith I, Ishitsuka H. Intranasal chalcone, Ro 09-0410, as prophylaxis against rhinovirus infection in human volunteers. J Antimicrob Chemother 1987; 20:887–892.
9. Phillpotts RJ, Higgins PG, Willman JS, Tyrrell DA, Lenox-Smith I. Evaluation of the antirhinovirus chalcone Ro 09-0415 given orally to volunteers. J Antimicrob Chemother 1984; 14:403–409.
10. Gwaltney JM Jr, Hayden FG. Prophylactic efficacy of intranasal RMI 15731 in experimental rhinovirus infection [Abst. 931]. 23rd Interscience Conference on Antimicrobial Agents and Chemotherapy, Las Vegas, ASM, 1983.
11. Turner RB, Dutko FJ, Goldstein NH, Lockwood G, Hayden FG. Efficacy of oral WIN 54954 for prophylaxis of experimental rhinovirus infection. Antimicrob Agents Chemother 1993; 37:297–300.
12. Al-Nakib W, Higgins PG, Barrow GI, Tyrrell DA, Andries K, Vanden Bussche G, Taylor N, Janssen PA. Suppression of colds in human volunteers challenged with rhinovirus by a new synthetic drug (R61837). Antimicrob Agents Chemother 1989; 33:522–525.
13. Barrow GI, Higgins PG, Tyrrell DAJ, Andries K. An appraisal of the efficacy of

the antiviral R 61837 in rhinovirus infections in human volunteers. Antiviral Chem Chemother 1990; 1:279–283.

14. Hayden FG, Andries K, Janssen PA. Safety and efficacy of intranasal pirodavir (R77975) in experimental rhinovirus infection. Antimicrob Agents Chemother 1992; 36:727–732.

15. Korant BD, Kauer JC, Butterworth BE. Zinc ions inhibit replication of rhinoviruses. Nature (London) 1974; 248:588–590.

16. Al-Nakib W, Higgins PG, Barrow I, Batstone G, Tyrrell DA. Prophylaxis and treatment of rhinovirus colds with zinc gluconate lozenges. J Antimicrob Chemother 1987; 20:893–901.

17. Farr BM, Conner EM, Betts RF, Oleske J, Minnefor A, Gwaltney JM, Jr. Two randomized controlled trials of zinc gluconate lozenge therapy of experimentally induced rhinovirus colds. Antimicrob Agents Chemother 1987; 31:1183–1187.

18. Smith DS, Helzner EC, Nuttall CE Jr, Collins M, Rofman BA, Ginsberg D, Goswick CB, Magner A. Failure of zinc gluconate in treatment of acute upper respiratory tract infections. Antimicrob Agents Chemother 1989; 33:646–648.

19. Mossad SB, Macknin ML, Medendorp SV, Mason P. Zinc gluconate lozenges for treating the common cold: a randomized, double-blind, placebo-controlled study. Ann Intern Med 1996; 125:81–88.

20. Eby GA, Davis DR, Halcomb WW. Reduction in duration of common colds by zinc gluconate lozenges in a double-blind study. Antimicrob Agents Chemother 1984; 25:20–24.

21. Merrigan TC, Hall TS, Reed SE, Tyrrell DAJ. Inhibition of respiratory virus infection by locally applied interferon. Lancet 1973; i:563–567.

22. Douglas RM, Moore BW, Miles HB, Davies LM, Graham NM, Ryan P, Worswick DA, Albrecht JK. Prophylactic efficacy of intranasal alpha 2-interferon against rhinovirus infections in the family setting. N Engl J Med 1986; 314:65–70.

23. Hayden FG, Gwaltney JM Jr. Intranasal interferon alpha 2 for prevention of rhinovirus infection and illness. J Infect Dis 1983; 148:543–550.

24. Hayden FG, Gwaltney JM Jr. Intranasal interferon-alpha$_2$ treatment of experimental rhinovirus colds. J Infect Dis 1984; 150:174–180.

25. Hayden FG, Albrecht JK, Kaiser DL, Gwaltney JM Jr. Prevention of natural colds by contact prophylaxis with intranasal alpha 2-interferon. N Engl J Med 1986; 314: 71–75.

26. Monto AS, Shope TC, Schwartz SA, Albrecht JK. Intranasal interferon-α2b for seasonal prophylaxis of respiratory infection. J Infect Dis 1986; 154:128–133.

27. Samo TC, Greenberg SB, Couch RB, Quarles J, Johnson PE, Hook S, Harmon MW. Efficacy and tolerance of intranasally applied recombinant leukocyte A interferon in normal volunteers. J Infect Dis 1983; 148:535–542.

28. Scott GM, Phillpotts RJ, Wallace J, Gauci CL, Greiner J, Tyrrell DA. Prevention of rhinovirus colds by human interferon alpha-2 from *Escherichia coli*. Lancet 1982; 2:186–188.

29. Samo TC, Greenberg SB, Palmer JM, Couch RB, Harmon MW, Johnson PE. Intranasally applied recombinant leukocyte A interferon in normal volunteers. II. Determination of minimal effective and tolerable dose. J Infect Dis 1984; 150:181–188.

30. Phillpotts RJ, Higgins PG, Willman JS, Tyrrell DA, Freestone DS, Shepherd WM.

Intranasal lymphoblastoid interferon (''Wellferon'') prophylaxis against rhinovirus and influenza virus in volunteers. J Interferon Res 1984; 4:535–541.

31. Phillpotts RJ, Scott GM, Higgins PG, Wallace J, Tyrrell DA, Gauci CL. An effective dosage regimen for prophylaxis against rhinovirus infection by intranasal administration of HuIFN-alpha 2. Antiviral Res 1983; 3:121–136.

32. Hayden FG, Mills SE, Johns ME. Human tolerance and histopathologic effects of long-term administration of intranasal interferon-α2. J Infect Dis 1983; 148:914–921.

33. Scott GM, Onwubalili JK, Robinson JA, Dore C, Secher DS, Cantell K. Tolerance of one-month intranasal interferon. J Med Virol 1985; 17:99–106.

34. Hayden FG, Kaiser DL, Albrecht JK. Intranasal recombinant alfa-2b interferon treatment of naturally occurring common colds. Antimicrob Agents Chemother 1988; 32:224–230.

35. Sperber SJ, Levine PA, Sorrentino JV, Riker DK, Hayden FG. Ineffectiveness of recombinant interferon-beta serine nasal drops for prophylaxis of natural colds. J Infect Dis 1989; 160:700–705.

36. Higgins PG, Al-Nakib W, Willman J, Tyrrell DA. Interferon-beta ser as prophylaxis against experimental rhinovirus infection in volunteers. J Interferon Res 1986; 6:153–159.

37. Higgins PG, Al-Nakib W, Barrow GI, Tyrrell DA. Recombinant human interferon-gamma as prophylaxis against rhinovirus colds in volunteers. J Interferon Res 1988; 8:591–596.

38. Hayden FG, Gwaltney JM Jr. Prophylactic activity of intranasal enviroxime against experimentally induced rhinovirus type 39 infection. Antimicrob Agents Chemother 1982; 21:892–897.

39. Levandowski RA, Pachucki CT, Rubenis M, Jackson GG. Topical enviroxime against rhinovirus infection. Antimicrob Agents Chemother 1982; 22:1004–1007.

40. Phillpotts RJ, Wallace J, Tyrrell DA, Tagart VB. Therapeutic activity of enviroxime against rhinovirus infection in volunteers. Antimicrob Agents Chemother 1983; 23:671–675.

41. Zerial A, Werner GH, Phillpotts RJ, Willmann JS, Higgins PG, Tyrrell DA. Studies on 44 081 R.P., a new antirhinovirus compound, in cell cultures and in volunteers. Antimicrob Agents Chemother 1985; 27:846–850.

42. Togo Y, Schwartz AR, Hornick RB. Antiviral effect of 3, 4-dihydro-1-isoquinoline-acetamide hydrochloride in experimental human rhinovirus infection. Antimicrob Agents Chemother 1973; 4:612–616.

43. Reed SE, Bynoe ML. The antiviral activity of isoquinoline drugs for rhinoviruses in vitro and in vivo. J Med Microbiol 1970; 3:346–352.

44. Reed SE, Craig JW, Tyrrell DAJ. Four compounds active against rhinovirus: comparison in vitro and in volunteers. J Infect Dis 1976; 133:A128–A135.

45. Abraham G, Colonno RJ. Many rhinovirus serotypes share the same cellular receptor. J Virol 1984; 51:340–345.

46. Colonno RJ, Callahan PL, Long WJ. Isolation of a monoclonal antibody that blocks attachment of the major group of human rhinoviruses. J Virol 1986; 57:7–12.

47. Greve JM, Davis G, Meyer AM, Forte CP, Yost SC, Marlor CW, Kamarck ME,

McClelland A. The major human rhinovirus receptor is ICAM-1. Cell 1989; 56: 839–847.

48. Staunton DE, Merluzzi VJ, Rothlein R, Barton R, Marlin SD, Springer TA. A cell adhesion molecule, ICAM-1 is the major surface receptor for rhinoviruses. Cell 1989; 56:849–853.

49. Marlin SD, Staunton DE, Springer TA, Stratowa C, Sommergruber W, Merluzzi VJ. A soluble form of intercellular adhesion molecule-1 inhibits rhinovirus infection. Nature 1990; 344:70–72.

50. Crump CE, Arruda E, Hayden FG. In vitro inhibitory activity of soluble ICAM-1 for the numbered serotypes of human rhinovirus. Antiviral Chem Chemother 1993; 4:323–327.

51. Condra JH, Sardana VV, Tomassini JE, Schlabach AJ, Davies ME, Lineberger DW, Graham DJ, Gotlib L, Colonno RJ. Bacterial expression of antibody fragments that block human rhinovirus infection of cultured cells. J Biol Chem 1990; 265:2292–2295.

52. de Arruda E, Crump CE, Marlin SD, Merluzzi VJ, Hayden FG. In vitro studies of the antirhinovirus activity of soluble intercellular adhesion molecule-1. Antimicrob Agents Chemother 1992; 36:1186–1191.

53. Hayden FG, Gwaltney JM Jr, Colonno RJ. Modification of experimental rhinovirus colds by receptor blockade. Antiviral Res 1988; 9:233–247.

54. Turner RB, Wecker MT, Pohl G, Witek TJ, Marlin S, McNally E, Hayden FG. Efficacy of soluble ICAM-1 (sICAM) for prevention of rhinovirus infection and illness. 37th Interscience Conference on Antimicrobial Agents and Chemotherapy, Toronto, American Society for Microbiology, 1997.

55. Smith MBH, Feldman W. Over-the-counter cold medications. A critical review of clinical trials between 1950 and 1991. J Am Med Assoc 1993; 269:2258–2263.

56. Akerlund A, Klint T, Olen L, Rundcrantz H. Nasal decongestant effect of oxymetazoline in the common cold: An objective dose-response study in 106 patients. J Laryngol Otol 1989; 103:743–746.

57. Doyle WJ, Riker DK, McBride TP, Hayden FG, Hendley JO, Swarts JD, Gwaltney JM Jr. Therapeutic effects of an anticholinergic-sympathomimetic combination in induced rhinovirus colds. Ann Otol Rhinol Laryngol 1993; 102:521–527.

58. Sperber SJ, Sorrentino JV, Riker DK, Hayden FG. Evaluation of an alpha agonist alone and in combination with a nonsteroidal antiinflammatory agent in the treatment of experimental rhinovirus colds. Bull NY Acad Med 1989; 65:145–160.

59. Curley FJ, Irwin RS, Pratter MR, Stivers DH, Doern GV, Vernaglia PA, Larkin AB, Baker SP. Cough and the common cold. Am Rev Respir Dis 1988; 138:305–311.

60. Sakchainanont B, Chantarojanasiri T, Ruangkanchanasetr S, Tapasart C, Suwanjutha S. Effectiveness of antihistamines in common cold. J Med Assoc Thai 1990; 73: 96–101.

61. Howard JC, Jr., Kantner TR, Lilienfield LS, Princiotto JV, Krum RE, Crutcher JE, Belman MA, Danzig MR. Effectiveness of antihistamines in the symptomatic management of the common cold. J Am Med Assoc 1979; 242:2414–2417.

62. Gaffey MJ, Gwaltney JM, Jr., Sastre A, Dressler WE, Sorrentino JV, Hayden FG. Intranasally and orally administered antihistamine treatment of experimental rhinovirus colds. Am Rev Respir Dis 1987; 136:556–560.

63. Doyle WJ, McBride TP, Skoner DP, Maddern BR, Gwaltney JM Jr, Uhrin M. A double-blind, placebo-controlled clinical trial of the effect of chlorpheniramine on the response of the nasal airway, middle ear and eustachian tube to provocative rhinovirus challenge. Pediatr Infect Dis J 1988; 7:229–238.

64. Gwaltney JM Jr, Park J, Paul RA, Edelman DA, O'Connor RR, Turner RB. Randomized controlled trial of clemastine fumarate for treatment of experimental rhinovirus colds. Clin Infect Dis 1996; 22:656–662.

65. Gwaltney JM Jr, Druce HM. Efficacy of brompheniramine maleate for the treatment of rhinovirus colds. Clin Infect Dis 1997; 25:1188–1194.

66. Gaffey MJ, Kaiser DL, Hayden FG. Ineffectiveness of oral terfenadine in natural colds: evidence against histamine as a mediator of common cold symptoms. Pediatr Infect Dis J 1988; 7:223–228.

67. Berkowitz RB, Tinkelman DG. Evaluation of oral terfenadine for treatment of the common cold. Ann Allergy 1991; 67:593–597.

68. Gaffey MJ, Hayden FG, Boyd JC, Gwaltney JM Jr. Ipratropium bromide treatment of experimental rhinovirus infection. Antimicrob Agents Chemother 1988; 32:1644–1647.

69. Duckhorn R, Grossman J, Posner M, Zinny M, Tinkleman D. A double-blind, placebo-controlled study of the safety and efficacy of ipratropium bromide nasal spray versus placebo in patients with the common cold. J Allergy Clin Immunol 1992; 90:1076–1082.

70. Diamond L, Dockhorn RJ, Grossman J, Kisicki JC, Posner M, Zinny MA, Koker P, Korts D, Wecker MT. A dose-response study of the efficacy and safety of ipratropium bromide nasal spray in the treatment of the common cold. J Allergy Clin Immunol 1995; 95:1139–1146.

71. Hayden FG, Diamond L, Wood PB, Korts DC, Wecker MT. Effectiveness and safety of intranasal ipratropium bromide in common colds: a randomized, double-blind, placebo-controlled trial. Ann Intern Med 1996; 125:89–97.

72. Gaffey MJ, Gwaltney JM Jr, Dressler WE, Sorrentino JV, Hayden FG. Intranasally administered atropine methonitrate treatment of experimental rhinovirus colds. Am Rev Respir Dis 1987; 135:241–244.

73. Gustafson M, Proud D, Hendley JO, Hayden FG, Gwaltney JM Jr. Oral prednisone therapy in experimental rhinovirus infections. J Allergy Clin Immunol 1996; 97:1009–1014.

74. Farr BM, Gwaltney JM, Jr., Hendley JO, Hayden FG, Naclerio RM, McBride T, Doyle WJ, Sorrentino JV, Riker DK, Proud D. A randomized controlled trial of glucocorticoid prophylaxis against experimental rhinovirus infection. J Infect Dis 1990; 162:1173–1177.

75. Sperber SJ, Hendley JO, Hayden FG, Riker DK, Sorrentino JV, Gwaltney JM Jr. Effects of naproxen on experimental rhinovirus colds. A randomized, double-blind, controlled trial. Ann Intern Med 1992; 117:37–41.

76. Higgins PG, Barrow GI, Tyrrell DA. A study of the efficacy of the bradykinin antagonist, NPC 567, in rhinovirus infections in human volunteers. Antiviral Res 1990; 14:339–344.

77. Aberg N, Aberg B, Alestig K. The effect of inhaled and intranasal sodium cromogly-

cate on symptoms of upper respiratory tract infections. Clin Exp Allergy 1996; 26: 1045–1050.

78.  Barrow GI, Higgins PG, Al-Nakib W, Smith AP, Wenham RB, Tyrrell DA. The effect of intranasal nedocromil sodium on viral upper respiratory tract infections in human volunteers. Clin Exp Allergy 1990; 20:45–51.

79.  Chalmers TC. Effects of ascorbic acid on the common cold: an evaluation of the evidence. Am J Med 1975; 58:532–536.

80.  Dykes MHM, Meier P. Ascorbic acid and the common cold: evaluation of its efficacy and toxicity. J Am Med Assoc 1975; 231:1073–1079.

81.  Hemila H. Does vitamin C alleviate the symptoms of the common cold?—A review of current evidence. Scand J Infect Dis 1994; 26:1–6.

82.  Gwaltney JM Jr. Combined antiviral and antimediator treatment of rhinovirus colds. J Infect Dis 1992; 166:776–782.

83.  Turner RB, Felton A, Kosak K, Kelsey DK, Meschievitz CK. Prevention of experimental coronavirus colds with intranasal α-2b interferon. J Infect Dis 1986; 154: 443–447.

84.  Higgins PG, Phillpotts RJ, Scott GM, Wallace J, Bernhardt LL, Tyrrell DAJ. Intranasal interferon as protection against experimental respiratory coronavirus infection in volunteers. Antimicrob Agents Chemother 1983; 24:713–715.

85.  Murray RS, Brown B, Brian D, Cabirac GF. Detection of coronavirus RNA and antigen in multiple sclerosis brain. Ann Neurol 1992; 31:525–533.

86.  Murray RS, Cai G-Y, Hoel K, Zhang J-Y, Soike KF, Cabirac GF. Coronavirus infects and causes demyelination in the primate central nervous system. Virology 1992; 188:274–284.

87.  Myint S, Harmsen D, Raabe T, Siddell SG. Characterization of a nucleic acid probe for the diagnosis of human coronavirus 229E infections. J Med Virol 1990; 31:165–172.

# AUTHOR INDEX

*Page numbers in italics refer to the reference section at the end of each chapter.*

# SUBJECT INDEX

## A

Acute respiratory infections (ARIs), 2
  classification of, 2–3
    lower respiratory tract infection, 2–3
    upper respiratory tract infection, 2
  etiology of, 3–7
  role of ARIs in developing countries,
      15–19
  role of various risk factors on the oc-
      currence of ARI, 13–15
    age of the host, 13
    anatomical abnormalities, 14
    breast feeding, 14–15
    crowding, 13
    gender, 14
    immunological deficiencies, 14
    inhaled pollutants, 14
    metabolic and genetic diseases, 14
    nutrition, 14–15
    social and economic factors, 15
  role of viruses and bacteria as causes
      of, 7–13
    lower respiratory tract, 8–13
    upper respiratory tract, 7–13
Adenovirus, 27, 90, 210
  in children, 63
  key features of, 25

Adenitis, 3
Adrenergic agents, 263
Adults,
  studies of viral respiratory tract infec-
      tions in exacerbation of asthma,
      48
    cohort studies, 55–56
    hospital-based incidental studies,
        52
    studies utilizing polymerase chain
        reaction, 58
  viral infections' influence on airway
      function and asthma in, 156–
      157
Age,
  incidence of lower respiratory tract in-
      fections and, 8–10
  incidence of upper respiratory tract in-
      fections and, 37–38
  risk of acute respiratory infections
      and, 13
Air pollution as risk factor for wheezing
    in children, 78
Airway hyperresponsiveness,
  to histamine and histamine release,
      130–132
  *see also* Allergy and airway hyper-
      responsiveness

*303*